P9-BYL-842

Mellissa Sevigny

keto for life

Look better, feel better, and
watch the weight fall off
with 160+ delicious
high-fat recipes

Victory Belt Publishing Inc.
Las Vegas

First Published in 2018 by Victory Belt Publishing Inc.

Copyright © 2018 Mellissa Sevigny

All rights reserved

No part of this publication may be reproduced or distributed in any form or by any means, electronic or mechanical, or stored in a database or retrieval system, without prior written permission from the publisher.

ISBN-13: 978-1-628602-89-0

The author is not a licensed practitioner, physician, or medical professional and offers no medical diagnoses, treatments, suggestions, or counseling. The information presented herein has not been evaluated by the U.S. Food and Drug Administration, and it is not intended to diagnose, treat, cure, or prevent any disease. Full medical clearance from a licensed physician should be obtained before beginning or modifying any diet, exercise, or lifestyle program, and physicians should be informed of all nutritional changes.

The author/owner claims no responsibility to any person or entity for any liability, loss, or damage caused or alleged to be caused directly or indirectly as a result of the use, application, or interpretation of the information presented herein.

Cover Design by Charisse Reyes

Interior Design by Justin-Aaron Velasco

Illustrations by Elita San Juan

Printed in Canada

TC 0519

Table of Contents

PART 1:

introduction / 4

Now Let's Talk About You / 6

How Keto Works / 8

Keto 411 / 14

Keto 911 / 21

Keto Tips and Tricks / 22

Keto Pantry Basics / 31

Supplements and Extras / 39

Get Equipped / 43

PART 2:

4-week basic keto meal plan & weekly shopping lists / 49

Week 1 / 50

Week 2 / 54

Week 3 / 58

Week 4 / 62

Guide to the Recipes / 65

PART 3:

the recipes / 67

Basics / 69

Fermented Foods / 109

Breakfast / 125

Chicken / 149

Beef / 175

Pork / 199

Seafood / 221

Veggie Mains & Sides / 247

Snacks & Appetizers / 283

Cocktails / 305

Desserts / 323

With Gratitude / 358

Resources / 360

Recipe Index / 362

Allergen Index / 370

General Index / 373

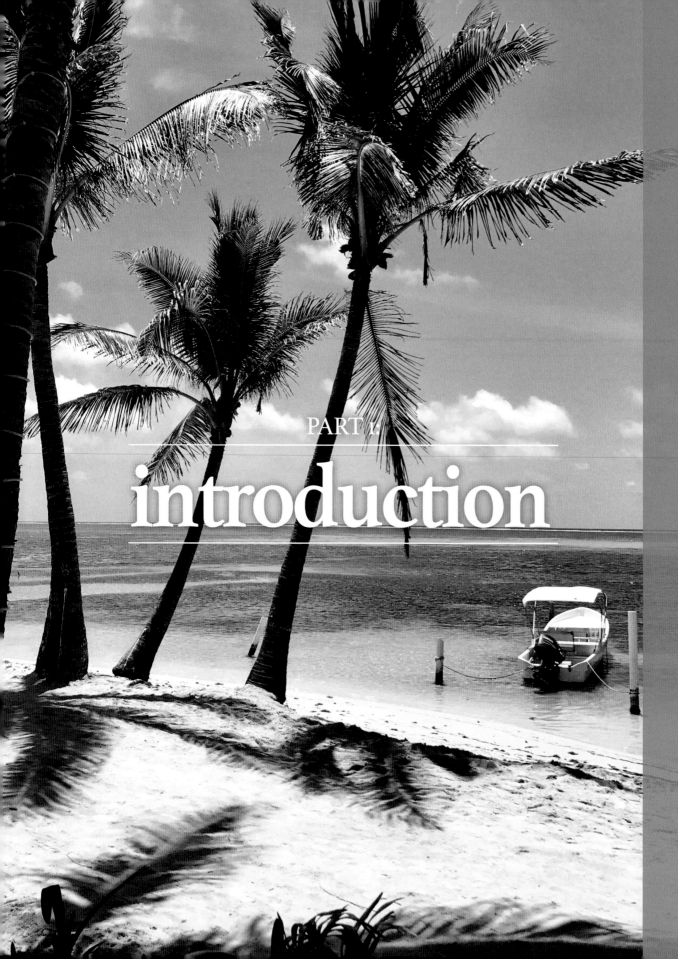

PART I:

introduction

As I sit here beginning this, my first "real" cookbook, several things are true. I'm turning forty-five this summer, I have a wonderful husband and son (aka Mr. Hungry and Hungry Junior), we live on the beach on a tropical island in Central America, and I'm very happy with my life in general.

It's also true that I'm not currently at the weight I want to be—but I'm going to get back there. In fact, it's a very real possibility that by the time you read this book, I already will have: at least six months will have passed since I wrote it.

I feel comfortable making this claim because I have complete confidence that getting back on the keto diet for a few months will take off the pounds and that my newly revisited morning workout routine will firm up the saggy bits. (I'm looking at you, batwings.)

I know this because I've done it before, and the keto diet has never failed me. And it's not just me—the keto diet is rapidly gaining in popularity because it just plain works. Thousands of people have had success using the keto recipes and meal plans on my blog, *I Breathe I'm Hungry*. And when I behave myself and follow them, too, I feel better, I definitely look better, and the weight falls off.

So, if keto is so great, why do people lose weight on it and then sometimes gain it back, as I did? Because the keto diet is like any other plan—if you stop doing it and go back to your old unhealthy eating habits, you'll gain weight. Annoying, but unavoidably true. I'd love to tell you that I have some hack whereby you can eat whatever you want and the weight will stay off—but I don't. Nobody does, and if someone claims that they do, then they are flat-out lying.

So why this book, then? Why even listen to me? I'm not a nutritionist or a doctor, and I'm not some hard-body trainer or life coach. Who am I to be telling you how to succeed on the keto diet?

I'm someone who's been where you are. Whether you are just starting out, you've started and stalled, or you had success but then gained it all back—I know how you're feeling, and I've gotten to the other side. Also, and perhaps more importantly, I'm good at food, and I know how to make living the keto life both easy and delicious.

Now Let's Talk About You

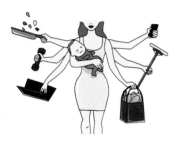

I'm guessing you're holding this book because in one way or another you want to lose weight, and you're hoping this book will help you do it. Or you're my mom and you just bought out the entire store. (Hi, Mom! I know you're excited, but stop buying all the books, okay? Leave some for everyone else!)

If I can be so forward, I'm going to assume that you are likely overweight, tired, frustrated, sick of feeling bad about yourself, and weary of diets that promise quick results but aren't sustainable in the long term. Maybe you've done them all and you're still not happy with your body.

Maybe you are a wife and/or mother who is wondering how to take care of everybody else and still take care of you. Perhaps you haven't been doing so well in that regard, and you're hoping for a change. You desperately want to be like all those "fitspo" moms you follow on Instagram—you know who they are! Dressed in the smallest sizes and the latest fashions, looking amazing with their flowing hair and carefree smiles. And let's not forget their handsome, adoring husbands and beautiful, well-behaved children.

We all want to believe that those enviable people exist—arranging peonies in their pristine white kitchens, doing yoga with their toddlers, feeding their appreciative families kale smoothies and steamed fish with a side of broccoli while their kids smile and say, "You're the best, Mom!" Because if they can do it, maybe we can, too.

Perfect moms everywhere (anywhere?), we salute you.

But let's get real—if that were you (or me!), you wouldn't need this book. The reality is probably more like this: You get up at the crack of dawn, get the kids off to school, go to work all day, come home, and schlep dinner onto the table to complaints of "Not this again!" or "You know I hate broccoli! Can't we order pizza?!" You've been "good" all day with your rice cakes and cucumber slices and lemon water and sadness, and you're tired. *(So. Very. Tired.)* There are questionable stains on your shirt, and you still have to help the kids do their homework and get them bathed before you can even think about getting some much-needed sleep. Let's not forget laundry, cleaning, and, oops, your little darling just reminded you that his diorama of the Second Continental Congress, complete with a miniature handwritten Declaration of Independence, is due tomorrow, and you haven't even started it!

Next thing you know, it's GET ME ALL THE CHOCOLATE AND WINE, STAT!

Boom, another day ends with you feeling like a failure because you couldn't stick to your diet.

Isn't it strange that when we're overweight and frustrated about it, no matter what amazing things we accomplish in a day, we still feel like we've failed when we give in to food? Food is supposed to bring us pleasure, but we're taught that we aren't allowed to enjoy it if we're fat. Like we've given up the right to enjoy eating and must deprive ourselves so that we can be thin—*as we should be.*

If asked how others would describe us, we might imagine them saying, "She's a great wife and/or mom, a hard worker, generous, successful at her job," etc., etc., but in our minds, it always ends with, *"Too bad she's fat."* Am I right?

So we think that if only we were skinny, people would like us more, they'd respect us more, and we'd be happier, kinder, better. That's just how the world works, isn't it?

The thing is, most of that narrative is in our own heads. Oh, sure, random people might judge us by the pound—but the ones who know and care about us see more than just our physical appearance. And for the record, I've known a lot of people with near-perfect bodies who are miserably unhappy. So, just like money can't buy happiness, neither can a six-pack—no matter what social media might be trying to make you believe.

"Wait … Is Mellissa *thin-shaming* now?! Is she telling me that I shouldn't want to lose weight and get into those size-four jeans I've been holding on to for twenty-two years?"

No. I'm not saying that at all. (Okay, maybe get rid of those jeans, though, because even when you do lose the weight, high-waisted mom jeans are never coming back into style, m'kay?) What I am telling you is that you don't need to be skinny to be good enough. You're already good enough. You have value no matter what your size, so don't let that jerky voice in your head tell you otherwise.

That being said, if losing weight is your goal, you *can* accomplish it, and the keto diet can help you do it. Not only can you do it, but you can do it while eating delicious food (that even your picky family will enjoy) and without slaving for hours in the kitchen or feeling hangry all the time.

In fact, once you become fat-adapted, you will have more energy than ever before. That means you'll be more productive at work and at home, leaving you with plenty of quality time to spend with your family and friends (and if one of those friends happens to be Netflix, then we've got a lot in common, I'm just saying).

Oh, and that chocolate and wine? You can still have it, just with a few small tweaks …

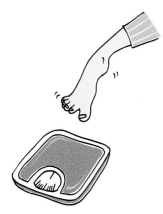

How Keto Works

So many people who have reached out via email and comments on my blog have told me that they struggled with their weight for years and then lost it almost effortlessly when they discovered and started the keto diet. How is that possible? What makes keto so different from other weight-loss plans?

Keto Is Like Snorkeling

I laughed to myself when I typed that heading because I know you're going to think I'm crazy, but bear with me for a moment while I explain this analogy.

Living on a small island in the Caribbean, we do a lot of snorkeling (because seriously, there isn't a lot else to do around here—and also, it's pretty amazing).

When we first moved to Belize and went snorkeling out on the reef, I was using a cheap pair of short fins that came in a snorkeling kit that cost around $30. I did fine when we swam out with the current, but when it came time to turn around and swim against the current, I struggled. I was getting it done, but I was *just so tired* by the time we got back to the boat.

Mr. Hungry suggested that I upgrade to a pair of fins that would move more water with each kick. When I did, the difference was incredible. I was able to swim long distances, even against the current, with what felt like almost no effort! Now, if I stopped kicking, I'd lose ground against the current, so I was still doing the work, but with the help of the bigger fins, I was getting a much greater return for my efforts.

On one of our recent snorkeling trips, the current was pretty strong, and we jumped off a catamaran with no flippers on to swim with the nurse sharks. It had been a long time since I'd been in the water without fins, so I was really surprised at how difficult it was to stay near the anchored boat with the current working against us.

I was recording the sharks with my GoPro when a huge spotted eagle ray (one of my favorites) came into view. If I had been wearing my fins, I easily could have gotten closer and gotten some great footage—but finless? I made zero progress, even while kicking madly and paddling with my arms. It was absolute futility. In fact, without my fins on, just swimming the thirty feet back to the boat against the current was a struggle. I made it, but I was exhausted by the effort.

So what does this have to do with keto?

Swimming Against the Current

I struggled with my weight from the time I hit puberty. When I was a senior in high school, I lost 70 pounds by taking diet pills, and I was miserable the entire time. I gained some of that weight back after I got married, but I didn't want to take the pills again because they made me so cranky and jittery that I feared for my marriage—and I'm only half kidding.

So I started working out and doing a popular low-calorie, low-fat plan. I lost some weight, but I was not where I wanted to be, even though I was running up to thirty miles per week and eating around 1,400 calories (or less) per day. And when I'd get tired or frustrated and eat whatever I wanted for a weekend, or when I cut back on my workouts in the slightest, I would gain instantly—as much as 8 pounds in as little as a week. It was so exhausting and discouraging that I eventually stopped trying, and in my thirties I gained about 65 pounds. I'd have spurts of trying to run and eat low-fat/low-calorie again, but I was miserable from the hunger and deprivation. Even my husband, though supportive, dreaded my dieting.

Meanwhile, I was pushing my workouts and getting injured because I was impatient to get back to where I'd been and wanted to see results quickly. It was a recipe for failure, and despite all that hard work, I was losing so slowly that it didn't seem worth it.

It felt like I could either be happy and live my life or be miserable in the pursuit of a perfect body. There didn't seem to be any middle ground for me. Why were so many of my friends drinking beer and wine, eating whatever they wanted, and still maintaining their enviable figures? It just didn't seem fair. It was like swimming against the current with no fins on and always being at the back of the pack.

Here's what I've learned.

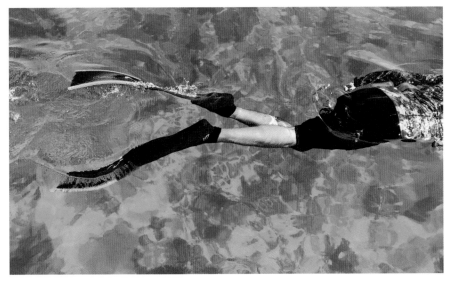

Keto Gives You Fins

Some people are born with fins—they put a little effort into it, true, but they don't have to work as hard as the rest of us to fight the current and stay fit. Maybe you are insulin resistant, have polycystic ovary syndrome (PCOS), or just seem prone to being heavier—genetically, you've got no fins. Maybe it sometimes feels like you don't even have limbs when it comes to fighting the current and losing weight. I've been there, and I know that feeling of hopelessness.

As you may already know, when you put on your keto fins, you suddenly gain ground—and it doesn't seem so hard! "Wait," you might think, "I'm losing weight while still eating delicious food? I'm not starving all the time? I don't hate life, and my family isn't tiptoeing around me because of my hangry-influenced hair trigger? And the scale keeps going down, and I feel like I really can do this? It's a miracle!"

Welcome to keto.

Now that's all well and good, but you might also be thinking, "Well, I tried keto, and it sort of worked, but I lost slowly and didn't have the amazing and fast results that I see others posting. I'm working hard, but I don't feel like I'm getting anywhere, so I'm frustrated."

Don't give up! What I've found is that not all fins are created equal, and not all fins work the same for every person. Maybe basic keto isn't the fins for you or, more importantly, for the sea you're swimming in.

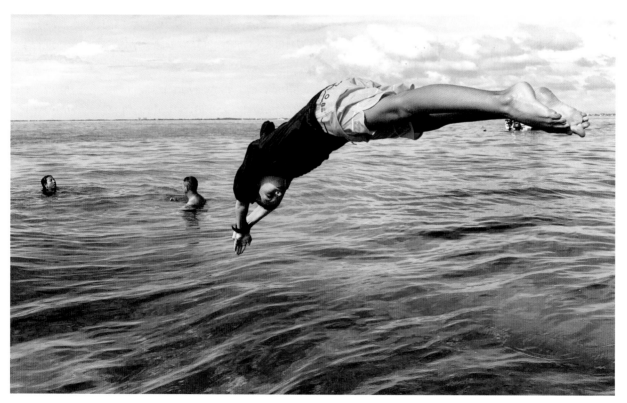

Keto Fins Aren't One-Size-Fits-All

So what do you do if regular keto hasn't worked for you? Try on some bigger fins. Different-shaped fins. More flexible fins. But how do you do that?

Since we moved to Belize, Mr. Hungry has gotten into spearfishing and free diving, so he's acquired several pairs of really long fins and fins made from different materials. Some are stiffer, and some are more flexible. When he goes out for the day, he grabs the fins that are best suited to the kind of swimming or fishing he's got planned and the conditions.

Like literal fins that come in many shapes, sizes, and materials, keto can be modified in many ways for better results based on the individual: intermittent fasting, dairy-free, sweetener-free, nut-free, gluten-free, lower protein, or any combination of those modifications and others. There are many variables that can make a huge difference. So if you're doing keto and it still feels like you're swimming against the current instead of with it, I encourage you to upgrade your fins.

After having successfully lost and kept off more than 70 pounds for almost two years on keto, I gained weight unexpectedly while taking huge doses of steroids for allergies in South Carolina a few years ago. We eventually moved to New York to get away from the pollen that was causing my allergies, and I was finally able to get off of all the medication I had been taking and start functioning like a normal person again.

I thought I'd be able to lose the weight easily like I had before, so I started with a vengeance. I was surprised to find that even though I was being super strict with my macros (ratios of fat, protein, and carbohydrates), I still wasn't losing—it was like someone had stolen my fins. I was getting really frustrated!

Then I gave up and ate cannoli and pizza every day for about a month. As you can imagine, that didn't help my weight situation or my self-esteem.

So I did some research on the possible reasons for my inability to lose weight even while doing keto and found that there are many factors that can affect each person differently. Since I was also struggling with digestion issues, I started experimenting with fermented foods to improve my gut health. I gave up alcohol, dairy, and sweeteners for a while to decrease inflammation and ate only eggs as my protein because they are so easy to digest. Lo and behold, I lost 12 pounds in two weeks! My macros were the same, but with those small changes I felt like I was back in control again.

Then we moved to Belize and life got a little crazy, so I maintained but didn't lose any more weight for a while.

After we had adjusted to life on a tiny island in a third-world country (which wasn't easy, believe it or not), I started keto again. It was slow going. Here I am in my forties, and with menopause on the horizon, that current is even stronger. I wasn't ready to throw in the towel, but I was discouraged.

I had given up all my favorite carb-heavy Caribbean foods (mango mojitos, I miss you so), I was strictly staying below my daily limit of 20 grams of net carbs, and I was definitely in ketosis, yet I lost only 7 pounds in almost three months. And it felt so *hard*. The keto fins that had worked well for me in the past weren't as effective anymore. I was older and navigating tougher currents—I needed to upgrade my fins again.

Out of desperation and thinking that my problem might be hormone related, I tried John Kiefer's Carb Nite Solution—where you eat keto all week and then have a ton of carbs within a few hours one night every seven to ten days. The very simplified explanation is that this approach is supposed to regulate your hormones so that your body doesn't catch on and stop responding to keto. It sounded awesome, and a lot of people were having great success with it, but to me, the two days after each carb binge felt like death, and I wasn't losing any faster. I gave up after a month.

Then I bought the book *The Complete Guide to Fasting*, by Dr. Jason Fung and Jimmy Moore. It is an incredible read and made so much sense to me! One quote from the book that I love is, "There is nothing easier than fasting, because fasting involves doing nothing." And it's true! Especially after all the confusion about what I should eat to get the best results— dairy or no dairy, nuts or no nuts, beef or chicken or fish?—I found the simplicity of this approach so refreshing.

So I decided to try it out. If I was traveling and I knew I wasn't going to be super strict with keto or wasn't going to have a lot of keto-friendly options, I just skipped breakfast and didn't eat until 1 p.m. I found that even if I ate a big lunch that included carbs and a light dinner that didn't, I wasn't gaining weight like I normally would have!

We went to Roatán, Honduras, for three weeks in June. I didn't eat keto, but I kept my carbs at an average of less than 100 grams per day. I also fasted almost every morning and ate only during a six-hour window. I got home and weighed myself, and I was down 4 pounds. It didn't seem possible!

I figured that if I could lose weight on vacation while not eating keto but while practicing intermittent fasting, even better things might happen if I combined the two. I tried it and lost 7 pounds in one week, and I never once felt hungry. I had found my new keto fins, and they were working!

Now, that doesn't mean that if you do exactly what I did, you will see the same results. You might—and that's great. But if *my* perfect fins aren't *your* perfect fins, you'll just have to experiment to find what's right for you—and that right fit can change over time, so you may have to continue making adjustments.

You might try a fat fast (where you eat only fats for three to five days) or even an egg fast (where you eat only eggs and fats for three to five days) to achieve better results. I have a free five-day egg fast meal plan on my website, and thousands of people have lost huge amounts of weight on it. Some have chosen to do an egg fast a couple of times a month, combined with regular keto, until they reached their goal—and then use the egg fast occasionally for maintenance.

Missing your veggies and don't have time for a lot of cooking? Try my 5-Day Keto Soup Diet (also on my website), which has no dairy, nuts, or sweetener and is loaded with veggies, nutrients, and satiating fat! This diet is blasting thousands of people past their plateaus, and they are consistently losing up to (and sometimes more than) 10 pounds a week on it.

And then there are a few people who have tried these plans and reported that they lost nothing. It doesn't mean that the plans don't work; they just aren't the right keto fins for those people.

Find Your Fins

It might take some experimentation to find the right fins for your body and your metabolism, but once you do, you'll be able to chase down your goals, and it will feel amazing. You will still have to keep swimming, but the amount of reward for your efforts will finally be worth it.

And, like Mr. Hungry, you might need an entire closetful of fins to pick from depending on your "current" situation. (See what I did there?) Had a celebration weekend or a weeklong vacation binge and need to get back on track? Pull out your aggressive "five-day plan" fins and use them to gain some ground. Hormones and/or health problems and medications making it harder to lose or maintain? Don your intermittent fasting (or other) fins and start seeing results again.

I can't tell you which fins are right for you—you need to try them on and swim around a bit to see which ones work best. But I can guarantee you that swimming with *any* keto fins is better than swimming with none—or not swimming at all.

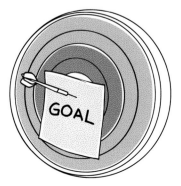

Keto 411

This section contains the bare minimum of what you need to know to begin a keto diet. If you read only one portion of the introduction, make it this one, because it gives you everything you need to get started.

How Long Will It Take Me to Get into Ketosis?

For most people, it takes about three days to get into ketosis, but it can take as many as four or five days.

How Many Carbs Should I Eat?

Eat less than 20 grams of net carbs per day to experience the benefits of ketosis. You calculate net carbs by subtracting grams of fiber (or sugar alcohols in some cases) from total grams of carbohydrate. Don't guess—you'd be surprised at how many grams of carbs there are in some foods you might once have considered "free," like onions, garlic, tomatoes, and kale, just to name a few. (More on that later.)

Some people believe that net carbs are a farce and that you should count total carbs on a keto diet. Personally, I find that approach way too restrictive because it unnecessarily limits your veggie intake and the variety of foods you can consume. My advice is to start with 20 grams of net carbs per day. If you are successful, then continue on, but if you're having trouble losing weight, then experiment with counting total carbs and see if it makes a difference for you.

Which Foods Are Not Acceptable on Keto?

I get this question a lot on the blog. The fact is that very few foods are *not* keto because pretty much anything that keeps you below 20 grams of net carbs per day can be included on a keto diet.

Fruit is a great example. People get dogmatic and leave comments on some of my blog recipes like "Pineapple isn't keto; therefore, this cake made with ¼ cup of crushed pineapple is not keto." That's simply not true. A moderate amount of fruit, or even a tablespoon of molasses for flavor, doesn't automatically make a recipe "not keto." If a serving of that recipe is within your carb budget for the day, then you absolutely can eat it.

Doing keto long-term doesn't mean that you can't ever have fresh fruit again. There are ways to fit it into your carb budget in moderation—and you should, because fruit is enjoyable and can be very nutritious. A low-carb tortilla has around 6 grams of net carbs and no nutritional value, whereas a Kefir Strawberry Smoothie (page 127) is loaded with pre- and probiotics, phytonutrients, antioxidants, and delicious flavor. Sometimes you want a sandwich, and I get that, but just as you might budget a carb-heavy tortilla or a slice of real bread into your day, you can make room for occasional fruits and fermented foods a few times a week. Your gut will thank you.

Some people prefer to eat almost no carbs the entire day and then use their entire daily carb budget on one small potato with dinner or half a chocolate bar for dessert. Others spread out their carbs equally over three meals, shooting for 6 to 7 grams of net carbs per meal. How you structure your day and budget your carbs is really up to you. You can only budget effectively, though, if you familiarize yourself with the carb counts of the foods you eat often or track what you eat with an app. The following are some common foods that a low-fat or low-calorie dieter might consider "free" but that are surprisingly high in carbs and can knock you out of ketosis without your even realizing it. Consume them sparingly, or try the suggested lower-carb alternatives instead.

Surprisingly High-Carb Foods and Their Substitutes		
Food	Net Carbs	Use Instead
Lemon/lime juice (1 tablespoon)	1.3g	Grated lemon or lime zest (0.4g per tablespoon)
Garlic powder (1 teaspoon)	2g	Minced garlic (1g per teaspoon)
Oyster or shiitake mushrooms (1 cup)	3.6g or 4.1g	White mushrooms (1.6g per cup) or cremini mushrooms (2.2g per cup)
Kale (1 cup chopped)	5g	Collard greens or Swiss chard (0.7g per cup)
Onions (1 cup chopped)	14g	Scallions (4.7g per cup) Dried onion flakes (3.7g per tablespoon) Shallots (3.4g per 2 tablespoons)
Potatoes (1 cup diced)	23g	Daikon (2.5g per cup) Cauliflower (3g per cup) Jicama (5g per cup) Celery root (11.6g per cup)

While many people believe that you must give up vegetables on a keto diet, that is simply not true. Lots of tasty and nutritious veggies are perfectly suited to a diet that restricts carbohydrates. The following are some of my favorites:

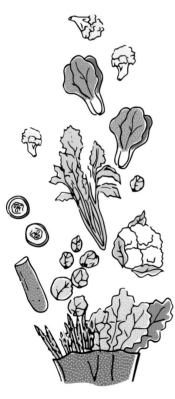

Ingredient	Net Carbs in 1 Cup Raw
Butter lettuce	0.3g
Arugula	0.4g
Spinach	0.4g
Green leaf lettuce	0.5g
Romaine lettuce	0.5g
Spring greens	0.7g
Bok choy	0.8g
Iceberg lettuce	0.9g
Romaine hearts	1.3g
Cucumbers	1.8g
Celery	1.9g
Red radishes	2.4g
Asparagus	2.5g
Daikon	2.5g
Cauliflower	3g
Green cabbage	3.2g
Broccoli	3.5g
Brussels sprouts	4.6g
Red cabbage	4.7g
Jicama	5g

What Are Ketostix, and Do I Need Them?

I do recommend getting some ketone test strips (aka Ketostix) if you're just starting out. You can purchase them online or at a regular pharmacy (look in the aisle where diabetic supplies are sold) for around $10 for a pack of fifty. You can cut them in half before using them to make them last even longer if you like.

These strips confirm whether ketones are being excreted through your urine. That's all. They won't change color if you aren't excreting any ketones; then they turn light pink if there is a trace of ketones, and it goes up from there to dark purple. The darkness of the strip doesn't matter; as long as you are showing even trace amounts, you are in ketosis and good to go. In fact, if your strip is really dark, you may be dehydrated and need to drink more water.

Here's a pro tip: Don't post pictures of your purple pee sticks on the internet. No matter how excited you are about getting into ketosis, nobody wants to see that.

You don't technically *need* Ketostix, but when you are suffering as much as you are likely to be in the first few days, it's nice to get validation that your change in diet is working and that you've gotten into ketosis. And if you aren't losing weight, sometimes testing your ketones and finding out that you aren't even in ketosis is a wake-up call that you might be consuming hidden carbs or doing something else wrong.

What About Sodium? Isn't Too Much Salt Bad for You?

When you eat low-carb, your body doesn't retain water in the same way, so sodium and other important electrolytes get flushed out quickly. You need to replenish these electrolytes or you will feel awful—you might even experience heart palpitations, cramps, panic attacks, and other scary things.

It is crucial to get a lot of sodium on a ketogenic diet—much more than you're used to, probably. Don't be alarmed, and don't try to cut back; the salt is important. Salted bone broth or stock is a great way to replenish electrolytes. In addition, you should supplement with potassium and magnesium to avoid unpleasant symptoms like light-headedness, cramps, and headaches.

Some people like to drink pickle juice or zero-carb sports drinks to get their electrolytes. However you choose to replenish them, it's important that you do. I discuss supplements later (see pages 39 to 42).

How Much Water Do I Need to Drink?

A *lot.* Aim for at least 100 ounces a day—especially in the first couple of weeks as your body adjusts to the natural diuretic effect of being in ketosis. Then you can lower it to 99 ounces a day if you're feeling confident.

What Is This Keto Flu I Keep Hearing About?

If this is your first time following a low-carb or ketogenic diet, you may be blindsided by the detox symptoms. I'm not going to lie: depending on how carb-heavy your diet was before you started keto, you may wish you were dead by day three.

Don't panic.

Headaches, bone-deep fatigue, irritability, dizziness, and more could be coming at you depending on how addicted your body is to carbs. Hang in there! The first three days are the hardest. Some of you have done it before and know to just ride it out. It will all get better soon.

Those of you who are new to the "keto flu" might panic, thinking your death is imminent. I can assure you, it is highly unlikely that you will die from sugar/carb withdrawal—but just to be sure, it's always wise to consult with your doctor before you embark on any new eating plan. If something feels truly off and you are concerned, it's better to be safe than sorry—seek medical attention.

Just remember, most keto flu symptoms can be alleviated by replenishing electrolytes (sodium, potassium, and magnesium) and drinking plenty of water.

How Much Protein and Fat Should I Eat?

Don't think you're going to cheat the system and lose weight faster by restricting carbs and fat and eating a lot of protein—you will feel (even more) awful, and, after an initial drop in water weight, your weight loss can be inhibited.

WARNING: Keto is not a high-protein diet! Your body can convert excess protein into glucose, and you don't want that. You want your body to learn to use fat for energy—that is the secret to unlocking your fat stores and losing weight almost effortlessly on a low-carb plan.

Remember: Keto is a low-carb, moderate-protein, high-fat way of eating.

You'll hear a lot of talk about macros on the keto diet. As mentioned earlier, that term refers to the ratios of macronutrients (fat, protein, and carbohydrates) you should be eating for optimal results. Typically, a reasonable breakdown to shoot for is 70 percent of your calories coming from fat, 25 percent from protein, and 5 percent from carbohydrates.

To determine how much fat and protein you personally should be eating, there are lots of free macro calculators available online that do the math for you based on your body mass and activity level. See the Resources section on page 360 for a list.

This Is Starting to Sound Complicated. Do I Have to Start Tracking Everything I Eat Now?

While some people love the process of tracking everything they eat with apps like MyFitnessPal, I find it tedious and frustrating. If you love charts and graphs and the confidence that every gram of food that passes your lips is accounted for, then by all means, track away. On the other hand, if you're like me and would rather shave your legs with a cheese grater while chewing on aluminum foil than spend an hour a day tracking and logging all your meals, you can rest easy knowing that it's not necessary. The only thing you really need to worry about (unless you run into a stall) is keeping your net carbs at or under 20 grams per day.

In that same vein, when you're first starting out, don't obsessively plan everything so that keto feels harder and more overwhelming than it has to. This statement may seem controversial to some, but I'm here to tell you not to worry about calories, or nitrates, or omega-3 versus omega-6 fats, or whether the meat you're eating skipped about on acres of lush pastureland while being fed organic vegan feed by the tiny, perfect hands of a thousand virgin milkmaids.

Get into ketosis. Give your body time to adapt so that you can function. *Then* you can worry about fine-tuning and all the other stuff. Seriously.

The basic strategy when starting keto is to (a) never get too hungry, and (b) stuff your face full of delicious high-fat, very-low-carb foods. If you open the door to hunger, your resolve can fly right out the window, and you're back to square one. (Sadly, I speak from experience on this.)

I Heard That Keto Can Make My Uterus and My Hair Fall Out. Is This True?

This one is strictly for the ladies.

In the first month or two on keto, you might experience some strange periods. Don't be alarmed. When you lose weight and your body detoxes from sugar and excess carbs, all kinds of hormonal changes can occur.

Initially, you might experience much heavier (and longer) periods than normal and/or more extreme PMS symptoms. This is common, and though it's inconvenient, it shouldn't last more than a few months at most.

If your weight loss is rapid on keto (and let's hope that it is), you might also lose more hair than normal for a month or two. Hair loss can be disconcerting, but it's not permanent and will stop when your hormones regulate.

I have experienced both of these effects on keto, and I can promise you that the increased energy, lost weight, clearer skin, and other pros far outweigh these temporary issues. Stay the course unless something seems really wrong, in which case you should talk with your doctor just to be on the safe side.

Will Intermittent Fasting Maximize My Results?

There is a vast wealth of information about the benefits of intermittent fasting written by actual doctors and scientists—which I am not. So if you're curious about how and why intermittent fasting works and what the health and weight-loss benefits are, I encourage you to look into it. I've provided a list of reliable websites and books about intermittent fasting in the Resources section on page 360.

In the meantime, you can give intermittent fasting a try simply by not eating within four hours of bedtime. If you go to bed at 10 p.m., for example, have your last meal at 6 p.m. Then sleep for eight hours, and when you get up and eat breakfast, you'll have fasted for twelve hours. Bonus points if you can wait four or even six hours before eating your first meal. (Coffee is okay if you must, and I do.) If you can accomplish that, you'll have fasted for at least sixteen hours. It wasn't even that hard, was it?

Try it and see how you do—you might find that you lose weight much faster when you shorten your daily eating window to six hours or less. Be sure to track your progress.

How to Keto: In Summary

Consume 20 grams or less of net carbs per day, not too much protein, and lots of fat. Drink at least 100 ounces of water per day, get plenty of salt, and supplement with potassium and magnesium. Boom, three days later you're in ketosis (which you can measure with your Ketostix) and on your way!

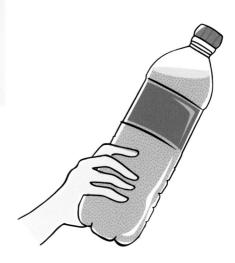

Keto 911

So you woke up on Monday morning amidst empty ice cream cartons and donut boxes, with frosting in your hair. Don't go into a tailspin! After you've gone off keto for a meal (or several), pull yourself together and take the following steps, stat.

- **Don't beat yourself up.** This is real life, and you need to enjoy it. Don't worry about one bad meal, or even a weekend of bad meals, as long as you're still making progress and not making a habit of straying.

- **Remind yourself of what keto has done for you:** better health, more energy, clearer skin, a more youthful appearance, a thinner physique, better-fitting clothes, improved self-esteem, and so on, which make it all worthwhile!

- **Relive your successes mentally**—like how good it felt that time your ex's eyes bugged out when you ran into him at the grocery store and he saw how great you looked.

- **Look at old photos of a heavier you** (keep some on your phone)— not to beat yourself up, but to remind yourself of what it felt like to be in that skin and how much better you feel now.

- **Get back on track ASAP!** Returning to keto will get harder with every passing day—you'll think (and believe me, I speak from experience), "Well, I'm already out of ketosis, so tomorrow I'll eat all the things I've been missing and then I'll get back on keto." (Trust me, you won't.) Or, "I have a party coming up this weekend anyway; I might as well wait until the day after to start keto again." (Love your optimism ... but nope.)

Also, it's important to be honest with yourself about potential pitfalls and temptations that you are unlikely to be able to resist. Keto is a means to an end that can help you reach your personal health and weight-loss goals, but you need to live your life.

If you are going to be attending an event or celebrating a special occasion and you are likely to cheat, have a plan for doing that. Then you can fast until noon the next day to get the glucose out of your system and resume keto with an extra-fatty, extra-low-carb lunch.

Don't be in denial about the potential for cheating and then let it derail you indefinitely. Plan for it in advance so that you can enjoy your brief hiatus and get right back to keto afterward. Cheating can be a slippery slope, though, so try to keep it to once a month or less to avoid hindering your overall progress.

Keto Tips and Tricks: How to Make It Work for You

Dealing with a Picky Family

I consider myself an authority on picky family members. Mr. Hungry will eat only about five vegetables, and of those, he will eat only two cooked—and even then only sparingly. He and my son abhor broccoli and cauliflower, both of which I love. Initially, they barely tolerated zucchini noodles, although they are finally getting used to them.

I've learned to make meals that we all can enjoy by keeping certain components separate. I generally make a simple salad, a keto-friendly protein that everybody likes, and then a starchy side of potatoes, bread, or pasta for them with a corresponding keto version for myself.

Here are some of the easy side-dish swaps that I rely on:

Mashed or baked potatoes → **Cheesy Cauliflower Puree (page 272)**

Rice → **Basic Cauliflower Rice (page 250)**

Pasta → **Basic Zucchini Noodles (page 252) or Cream Cheese Noodles (page 72)**

French fries → **Spicy Jicama Shoestring Fries (page 280)**

Tortillas → **Cream Cheese Wraps (page 70)**

Put enough fat and flavor into your keto-friendly side dishes and you may find, as many of my blog readers have, that your family only *thinks* they don't like certain veggies; sometimes it's more about texture than flavor. There are very few people who can resist my Cheesy Cauliflower Puree (page 272)—and if you can get your family to eat that, then you can use it as a base for all sorts of meals.

Broccoli Cheddar Puffs (page 296) are downright addicting if you can get your family past the idea of broccoli and trying that first bite.

My guys love jicama fries (see page 280 for my Spicy Jicama Shoestring Fries recipe), so I don't have to make two kinds of fries anymore. And since they'll tolerate zoodles, I almost never make pasta. When covered in Alfredo sauce or used to make Vegetable Lasagna (page 260), the Cream Cheese Noodles (page 72) are close to impossible to distinguish from the real thing—my guys will eat those no problem.

Winning over picky family members to keto-friendly foods can take time, so don't try to implement huge changes cold turkey. Make both versions the first time and have them sample yours.

Pro Tip: Season to Your Advantage

When serving both keto and nonketo versions of a dish, season the nonketo version a little less, making it a little less delicious than usual. That way, the cauliflower puree will really stand out as amazing compared to the mashed potatoes.

Instead of announcing, "WE'RE ALL GOING TO START EATING HEALTHIER AROUND HERE, SO YOU'D BETTER GET ON BOARD," ease them into it. Start by making the recipes from this book that you know right away your family might like. Only you will know which ones might appeal the most to your tribe, but here are a few suggestions:

► Cajun Pork Chops with Aioli (page 200)

► Chili con Carne (page 182)

► Easy Nacho Dip (page 294)

► Easy Salsa Chicken (page 158)

► Meatballs alla Parmigiana (page 192)

► Pecan-Crusted Chicken Fingers (page 152)

► Shrimp Fajitas (page 240)

► Snickerdoodle Crepes (page 132)

Within a few weeks, once they've got their favorites, you may find that eating keto is getting a whole lot easier. You can still order pizza for the family on pizza night and just eat the toppings if that's your tradition, but it doesn't have to be every night. With this more gradual approach, they won't feel deprived and like your "horrible diet" is ruining their lives.

Little treats like the Cinnamon Walnut Streusel Muffins (page 128) are great to have on hand—my guys will ask if they can have one of mine for breakfast. The muffins are easy to make and taste great. If you make them available, you may find that your family will default to the tasty keto versions on their own. Or you may not want to share, and that's okay, too. Even if you can only get everybody on board with dinner, your life will be so much easier—and so will meal planning.

Speaking of meal planning, I put together four weeks of keto meal plans and shopping lists to make your first month pretty much foolproof! See pages 50 to 64.

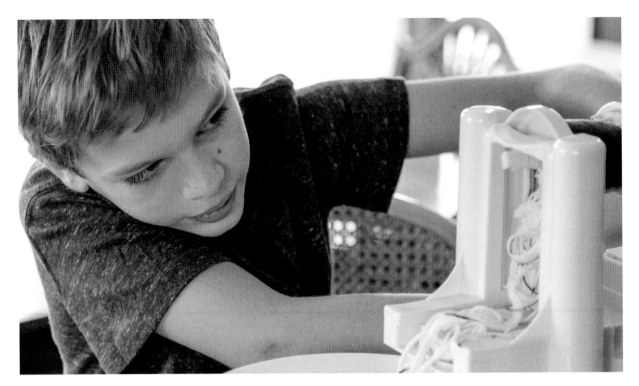

Getting the Kids Involved

Getting your kids involved in the kitchen while they're young is great: not only will they love spending the time with you, but they will be more invested in trying the food you make together. It will also teach them cooking skills that will enable them to live healthier once they are on their own—rather than defaulting to pizza and the drive-thru because they don't know how to cook.

Start your kids off with fun tasks like making zucchini noodles, ricing cauliflower, and blending smoothies. Before you know it, they'll be making eggs, cream cheese pancakes, and maybe even muffins and no-chop chili—with the added bonus that your own cooking time for the family will be cut way back.

Making It Easy: Shortcuts

Here are some items you can buy already prepared in the produce aisle or at the deli counter to save time preparing meals at home or when traveling or out for the day:

- ► cauliflower crumbles
- ► celery sticks
- ► cheese crisps
- ► chicken salad
- ► cooked salmon
- ► grilled chicken
- ► peeled hard-boiled eggs
- ► pickles
- ► pork rinds
- ► rotisserie chickens
- ► tuna packets (you can squeeze mayonnaise packets into them)

Beware of hidden carbs and sugars, and don't be afraid to ask for an ingredient list before buying something from a deli counter in a grocery store.

A Note About Snacking

As a rule, try not to snack after you've become fat-adapted. You'll find that ketosis is a natural appetite suppressant anyway, so don't force yourself to snack out of habit. The longer you go without eating, the less insulin your body will produce and the faster you'll lose weight. Don't freak out every time you feel a little bit hungry—it's not a bad thing to make your body wait for a meal (unless you have a medical condition, of course), and your life will be easier if you aren't planning snacks in addition to meals. Not snacking also keeps your calories down. But if you find yourself needing some quick keto snacks that you can take on the go, the following are some options that don't require refrigeration:

- ▶ 12 almonds—Count them out; don't eat almonds without paying attention to the number or you could inadvertently go over your carb budget.

- ▶ Ripe avocado—Even in your car, you can use a plastic knife and fork to cut it open; if it comes with a napkin and tiny paper packets of salt and pepper, you're in business.

- ▶ Epic bars—They aren't cheap, but they are made from wholesome ingredients and have very few carbs.

- ▶ Celery sticks with almond butter or peanut butter—Prepare this snack ahead of time in preportioned sizes.

- ▶ Homemade beef jerky or sugar-free beef jerky—Don't overdo it or you could get too much protein.

- ▶ Pistachios in the shell—Shelling them takes time, so you'll eat less, but to be safe, make sure you have them preportioned.

- ▶ Pork rinds—These are pretty much zero-carb and great for when you want something crunchy to nosh on. They also come in snack-sized bags, so they are easy to keep at your desk or in the car.

- ▶ Parmesan Crisps (page 298)

- ▶ Keto Seed Crackers (page 300)

- ▶ Buffalo Mixed Nuts (page 301)

- ▶ No-Bake Sesame Cookies (page 338)

Eating Out on Keto

One reason I was having trouble losing the weight I'd gained while on steroids for my allergies was that we were traveling a ton for a project my husband was doing at the time—and that meant a lot of eating out. I love food, and I *really* love when other people cook it for me. Eating out once in a while is okay, but we got to the point where we were eating out at least five times a week.

Even when you're doing your very best to adhere to keto at a restaurant, there are hidden carbs everywhere—you just can't see what the cooks are putting in your food. Chances are you're getting kicked out of ketosis, or close to it, almost every time you eat at a restaurant. If it's only once in a while, you'll get back on track quickly and resume losing, but if you eat out frequently, you're likely to find yourself stalled and not making progress.

For best results, try to eat out as little as possible when in weight-loss mode—once a week or less. That puts you firmly in the driver's seat of what's going into your food and how many carbs you're *really* getting. Another upside is that you'll enjoy eating out even more when you do, because you won't be doing it all the time.

If your job or lifestyle requires you to eat out a lot, it doesn't mean you can't be successful on keto; you'll just have to be extra diligent to avoid hidden carbs. The following are some tips for eating out on keto:

▶ Scope out the restaurant online if possible. Take your time perusing the menu in private and figure out what you're going to order in advance. Lots of bad decisions are made on the fly when everyone else has ordered and you feel pressured. Go in with a plan.

▶ Don't be afraid to ask—very nicely—for substitutions (for example, steamed broccoli with butter instead of fries, or a double portion of side salad instead of mashed potatoes) or to get details about the ingredients used. Is this dressing made with sugar or honey? Is the chicken breaded? Is the sauce thickened with flour? Briefly tell your server why you're asking. Most will want to help, because if they find you pleasant, they will be invested in your success.

▶ If you frequent the restaurant often, always be friendly and courteous—and be sure to tip well (you should anyway) so that the servers and chef, once they know your preferences, will go the extra mile to make sure that you're not getting extra carbs. They may even comment on your weight loss over time, and that's always fun.

▶ When in doubt, keep it simple! The fewer components to your dish, the better off you'll be. Dressings, garnishes, sauces, and the like are a minefield of potential carbs—and way more carbs than you might think. You can't go wrong with a bunless burger, steak (without sweet sauces), grilled fish or chicken with sauce on the side, and broccoli, zucchini, or cauliflower with butter and salt.

▶ Have your town mapped out mentally and know where to get keto-friendly fast food if you're on the go and find yourself without snacks. My go-to when we lived in the States was the McDonald's McDouble. It was on the dollar menu at the time and had two patties with cheese. I'd order two of them for $2, and those four patties would keep me full and satisfied for hours. I know it's not health food, but it's better than caving in to carbs when you're ravenous and pressed for time. You do what you have to do to get through those moments, even if you usually prefer grass-fed everything.

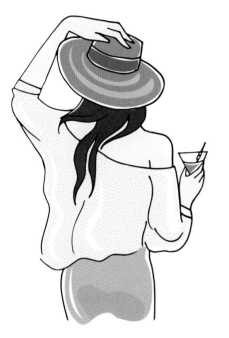

Tips for Staying Keto While Traveling or Vacationing

- *Don't let yourself get desperately hungry!*

- *Bring keto-friendly snacks with you (see page 25).*

- *Scope out keto-friendly options at or near your hotel ahead of time. (Yelp is your friend.)*

- *Budget your carbs for the day so that you can enjoy a few french fries or a couple of bites of your spouse's cake at dinner—you'll still feel like you're celebrating or having a special night out, and it won't hinder your progress.*

- *Avoid foods you know will trigger a full-on binge. For me, it's tortilla chips and salsa or nachos. They're my keto kryptonite! Once I start eating them, it's over.*

Entertaining on Keto

When I dieted in the past, I tended to avoid people and social situations that might have led me to cheat. As humans, so many of our recreational activities and especially our celebrations revolve around eating and drinking. One could argue that they shouldn't and that we should find other ways to spend time together, but that isn't realistic for most of us.

Cutting yourself off from social interactions because you're trying to lose weight is just not sustainable long-term. You'll get lonely and feel like you're giving up too much in the pursuit of better health or a trimmer figure—and eventually you'll fail.

The good news is that you don't have to live like a hermit in order to lose weight on keto. It's true that meeting up at a restaurant can be rife with temptations, but as discussed on page 26, there are many strategies you can employ to stay keto while eating out.

What if you're going to someone's house, though? That can be a tough situation. It's not like you can just order something keto off the menu—generally you're going to eat what your host is serving. After all, when someone cooks for you, it's usually a labor of love, and they want you to enjoy the food. Because it would be rude to show up and not eat, you face a lot of pressure to go off plan. There are a few ways to make this work for you and not lose a friend in the process.

If you've been invited to a gathering and you anticipate going over your carb budget, plan for success by eating something keto before you go—you'll be less hungry. Enjoy the meal in moderate quantities (read: don't go hog wild). Plan to fast the next morning with just coffee, tea, or water, and then have a very-low-carb, high-fat lunch at around noon. You'll be back in ketosis with barely a hitch.

If you don't want to risk getting kicked out of ketosis, you can tactfully inquire as to what your host is planning to serve and, if appropriate, offer to bring something to complement the meal. A side dish is usually a good bet because if the main course is a protein you can have, then your own keto-friendly side and a simple salad, if they have one, is a relatively safe meal.

If the host is planning to serve pasta, you can ask to bring your own zucchini noodles (see page 252) to go with their sauce. It never hurts to bring some keto cookies to share; then you can avoid whatever sugar-laden dessert is being offered and show your fellow diners that keto cookies (my Pecan Shortbread Cookies on page 340 would be a great option) are in fact delicious.

But what works best for me is to host plenty of gatherings myself. People love getting invited over, you're in full control of the menu, and you don't have to drive home afterward, so you can be in your pj's forty-eight seconds after the last guest leaves. There's really no downside here, I'm just saying.

With that in mind, I've put together a few menus for entertaining using recipes in this book that are delicious and relatively easy to prepare. This way, you can stay keto while having fun with your friends and family—and the entire neighborhood will be begging for an invite.

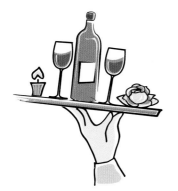

ROMANTIC DINNER FOR TWO

Old-Fashioned (page 309)

Spicy Tuna Cakes (page 228)

Creamy Lobster Risotto (page 242)

Triple Chocolate Cheesecake (page 346)

GIRLS' NIGHT

Pink Grapefruit Martini (page 306)

Wasabi & Ginger Cauliflower Hummus (page 288)

Faux-lafel (page 266)

Pecan Shortbread Cookies (page 340)

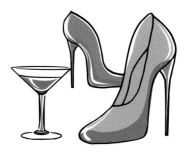

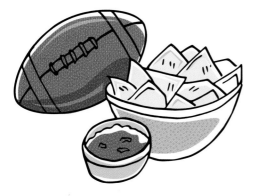

GAME DAY

Caipirinha (page 310)

Buffalo Mixed Nuts (page 301)

Easy Keto Guacamole (page 293)

Easy Nacho Dip (page 294)

Chili con Carne (page 182)

Bacon & Cheddar Cornless Muffins (page 302)

Snickerdoodle Haystack Cookies (page 342)

BRUNCH BUFFET

Prosecco

Spanish Tortilla with Chorizo (page 130)

Spicy Shrimp-Stuffed Avocados (page 244)

Smoked Salmon Stacks (page 234)

Lemon Sour Cream Bundt Cake (page 334)

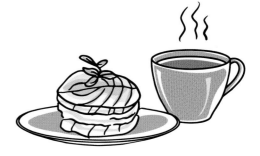

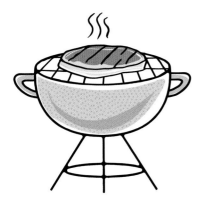

CASUAL DINNER WITH FRIENDS

Whiskey Sour (page 317)

Marinated Skirt Steak (page 178)

Cheesy Cauliflower Puree (page 272)

Sautéed Mushrooms (page 281)

Creamed Spinach (page 278)

Coconut Tarts (page 348)

PATIO PARTY

Margarita (page 318)

Chipotle Deviled Eggs (page 290)

Jerk Chicken (page 172)

Orange & Tarragon Coleslaw (page 276)

Bacon & Cheddar Cornless Muffins (page 302)

Coconut Paletas (page 350)

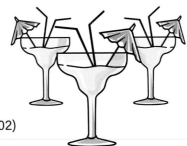

Alcohol on Keto

You may have noticed that all my entertaining menus include an optional cocktail. That doesn't mean I think you should drink every time you get together with friends, but because consuming alcohol is a common social practice, I've supplied you with some keto-friendly options for doing so.

Make no mistake, though: even keto-friendly spirits that don't contain any carbs will slow your weight-loss progress. The simple explanation is that your liver can't focus on helping you shed fat if it's otherwise occupied metabolizing alcohol. So during the hours you're drinking, and for as long as it takes your liver to clear the alcohol out of your system afterward, you aren't losing.

So why include drinks in a weight-loss cookbook at all? Whether or not you use these recipes is up to you—and you can certainly abstain completely. But for me, keto is a long-term strategy—not just to lose but also to maintain. I've found that being so restrictive that you never have any fun makes life on keto harder, and therefore less sustainable in the long term.

Having an occasional (and delicious) keto cocktail with friends is fun—so as long as you aren't overdoing it, you should still be able to lose weight consistently and maintain that loss indefinitely.

Keto Pantry Basics

The following are some keto-friendly ingredients that I always have on hand and that are used liberally throughout the recipes in this book. Some of them are perishable, such as dairy products, and are destined for the refrigerator shelf, but many will sit happily in your pantry for months, ready for you to use them when needed. For many of them, you'll find the best price and availability online, so I typically place a big Amazon order a few times a year to stock up.

Pro Tip: Add Flavor, Not Carbs

There are many ways to add flavor, not carbs, to your meals. While the old you might have relied on sugary sauces and condiments to add pizzazz to meats and veggies, you'll be happy to know that you don't have to sacrifice flavor on keto! In fact, fresh herbs, homemade dressings, and other keto-friendly condiments taste so much better than the store-bought stuff you're probably used to that you may find your food is tasting better than ever before!

- *One of my favorite products right now is truffle salt. I put it on steaks, on chicken, and especially in my cauliflower puree to make it truly next-level— and all it takes is a sprinkle. You can find it at specialty stores or order it online. A little goes a long way, so it's worth a splurge!*

- *Another of my secret weapons is mascarpone cheese. It makes the creamiest sauces, adding richness and a velvety mouthfeel that you typically get only from a flour-based roux. Think of it as solid heavy cream—it makes sauces thicker, makes desserts richer and creamier, and melts in seconds. All with almost no carbs.*

- *Compound butters (butter infused with herbs, aromatics, and potent flavors that pop) take just minutes to make, can be stored in the freezer for months, and add incredible flavor and richness to simply prepared meats and veggies.*

- *Herb-infused oils and simple syrups can bring bright, fresh flavors to both sweet and savory dishes and cocktails. To make herb-infused oils, wash and thoroughly dry the fresh herb or combination of herbs you will be using. Place in a clean glass jar and pour in enough olive oil to cover the herbs completely. About 1 cup should do. Cover and place in a sunny window for about a week, until the oil has absorbed the amount of flavor that you desire. Strain out the herbs and store in the refrigerator for up to three months to preserve the flavor.*

Almond Flour

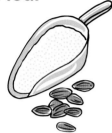

Useful for breading, as a filler, and especially in baked goods, almond flour has become indispensable to my keto kitchen. What you need to know before purchasing is that not all almond flour is created equal. Much of what you find in grocery stores (if you find it at all) is almond meal—almonds that have been coarsely ground with the skins still on. While this product can work fine as a filler in meatballs or as a breading, it's not going to give you the texture you're looking for in baked goods.

It's imperative that you use blanched (skins removed) almond flour in baked goods. For best results, I recommend that you purchase a superfine grind. It's a little pricier but produces baked goods that are very close in texture and flavor to the real wheat-flour-based thing. To get the cheapest price, I buy almond flour online in 5-pound bags and store it in my freezer so it stays fresh for months.

Coconut Flour

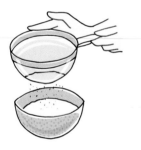

Coconut flour is high in fiber, so the net carbs are relatively low. It can be used in breading, for baking, and even to thicken sauces. It's highly absorbent and has a finer texture than almond flour, so it works well for breads and muffins. Because coconut flour is so absorbent, though, it cannot be substituted at a 1:1 ratio for other flours. For best results, I usually use a combination of almond flour and coconut flour in my baked goods recipes, so I recommend always having some of each on hand. If you are just starting out with keto baking, I implore you to follow the recipes as written until you've gotten familiar with the unique properties of these ingredients. Only then should you start experimenting with making substitutions on your own.

Sweeteners

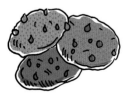

As the keto diet gains in popularity, more and more low-carb sweeteners are hitting the market—which is a good thing because it gives you options. Be aware, though, that many sugar substitutes contain bulking agents that add carbs. The labels can be misleading, because when they list the nutrition info for 1 teaspoon of sweetener, they say the net carbs are 0—yet 1 cup of that same sweetener could contain as much as 24 grams of net carbs, as is the case with Splenda.

For that reason, I prefer erythritol, specifically Swerve brand. It comes in both granulated and powdered forms; measures cup for cup like sugar, so it's easy to use in recipes; and naturally behaves like sugar, so it doesn't require help in the form of carb-heavy bulking agents like maltodextrin.

Because erythritol has a negligible impact on blood sugar levels, I do not include it in the net carb counts for the nutrition information in my recipes. I do, however, provide the erythritol carbs separately for those of you who are sticklers for counting total carbs.

If you choose to use a different sweetener and your brand also measures cup for cup like sugar, then following the recipes in this book will be easy—just use the same amount of your sweetener. Otherwise, go to the website of whatever sweetener brand you are using, and you should find a chart that tells you the equivalent measurement of your product against a list of sugar measurements. Because erythritol measures like sugar, just use the amount of your product that corresponds to the amount of sweetener called for in my recipes. For example, if my recipe calls for ½ cup of erythritol and you are using a different sweetener, go to your sweetener's website, find ½ cup of sugar on the chart, and use whatever amount of your sweetener is equivalent.

That being said, if you use a sweetener other than erythritol, I can't guarantee you will get the same results I did—the flavor and texture could turn out very different.

Dairy Products

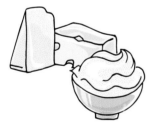

You can do a keto diet without dairy, but most people on keto rely heavily on dairy for fat, flavor, and texture. Also, cheese is amazing, am I right?

Commonly used dairy products on keto are heavy whipping cream, soft and hard cheeses like mozzarella and cheddar, full-fat cream cheese, mascarpone cheese, and, of course, butter.

When shopping for dairy ingredients, remember that not all brands are created equal. Sometimes (but not always), you have to pony up for the name brand over the generic because the carbs are lower. When buying heavy cream and cream cheese, choose organic if you can find it, because most nonorganic brands use thickeners that add carbs. Buy your mozzarella and cheddar cheeses in blocks or slices rather than in shreds—shredded cheese is coated with food starch to prevent clumping, which can add carbs.

Butter

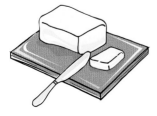

Not all butter is created equal. The quality of the cream used will determine the level of nutrients the butter contains as well as its flavor. For that reason, I prefer butter from grass-fed cows. One brand that is easy to find in the United States is Kerrygold, and that's what I used when I lived there. Another high-quality butter commonly available in the U.S. is Organic Valley Pasture Butter. There is a brand called Anchor that is from New Zealand, and I used that exclusively while living in Belize.

While it's not strictly necessary to use butter from grass-fed cows on a ketogenic diet, because you rely so heavily on fats, it's good to go with the best quality you can get. That being said, any brand of butter will work for the recipes in this book.

I use salted butter in most of my recipes, but occasionally you will see a recipe that specifies unsalted. For example, in the Bulletproof Pumpkin Spice Latte (page 126), salted butter would taste strange.

Nut Milks

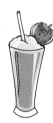

Because dairy milk is high in carbs due to its natural sugars, most people on keto avoid it. A great keto alternative is nut milks like almond and cashew milk. Commonly available in the dairy case, unsweetened nut milks are naturally low in carbs. They work great in ice creams and baking recipes, as well as in smoothies and keto cereals.

Pork Rinds

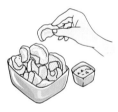

Pork rinds aren't everyone's cup of tea, but once you get used to their flavor and texture, they are handy for all sorts of things! I like dipping them in Easy Nacho Dip (page 294) or even Jalapeño & Cilantro Cauliflower Hummus (page 284). Pork rinds are great as a snack and, when ground up, are also very useful as a nut-free breading for fried foods or even as a filler for meatballs. I've seen people sprinkle pork rinds with cinnamon and sugar and eat them like cereal, but I'm not sure I'd go that far.

Chocolate and Cocoa Powder

If I'm going to eat chocolate, I want it to taste amazing. Your recipes will taste only as good as the chocolate or cocoa powder you use, so be sure to use the best quality you can find and afford. I like Dutch-processed cocoa powder for its less bitter taste. My favorite brand is Saco, which is available in some grocery stores and on Amazon. For baking chocolate, I like Valhrona, Guittard, Dagoba, and Scharffen Berger. You'll be amazed at the difference good-quality chocolate makes in your recipes.

Unsweetened Shredded Coconut

Also referred to as desiccated or dried coconut, this low-carb, high-fat ingredient can bulk up and add texture to cereals, cookies, ice creams, candies, and fat bombs. It can be toasted for a richer flavor and can be used to garnish both sweet and savory dishes.

Fresh Herbs

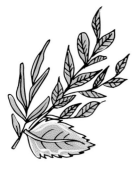

When it comes to adding flavor and brightness to a dish, there is no substitute for fresh herbs. Dried herbs have their place as well, but when recipes call for fresh herbs, do your best to obtain them. If you substitute dried herbs where fresh are called for, you will definitely not be tasting the dish at its best.

To keep costs down, try starting a garden or joining a co-op—then, when you have an abundance, you can chop and freeze your fresh herbs to use for months after the harvest. You can also infuse oils and simple syrups with fresh herbs to give soups, salads, meats, and veggies an added punch of flavor before serving (see page 84 for instructions).

Avocado Oil

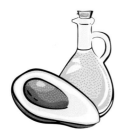

Avocado oil is my new favorite oil for frying and salads! It's got a high smoke point and a really light flavor. You can find it at warehouse stores like BJ's and Costco. I don't recommend stocking up at your local grocery store, since even a small bottle can be spendy. As always, Amazon is your friend if you don't live near a big box store to get the best price. In recipes where I call for avocado oil "or another light-tasting oil," you can substitute olive oil, grapeseed oil, or (sparingly because it's not good for you) regular vegetable oil in place of the avocado oil.

Olive Oil

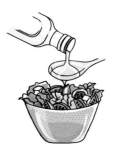

Extra-virgin olive oil is healthy for you, is easy to get, and has a distinctive flavor that makes it great in salads and other cold applications. You can cook with extra-virgin olive oil, too; just be careful not to let it get too hot or it will scorch. I prefer organic and purchase it at Costco when they have it, or on Amazon.

Coconut Oil

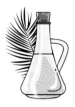

Although coconut oil got a bad rap in the 1980s and '90s, studies have shown that it's actually a very healthy and stable saturated fat. It's an excellent dairy-free replacement for butter, and the two can be used interchangeably in most recipes. Coconut oil has a low smoke point, so it isn't fantastic for frying; I use avocado oil instead. Always go organic and cold-pressed for the best health benefits.

Collagen Powder

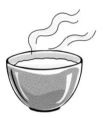

Collagen powder is amazing for your skin, hair, and nails, but it's also a fantastic thickener for smoothies, soups, and gravies. It dissolves completely and has no discernible flavor, so I sometimes add it to bulletproof coffee to make it even richer and frothier. I prefer the Great Lakes brand, which I purchase on Amazon. Collagen powder is also sometimes called collagen peptides or collagen hydrolysate.

Protein Powder

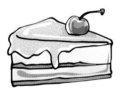

I try to keep my use of protein powder to a minimum because excess protein can be turned into glucose, and that can inhibit weight loss. That being said, for a quick breakfast on the go, it's hard to beat a tasty smoothie. I also use protein powder occasionally in desserts because it adds bulk and can improve texture. Be sure to read labels to make sure you aren't getting excess carbs in the form of sugars or fillers. I like Isopure zero-carb protein powder, which I purchase on (you guessed it!) Amazon. The Isopure brand is 100 percent whey protein and is available unflavored or flavored; currently they have fourteen flavors available, including Creamy Vanilla, Chocolate, Toasted Coconut, and even Mint Chocolate Chip!

Xanthan Gum

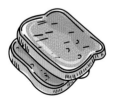

A natural low-carb thickener, xanthan gum might become your new best friend in the kitchen. It makes gravies and sauces thicker, makes liquids more syrupy, and gives gluten-free and keto-friendly baked goods an authentically springy texture. It's inexpensive, and a little goes a long way. I order mine online, but these days it's relatively common to find it in the baking aisle or gluten-free section of the grocery store as well. I've found that there isn't much difference from brand to brand, so I usually purchase whatever is cheapest. If you don't have or can't get xanthan gum, arrowroot powder or guar gum are both acceptable substitutes.

Wheat-Free Soy Sauce

Sometimes only soy sauce produces the umami flavor you want, and there are many wheat-free versions (often labeled as tamari) to choose from these days. A lot of grocery stores carry it in the Asian or gluten-free aisle, but if you can't find it locally, there is always the internet.

Sugar-Free Fish Sauce

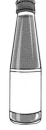

I use fish sauce in a lot of my Asian-inspired recipes because it adds a complex and authentic flavor without soy or wheat. In my opinion, Red Boat brand has hands-down the best flavor and no added sugar.

Flavored Extracts

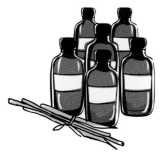

I use a lot of flavored extracts in drinks, candies, and baked goods to get the flavors that normally come from fruits and other ingredients, but without the high carbs. I don't have a brand preference, but I have found that Watkins offers a lot of hard-to-find flavors. There is a much larger variety online than you'll usually find in grocery stores. Some of my favorites are almond, mint, hazelnut, rum, cherry, and banana—but there are many, many more, even exotic flavors like pineapple and passionfruit. You are limited only by your imagination with the use of flavored extracts!

For best results, always use pure vanilla extract, not imitation. That being said, you may not be aware that a surprising number of premium pure vanilla extracts contain added sugars! When purchasing vanilla extract, be sure that it is unsweetened and free of glucose or cane syrup and unexpected carbs.

Sugar-Free Flavored Syrups

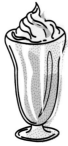

Sugar-free flavored syrups are great not just for coffee but also for flavoring ice creams, baked goods, dressings, and sauces. The most popular brands are Davinci and Torani, and you can find these in the coffee aisle of most grocery stores. The best selection can be found online, and many seasonal varieties are available only a couple of months per year.

Salt

My go-to salt for cooking is coarse kosher salt, usually Morton's brand. It has a nice flaky texture and a mild salt flavor. Please be aware that not all salt measures the same. Table salt or fine sea salt will pack a lot more sodium into a teaspoon than coarse kosher salt will.

When following my recipes, I recommend using kosher salt whenever salt is called for. (The Easy Lacto-Fermented Half-Sour Pickles recipe on page 112 is the sole exception in this book.) That being said, if you opt for a different salt, here's a handy reference to help you figure out how much to use. The less salt you're using, the closer in measurement they are.

Coarse Kosher Salt	Table Salt or Fine Sea Salt
½ teaspoon	½ teaspoon
1 teaspoon	¾ teaspoon
1 tablespoon	2¼ teaspoons

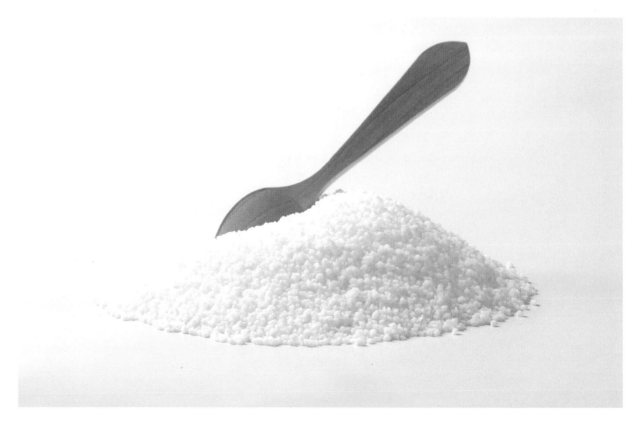

Supplements and Extras

There are entire stores and websites dedicated to selling vitamins and supplements, so figuring out how much (if any) we need to consume in order to be healthy can be a confusing process. Generally, I believe that a daily multivitamin (sugar-free, of course) is good enough to get the job done if you're eating a balanced diet and don't have any existing health problems. That being said, there are certain foods and supplements that I find beneficial in my day-to-day life and on keto, so I'm including a list of them here in case you can benefit from them as well.

Moringa

I first heard about moringa while living in Belize, where it grows abundantly and is available in many forms. A friend (who was not on keto) raved about how it works for her as an appetite suppressant and also stabilizes her blood sugar, so I started looking into it.

Turns out moringa is incredibly nutrient dense, specifically loaded with vitamins A, C, and E, plus calcium and potassium—all especially beneficial on a keto diet when you aren't consuming much fruit. Moringa is also very high in antioxidants and phenols that protect the liver, brain, and heart and can lower inflammation in the entire body. It has antimicrobial and antibacterial properties and promotes wound healing by improving blood clotting as well. Finally, moringa has been shown to reduce glucose levels in diabetic patients.

That is a short summary of moringa's benefits, but there are many more, so I encourage you to do your own research on this amazing plant!

I drink moringa tea a few times a week—it's great hot or iced, depending on the time of year. My Moringa Super Green Smoothie (page 147), made with moringa powder, is a delicious way to get some healthy moringa into your keto diet!

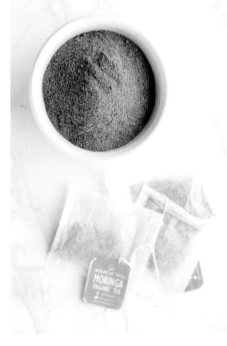

Prebiotics

Most people have heard of probiotics and know that they are good bacteria that live in your gut and promote regularity and a healthy immune system. Fewer people are aware that those bacteria feed on something called prebiotics, which are specific types of fiber that nourish your gut bacteria. Without prebiotics, your beneficial gut bacteria can die off and leave you vulnerable to infections, leaky gut, allergies, and other maladies.

Because the keto diet isn't as rich in fiber and carbohydrates that would typically feed your good bacteria, you have to seek out foods that will keep your bacteria in balance, with the good ones thriving. Here are some keto-friendly foods that are rich in prebiotic fiber:

- ▶ Asparagus (raw)
- ▶ Cacao nibs and powder
- ▶ Flax seeds
- ▶ Garlic (raw)
- ▶ Inulin fiber
- ▶ Jicama
- ▶ Konjac flour/glucomannan (found in shirataki noodles)
- ▶ Onions (raw or cooked)
- ▶ Seaweed

Try to get some of these prebiotic-rich foods into your diet at least a few times a week to keep your gut healthy.

Probiotics

A healthy level of beneficial bacteria in the gut is crucial to an effective immune system, is helpful in controlling candida overgrowth, and has even been linked to better moods and improvements in skin conditions like eczema. More and more research is being done on how probiotics can improve health, and the findings are pretty incredible.

There are tons of probiotic supplements on the market, but the best way to get a wide variety of probiotic bacteria into your system is to eat fermented foods. Sauerkraut, pickles, kefir, cultured vegetables, and kombucha are widely available even in mainstream grocery stores these days. Better yet, you can make your own fermented foods at home, which is cheaper and likely more potent.

I've provided a chapter of easy recipes for fermented foods in this book, beginning on page 109. They are delicious and will keep your gut bacteria thriving!

Oregano Oil

Oregano oil is a powerful essential oil that has antifungal, antibacterial, antimicrobial, and even antiviral properties. If you are struggling with candida overgrowth (common in people who have followed a sugar- and carb-heavy diet in the past), then oregano oil has been shown to be very effective in getting it under control.

At the first sign of a cold, I take a few drops of oregano oil under my tongue. If I catch it early enough, I can avoid getting sick even when everyone around me is coughing up a storm. Oregano oil is also fantastic if you suspect that you've eaten something off—it kills bacteria in the stomach quickly and usually resolves any problems within an hour or two.

Oregano oil is also antiparasitic, so we take it on the regular living in Central America. Because we don't want to kill off the good bacteria with the bad, we never take oregano oil for more than ten days at a time, and then afterward we eat lots of probiotic foods to repopulate any beneficial bacteria that might have been collateral damage.

Potassium

Potassium supplementation is crucial on a keto diet because you drink a lot of water and don't retain fluid, which results in a lot of lost electrolytes. An imbalance in sodium, potassium, and magnesium can wreak havoc on your body in the form of headaches, cramps, and even heart palpitations and dizzy spells. It can also cause moodiness.

A lot of natural sources of potassium, like bananas and potatoes, are off-limits on a keto diet—or at least in quantities high enough to make a difference. If you're seeking to boost your potassium intake without pills or powders, the following is a list of high-potassium foods that are keto-friendly:

▶ Avocado

▶ Romaine lettuce

▶ Salmon (fresh or canned)

▶ Spinach

▶ Swiss chard

▶ Tomato sauce

The easiest way to get your potassium on a keto diet is with a product called lite salt. It's half sodium and half potassium and tastes almost exactly like regular salt. Just ½ teaspoon per day spread out over your regular consumption of food will help immensely. That being said, it is possible to overdose on potassium and get hyperkalemia, so don't go crazy with lite salt, either. Just a few shakes a day and you should be fine. You can find lite salt in the spice aisle in most grocery stores, and it's pretty inexpensive.

Magnesium

Magnesium deficiency is also common on a keto diet. It can cause unpleasant symptoms like muscle spasms and cramps, heart palpitations, headaches, nausea, anxiety, and difficulty sleeping, just to name a few.

Getting enough magnesium on a keto diet is possible if you eat lots of magnesium-rich foods like these:

- Almonds
- Avocados
- Beet greens
- Bone broth
- Cashews
- Dark chocolate
- Hemp seeds

- Mineral water
- Pumpkin seeds
- Sardines
- Spinach
- Sunflower seeds
- Swiss chard

If you find that you are still suffering from symptoms of magnesium deficiency even after adding these foods to your diet, you can supplement with magnesium citrate, which is inexpensive and comes in pill or powder form. Beware of oversupplementation of magnesium citrate, which has a laxative effect.

An Epsom salt bath or foot soak also works wonders for a magnesium deficiency, as magnesium can be absorbed effectively through the skin. My favorite way to get magnesium is to dissolve a few tablespoons of Epsom salts in a small amount of water and then blend it with organic coconut oil and a drop of lavender essential oil to make a calming moisturizer that I apply before bed—it smells amazing, and I sleep like a baby.

Get Equipped

I firmly believe that you don't need thousands of dollars' worth of appliances to be a good cook, keto or otherwise. For the most part, you can get by with a good knife, some cutting boards, and a few decent pots. That being said, there are kitchen tools that make cooking easier and save you time, and I'm always a fan of that. The following are some of my favorite tools and gadgets that you may want to consider investing in.

Immersion Blender

Essential for making low-carb soups without having to transfer them to a countertop blender, an immersion blender also does a great job of making small batches of whipped cream super fast! I use this tool to make my bulletproof coffee, and it is creamy, frothy perfection!

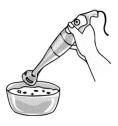

Slow Cooker

Everyone should have one of these. Set it and forget it. The end.

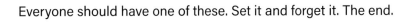

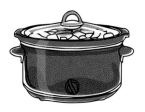

Personal-Sized Blender

I love this inexpensive small appliance for making Cream Cheese Pancakes (page 138), dressings, gravies, and even Cheesy Cauliflower Puree (page 272). My favorite is the Magic Bullet. It's easy to use and to clean for smaller batches.

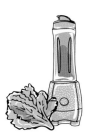

Blender, Preferably Commercial-Grade

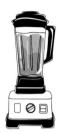

Though a commercial-grade blender isn't always required, sometimes you need a big workhorse of a blender for making your own nut flours, nut butters, and larger batches of soups, sauces, and so on. My favorite, the Vitamix, is so powerful that you can throw your raw ingredients into it and blend for five or six minutes, and it generates enough heat to cook your food while it's blending—leaving you with hot soup when you turn it off. Pretty amazing! It's also great for making smoothies and frozen cocktails in a flash. When a commercial-grade blender is particularly helpful in a recipe, I've noted that; however, nearly all of the recipes in this book can be made with a regular kitchen blender if that's what you've got.

Food Processor

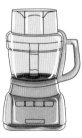

I don't use a food processor all the time, but it really comes in handy for blending chunky items that you don't want to liquefy, like my Roasted Red Pepper Cauliflower Hummus (page 286). Because I don't use it that often, the 8-cup size works just fine for me, but if you are cooking for a larger family, then you can get food processors with a capacity of up to 16 cups. They are sold in mini sizes as well, but I find that my Magic Bullet works fine for small batches on pulse mode. Also, some blenders, like the Ninja, come with both blender and food processor attachments that use the same power base to save space.

Ice Cream Maker

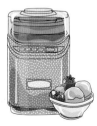

Obviously, nobody needs an ice cream maker to survive, but because homemade ice creams lend themselves so well to the keto diet, it's a nice appliance to have and also fun for kids to use. I love my trusty Cuisinart ice cream maker, which you can get in the 1.5-quart size for under $50.

Ice Pop Molds

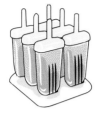

When you don't want to deal with the hassle of making ice cream, ice pops are an easier alternative—and always a hit with the kids as well! You can buy ice pop molds in a wide variety of shapes and sizes on Amazon; just remember that the more basic the shape, the easier it will be to fill and clean. The molds I used for my Coconut Paletas (page 350) hold about 3 ounces of liquid each, which is pretty standard.

Dutch Oven

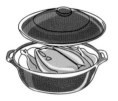

Awesome for simmering bone broths, soups, stews, and sauces, a Dutch oven also goes from stovetop to oven and back, making it super versatile for searing a piece of meat on the stovetop and then sending it to the oven to braise for a few hours. Mmm ... pot roast for dinner!

Spiral Slicer

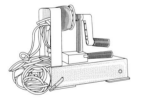

There is no end to the fun and delicious creations you can make with this inexpensive kitchen gadget! It turns all kinds of fruits and veggies, including zucchini, into tasty low-carb, gluten-free, and Paleo-friendly noodles for salads or to replace traditional pasta.

At Least One Great Knife

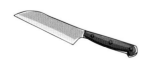

I use my chef's knife for almost everything, but a good paring knife also comes in handy sometimes. There are lots of great brands out there, but my absolute favorite knives are from Global. They are easy to clean and have no joints or crevices to harbor bacteria. They are an investment but will last a lifetime and stand up to endless sharpening.

Nonstick Cookware and Bakeware

Even though keto cooking is high-fat, you still can't beat nonstick pans and bakeware for easy removal and cleanup. I prefer ceramic for pans and silicone for bakeware—but any unscratched nonstick surface will work. You can find good deals on these items at almost every store, especially home stores like T.J.Maxx and HomeGoods.

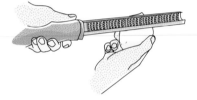

Microplane Grater

Microplane graters come in a variety of coarsenesses and are awesome for grating citrus zest, which I use a lot in my recipes to contribute a citrus flavor without the carbs found in citrus juice. I also use them to grate chocolate and Parmesan cheese on the regular.

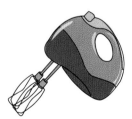

Electric Mixer

For years I got by with my trusty handheld mixer, but I dreamed of having a big KitchenAid stand mixer. When I finally got one, it was a beauty and I was really excited about it. I almost never used it, though, because the handheld mixer got the job done and was so much easier to clean and store! I eventually sold my stand mixer when we moved, and I never got another one. An electric mixer is crucial for beating egg whites and creaming butter and sweetener properly, but if you don't have a big stand mixer, an inexpensive handheld mixer will do the job just fine.

Kitchen Scale

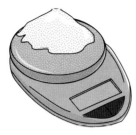

You can buy a kitchen scale for around $20. While I don't use mine all the time, it comes in handy for weighing meats and things like baking chocolate that can't easily be measured by volume.

Parchment Paper

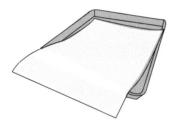

I'm listing parchment paper in essential kitchenware because I use it all the time! It's so helpful for baking, especially because it keeps things from sticking, makes baked goods easy to remove without breaking, and prevents the accumulation of baked-on gunk, which makes doing dishes a whole lot easier. I usually buy it in bulk at Costco, but you can order it online as well.

Instant Pot

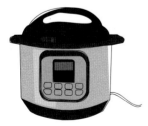

Though not necessarily essential, the Instant Pot is taking the world by storm, and for good reason. Primarily used as a pressure cooker, it also works as a slow cooker, has a sauté function, and even has presets for making rice and yogurt (which I never use). If you're intimidated by a traditional pressure cooker, then a multicooker like the Instant Pot is for you. Very easy to use and not scary at all, it can help you get even the toughest cuts of meat on the table in under an hour. It even makes cheesecake!

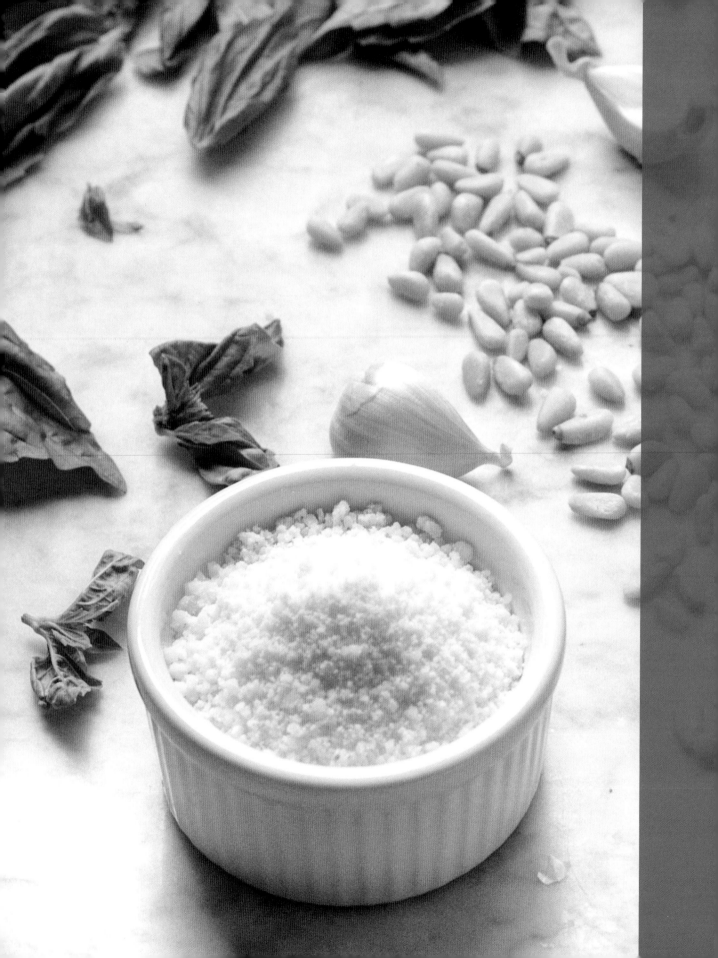

PART 2:

4-week basic keto meal plan & weekly shopping lists

These meal plans are meant to feed one person, so if you're doing keto for two, plan to double everything. The daily nutrition information assumes one serving as defined in each recipe. A weekly shopping list follows each week's meal plan.

Week 1

Prep Notes

☑ Make three batches of Cream Cheese Pancakes (page 138) at the beginning of the week and reheat in the microwave as needed to save time in the mornings.

☑ Make and freeze a batch of Snickerdoodle Haystack Cookies (page 342) to use throughout the four weeks of the plan. Defrost for at least 5 minutes before eating.

WEEK 1	BREAKFAST	LUNCH	
DAY 1	coffee w/ 2 tablespoons heavy whipping cream, Cream Cheese Pancakes w/ 1 tablespoon butter & sugar-free syrup	Easy No-Chop Chili, ¼ cup Easy Keto Guacamole, 2 tablespoons full-fat sour cream	
DAY 2	coffee w/ 2 tablespoons heavy whipping cream, 2 slices bacon, 2 eggs w/ 1 tablespoon butter	Easy Salsa Chicken, Basic Cauliflower Rice	
DAY 3	coffee w/ 2 tablespoons heavy whipping cream, Cream Cheese Pancakes w/ sugar-free syrup	Zoodles with Creamy Roasted Red Pepper Sauce	
DAY 4	coffee w/ 2 tablespoons heavy whipping cream, 2 slices bacon, 2 eggs w/ 2 tablespoons butter	Cajun Pork Chops with Aioli, 2 cups spring greens	
DAY 5	coffee w/ 2 tablespoons heavy whipping cream, Cream Cheese Pancakes w/ 1 tablespoon butter & sugar-free syrup	Easy No-Chop Chili, ¼ cup Easy Keto Guacamole, 2 tablespoons full-fat sour cream	
DAY 6	coffee w/ 2 tablespoons heavy whipping cream, 2 slices bacon, 2 eggs	Cajun Pork Chops with Aioli, 2 cups spring greens	
DAY 7	coffee w/ 2 tablespoons heavy whipping cream, 2 slices bacon, 2 eggs	Cajun Pork Chops with Aioli, 2 cups spring greens	

DINNER	DESSERT	MACROS	
Easy Salsa Chicken, Basic Cauliflower Rice, 2 cups spring greens, 2 tablespoons Bacon & Tomato Dressing	Snickerdoodle Haystack Cookie	calories	1575
		fat	117g
		protein	102g
		net carbs	16g
Zoodles with Creamy Roasted Red Pepper Sauce, 2 cups spring greens, 2 tablespoons Bacon & Tomato Dressing	Snickerdoodle Haystack Cookie	calories	1367
		fat	103g
		protein	76g
		net carbs	16g
Cajun Pork Chops with Aioli, 2 cups spring greens	Snickerdoodle Haystack Cookie	calories	1551
		fat	132g
		protein	72g
		net carbs	15g
Easy Salsa Chicken, Basic Cauliflower Rice, 2 cups spring greens, 2 tablespoons Bacon & Tomato Dressing		calories	1500
		fat	126g
		protein	132g
		net carbs	10g
Easy Salsa Chicken, Basic Cauliflower Rice, 2 cups spring greens, 2 tablespoons Bacon & Tomato Dressing	Snickerdoodle Haystack Cookie	calories	1568
		fat	117g
		protein	102g
		net carbs	16g
Beef Burrito Bowl	Snickerdoodle Haystack Cookie	calories	1549
		fat	116g
		protein	110g
		net carbs	12g
Beef Burrito Bowl	Snickerdoodle Haystack Cookie	calories	1549
		fat	116g
		protein	110g
		net carbs	12g

Shopping List

Produce

avocados, 4

cauliflower, 1 large head

cherry tomatoes, 5

cilantro, 1 bunch

garlic, 1 bulb

jalapeño pepper, 1

lemon, 1

lime, 1

parsley, 1 bunch

red onion, 1

romaine lettuce, 1 head

spring greens, 2½ pounds

yellow onion, 1

zucchini, 2 medium

Dairy

butter, 1 stick salted, ½ stick unsalted

cheddar cheese, 8 ounces

cream cheese, 8 ounces

heavy whipping cream, ½ pint

mascarpone cheese, 3 ounces

Parmesan cheese, ½ ounce

sour cream, full-fat, 1 cup

Protein

bacon, no sugar added, 1 pound

chicken cutlets, boneless, 6 (6 ounces each) (2¼ pounds total)

eggs, 15

ground beef (80/20), 1 pound

pork chops, bone-in, 4 (8 ounces each) (2 pounds total)

Grocery

roasted red peppers, 1 jar

unsweetened shredded coconut, 6 ounces

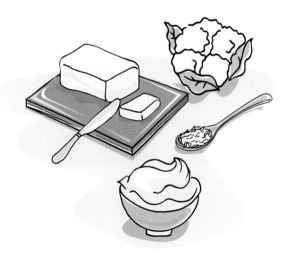

Check Your Fridge, Freezer, or Pantry For:

avocado oil

baking soda

Cajun Seasoning (page 76)

cayenne pepper

chipotle powder

coconut flour

coffee

Creole seasoning

garlic powder

granulated erythritol

ground black pepper

ground cinnamon

ground coriander

ground cumin

kosher salt

mayonnaise

onion powder

sugar-free pancake syrup

vanilla extract

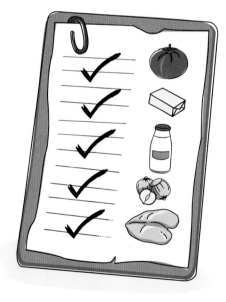

Week 2

Prep Notes

☑ Make the Cinnamon Walnut Streusel Muffins (page 128) at the beginning of the week and store them in the freezer to defrost as needed over the next couple of weeks. When you're ready to eat, defrost one on the counter for 10 minutes or microwave on high for 15 seconds.

WEEK 2	BREAKFAST	LUNCH	
DAY 1	coffee w/ 2 tablespoons heavy whipping cream, Cinnamon Walnut Streusel Muffin	Green Chicken Enchilada Cauliflower Casserole, 2 tablespoons sour cream	
DAY 2	coffee w/ 2 tablespoons heavy whipping cream, Cinnamon Walnut Streusel Muffin	Green Chicken Enchilada Cauliflower Casserole, 2 tablespoons sour cream	
DAY 3	coffee w/ 2 tablespoons heavy whipping cream, Cinnamon Walnut Streusel Muffin	Green Chicken Enchilada Cauliflower Casserole, 2 tablespoons sour cream	
DAY 4	coffee w/ 2 tablespoons heavy whipping cream, Cinnamon Walnut Streusel Muffin	Chicken Larb	
DAY 5	coffee w/ 2 tablespoons heavy whipping cream, Cinnamon Walnut Streusel Muffin	Chicken Larb	
DAY 6	coffee w/ 2 tablespoons heavy whipping cream, Cinnamon Walnut Streusel Muffin	Meatballs alla Parmigiana, 1 cup Basic Zucchini Noodles	
DAY 7	coffee w/ 2 tablespoons heavy whipping cream, Cinnamon Walnut Streusel Muffin	Meatballs alla Parmigiana, 1 cup Basic Zucchini Noodles	

DINNER	DESSERT	MACROS	
Chicken Larb	Snickerdoodle Haystack Cookie	calories	1115
		fat	84g
		protein	69g
		net carbs	15g
Chicken Larb	Snickerdoodle Haystack Cookie	calories	1115
		fat	84g
		protein	69g
		net carbs	15g
Meatballs alla Parmigiana, 1 cup Basic Zucchini Noodles	Snickerdoodle Haystack Cookie	calories	1366
		fat	107g
		protein	78g
		net carbs	17g
Meatballs alla Parmigiana, 1 cup Basic Zucchini Noodles	Cinnamon Walnut Streusel Muffin	calories	1295
		fat	99g
		protein	75g
		net carbs	19g
Green Chicken Enchilada Cauliflower Casserole, 2 tablespoons sour cream	Snickerdoodle Haystack Cookie	calories	1115
		fat	84g
		protein	69g
		net carbs	15g
Green Chicken Enchilada Cauliflower Casserole, 2 tablespoons sour cream		calories	1185
		fat	89g
		protein	76g
		net carbs	15g
Cauliflower Risotto with Sherry & Hazelnuts		calories	1226
		fat	98g
		protein	51g
		net carbs	16g

Shopping List

Produce

basil, 1 bunch

butter lettuce, 2 heads

cauliflower, 3 medium heads

cilantro, 1 bunch

ginger, 1 knob

lime, 1

mint, 1 bunch

red onion, 1

thyme leaves, 1 package

zucchini, 2 medium

Protein

chicken breasts, boneless, skinless, 1 pound

ground beef (80/20), 1 pound

ground chicken, 1 pound

Grocery

dry sherry, 1 bottle

hazelnuts, raw, 2 ounces

salsa verde, 4 ounces

walnuts, raw, 2 ounces

Dairy

butter, 1½ sticks + 1 tablespoon

cream cheese, full-fat, 4 ounces

heavy whipping cream, ½ pint

mascarpone cheese, 2 ounces

Parmesan cheese, 2 ounces

sharp cheddar cheese, 4 ounces

sour cream, full-fat, ½ pint

unsweetened vanilla-flavored almond milk, 1 carton

whole-milk mozzarella cheese, 4 ounces

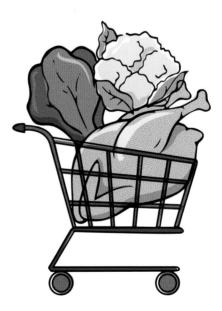

Check Your Fridge, Freezer, or Pantry For:

almond flour

baking powder

coconut flour

coconut oil

coffee

dried oregano leaves

fish sauce

garlic powder

granulated erythritol

ground black pepper

ground cinnamon

kosher salt

marinara sauce (store-bought or homemade, page 106)

onion powder

red pepper flakes

Sriracha sauce

vanilla extract

wheat-free soy sauce

xanthan gum

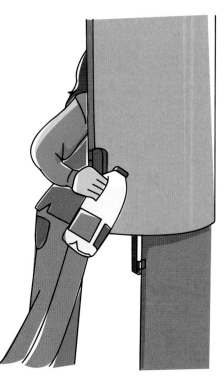

Week 3

Notes

You'll note that this week's plan does not include a dessert recipe. If you feel the need for something sweet, you may add 1 ounce of dark chocolate to each day. If you opt to do this, be sure the brand you are using contains less than 5g net carbs per ounce.

WEEK 3	BREAKFAST	LUNCH	
DAY 1	coffee w/ 2 tablespoons heavy whipping cream, 2 slices bacon, 2 eggs w/ 1 tablespoon butter	Cauliflower Risotto with Sherry & Hazelnuts (from Week 2)	
DAY 2	coffee w/ 2 tablespoons heavy whipping cream, 2 slices bacon, 2 eggs w/ 1 tablespoon butter	Chili con Carne, 2 tablespoons sour cream, Bacon & Cheddar Cornless Muffin	
DAY 3	coffee w/ 2 tablespoons heavy whipping cream, 2 slices bacon, 2 eggs w/ 1 tablespoon butter	Pecan-Crusted Chicken Fingers, 2 tablespoons Sweet Sriracha Dipping Sauce, 2 cups spring greens	
DAY 4	coffee w/ 2 tablespoons heavy whipping cream, Cinnamon Walnut Streusel Muffin	Chili con Carne, 2 tablespoons sour cream, Bacon & Cheddar Cornless Muffin	
DAY 5	coffee w/ 2 tablespoons heavy whipping cream, 2 slices bacon, 2 eggs w/ 1 tablespoon butter	Pork Fried Cauliflower Rice, 2 cups spring greens, 2 tablespoons Ginger Scallion Dressing	
DAY 6	coffee w/ 2 tablespoons heavy whipping cream, Cinnamon Walnut Streusel Muffin	Chili con Carne, 2 tablespoons sour cream, Bacon & Cheddar Cornless Muffin	
DAY 7	coffee w/ 2 tablespoons heavy whipping cream, 2 slices bacon, 2 eggs w/ 1 tablespoon butter	Pork Fried Cauliflower Rice, 2 cups spring greens, 2 tablespoons Ginger Scallion Dressing	

DINNER		MACROS	
Chili con Carne, 2 tablespoons sour cream, Bacon & Cheddar Cornless Muffin	182 / 302	calories	1452
		fat	118g
		protein	68g
		net carbs	13g
Pecan-Crusted Chicken Fingers, 2 tablespoons Sweet Sriracha Dipping Sauce, 2 cups spring greens	152 / 99	calories	1538
		fat	124g
		protein	90g
		net carbs	12g
Chili con Carne, 2 tablespoons sour cream, Bacon & Cheddar Cornless Muffin	leftover / leftover	calories	1538
		fat	118g
		protein	68g
		net carbs	13g
Pork Fried Cauliflower Rice, 2 cups spring greens, 2 tablespoons Ginger Scallion Dressing	204 / 88	calories	1341
		fat	110g
		protein	79g
		net carbs	15g
Pecan-Crusted Chicken Fingers, 2 tablespoons Sweet Sriracha Dipping Sauce, 2 cups spring greens	leftover / leftover	calories	1283
		fat	98g
		protein	82g
		net carbs	12g
Pork Fried Cauliflower Rice, 2 cups spring greens, 2 tablespoons Ginger Scallion Dressing	leftover / leftover	calories	1341
		fat	110g
		protein	79g
		net carbs	15g
Pecan-Crusted Chicken Fingers, 2 tablespoons Sweet Sriracha Dipping Sauce, 2 cups spring greens	leftover / leftover	calories	1283
		fat	98g
		protein	82g
		net carbs	12g

Shopping List

Produce

cauliflower, 1 medium head

cilantro, 1 bunch

garlic, 1 bulb

ginger, 1 knob

limes, 3

scallions, 1 bunch

spring greens, 1 pound

yellow onion, 1

Dairy

butter, 1 pound

heavy whipping cream, 1 pint

sour cream, full-fat, 1 pint

Protein

bacon, no-sugar-added, 1 pound

beef chuck, boneless, 2 pounds

chicken tenders or boneless, skinless
chicken breasts, 1 pound

eggs, 1 dozen

pork sirloin cutlets, boneless,
1 pound

Grocery

beef broth, 3 cups

chipotles in adobo sauce,
1 small can

pecans, raw, 8 ounces

Frozen

peas, 4 ounces

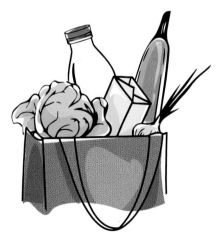

Check Your Fridge, Freezer, or Pantry For:

almond flour

apple cider vinegar

avocado oil

baking soda

cayenne pepper

chili powder

Cinnamon Walnut Streusel Muffins (left over from Week 2)

coconut flour

coconut oil

coffee

dried oregano leaves

dry sherry (left over from Week 2)

fish sauce

garlic powder

ginger powder

granulated erythritol

ground black pepper

ground cinnamon

ground coriander

ground cumin

kosher salt

mayonnaise

olive oil

onion powder

red pepper flakes

Sriracha sauce

toasted sesame oil

vanilla extract

wheat-free soy sauce

white vinegar

Worcestershire sauce

xanthan gum

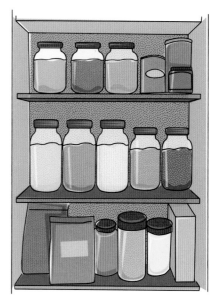

Week 4

WEEK 4	BREAKFAST		LUNCH	
DAY 1	coffee w/ 2 tablespoons heavy whipping cream, 2 slices bacon, 2 eggs w/ 1 tablespoon butter		Korean BBQ Beef Wraps	190
DAY 2	coffee w/ 2 tablespoons heavy whipping cream, Spanish Tortilla with Chorizo	130	Chicken Tetrazzini	leftover
DAY 3	coffee w/ 2 tablespoons heavy whipping cream, Spanish Tortilla with Chorizo	leftover	Chicken Tetrazzini	leftover
DAY 4	coffee w/ 2 tablespoons heavy whipping cream, Cinnamon Walnut Streusel Muffin	leftover	Korean BBQ Beef Wraps	leftover
DAY 5	coffee w/ 2 tablespoons heavy whipping cream, Spanish Tortilla with Chorizo	leftover	Korean BBQ Beef Wraps	leftover
DAY 6	coffee w/ 2 tablespoons heavy whipping cream, Spanish Tortilla with Chorizo	leftover	Chicken Tetrazzini	leftover
DAY 7	coffee w/ 2 tablespoons heavy whipping cream, Cinnamon Walnut Streusel Muffin	leftover	Sweet & Spicy Asian Meatballs, Basic Cauliflower Rice	leftover leftover

DINNER		DESSERT		MACROS	
Chicken Tetrazzini		Pecan Shortbread Cookie		calories	1307
				fat	96g
				protein	78g
				net carbs	16g
Korean BBQ Beef Wraps		Pecan Shortbread Cookie		calories	1359
				fat	99g
				protein	80g
				net carbs	17g
Sweet & Spicy Asian Meatballs, Basic Cauliflower Rice		Pecan Shortbread Cookie		calories	1473
				fat	116g
				protein	77g
				net carbs	17g
Chicken Tetrazzini		Pecan Shortbread Cookie		calories	1231
				fat	92g
				protein	58g
				net carbs	17g
Sweet & Spicy Asian Meatballs, Basic Cauliflower Rice		Pecan Shortbread Cookie		calories	1386
				fat	108g
				protein	77g
				net carbs	16g
Sweet & Spicy Asian Meatballs, Basic Cauliflower Rice		Pecan Shortbread Cookie		calories	1470
				fat	116g
				protein	77g
				net carbs	17g
				calories	773
				fat	77g
				protein	47g
				net carbs	8g

You've completed one month!
Celebrate with dinner out!

Shopping List

Produce

cauliflower, 2 large heads

celery root (celeriac), 1 medium

green leaf lettuce, 1 head

red bell pepper, 1

scallions, 1 bunch

white mushrooms, 4 ounces

yellow onion, 1

zucchini, 3 medium

Dairy

butter, 1½ sticks

heavy whipping cream, 1 pint

Manchego cheese, 2 ounces

Parmesan cheese, 2 ounces

Protein

beef sirloin, 1 pound

chicken thighs, boneless, skinless, 1 pound

chorizo, raw (fresh), 8 ounces

eggs, 1 dozen

ground pork, 1 pound

Grocery

chicken broth, 1 cup

water chestnuts, 1 (4-ounce) can

Check Your Fridge, Freezer, or Pantry For:

almond flour

avocado oil

cayenne pepper

coffee

dry sherry (left over from Week 2)

extra-virgin olive oil

frozen peas (left over from Week 3)

granulated erythritol

ground black pepper

ground nutmeg

kosher salt

pecans, raw (left over from Week 3)

red pepper flakes

Sriracha sauce

toasted sesame oil

unseasoned rice wine vinegar

vanilla extract

wheat-free soy sauce

xanthan gum

Guide to the Recipes

Now that you know the basics of how to succeed on a ketogenic diet, let's talk about my favorite part—the recipes! As many of you know, I have a blog called I Breathe I'm Hungry, where I post delicious keto recipes for free on a weekly basis. While this book contains a few reader favorites, like Cream Cheese Pancakes (page 138), Meatballs alla Parmigiana (page 192), and Green Chicken Enchilada Cauliflower Casserole (page 156), almost all of the recipes in this book are brand-new—and they're some of my favorites so far, if I do say so!

My goal when creating the recipes for *Keto for Life* was to give you a variety of interesting flavors and cuisines to choose from, but also to keep them family-friendly, relatively easy to execute, and, above all, delicious. According to the friends and family I've enlisted as taste-testers, these are indeed some of my best recipes yet!

All of the recipes in this book are gluten- and grain-free, mostly because I believe that those foods cause cravings and inflammation, which can slow your progress.

For those of you with allergies or intolerances, I've included handy icons that identify whether a recipe is dairy-free, egg-free, and/or nut-free. To help you with meal planning, there is an allergen index at the back of the book that enables you to see at a glance which recipes are dairy-free, egg-free, and/or nut-free. Please note that with regard to the allergen icons, coconut is not treated as a tree nut, so recipes that contain coconut products (but no tree nuts) are designated as nut-free.

For those of you who are vegetarian or are looking to limit your consumption of meat, you will find an icon identifying vegetarian recipes. To look up the vegetarian recipes in the book, turn to the allergen index.

Each recipe provides the yield, prep time, and cook time, as well as nutrition information and tips on storage and reheating for meal prep. I've also included Pro Tips and other tricks throughout the book to help you improve your efficiency and up your cooking game overall.

I hope that you and your family will love the recipes and find favorites in these pages that you will make for years to come!

I'd love it if you would snap a photo of your family cooking and/or enjoying the recipes and tag me on Instagram @ibreatheimhungry! If you're okay with me sharing them, too, be sure to hashtag them #IBIHketoforlife. I'll be on the lookout for your favorites and will get such a kick out of seeing your photos!

Now let's get cooking!

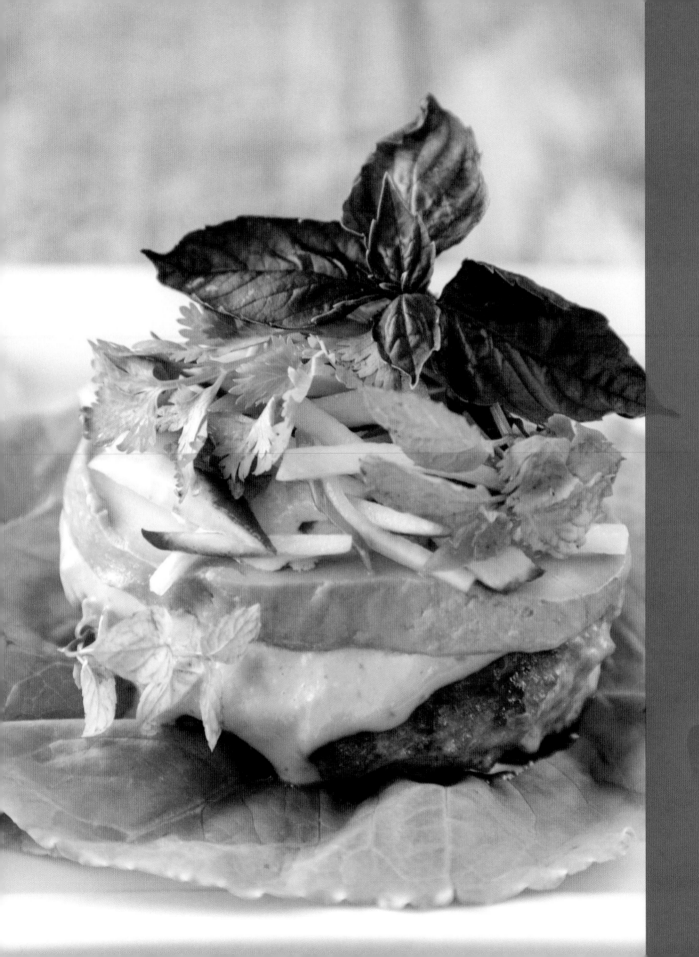

PART 3:

the recipes

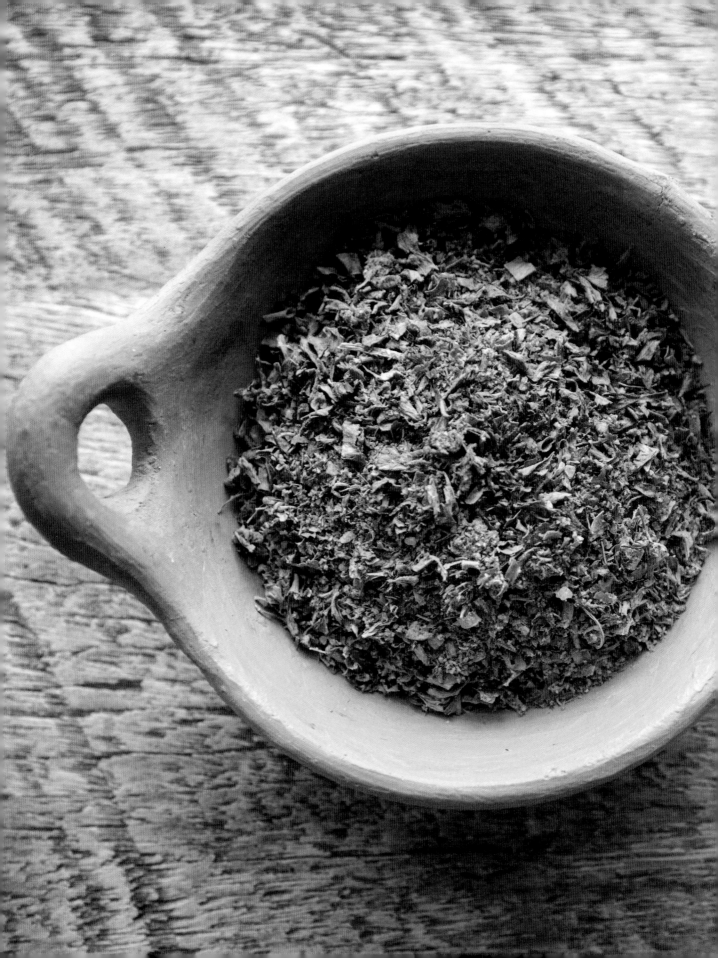

basics

Cream Cheese Wraps / 70

Cream Cheese Noodles / 72

Keto Breadcrumbs / 74

Basic Breading / 75

Cajun Seasoning / 76

Chicken Seasoning / 77

Blackening Seasoning / 78

Jerk Seasoning / 79

Beef Seasoning / 80

Fish and Seafood Seasoning / 81

Easy Chicken Bone Broth / 82

Simple Syrup—Basic and Flavored / 84

Creamy Basil-Parmesan Vinaigrette / 86

Strawberry Basil Vinaigrette / 87

Ginger Scallion Dressing / 88

Bacon & Tomato Dressing / 89

Creamy Blue Cheese Dressing / 90

Creamy Lemon Caper Dressing / 92

Tangy Feta & Dill Dressing / 93

Tahini Lemon Dressing / 94

Raspberry Coulis / 95

Easy Basil Pesto / 96

Basic Remoulade / 97

Cucumber Raita / 98

Sweet Sriracha Dipping Sauce / 99

Compound Butter / 100

Keto Ketchup / 102

Easy Keto BBQ Sauce / 104

Sweet Chili Sauce / 105

Easy No-Cook Marinara / 106

5-Minute Alfredo Sauce / 107

Cream Cheese Wraps

I keep my freezer stocked with these wraps at all times; they are great for sandwich-style wraps, fajitas, soft tacos, and even enchiladas. There is no end to what you can do with these wraps, and they can be thawed in the microwave in just a few seconds.

Yield: **4 wraps** • Serving Size: **1 wrap** • Prep Time: **5 minutes** • Cook Time: **12 minutes**

4 large eggs

3 ounces cream cheese (⅓ cup), softened

¼ teaspoon kosher salt

⅛ teaspoon ground black pepper

⅛ teaspoon garlic powder

1 tablespoon butter

1 Place all of the ingredients except for the butter in a small blender and blend for 30 seconds, or until smooth. Let the batter rest for 5 minutes.

2 Melt the butter in a 10- to 12-inch nonstick skillet over medium heat until bubbling. Pour ¼ cup of the batter into the pan and tilt the pan in a circular motion to create a round shape about 8 inches in diameter. Cook for 2 minutes, or until the center of the wrap is no longer glossy and wet looking.

3 Carefully flip the wrap and cook for 30 more seconds. Remove to a plate and repeat with the remaining batter, making a total of 4 wraps.

4 Store in an airtight container in the refrigerator for up to 5 days or in the freezer for up to 3 months.

Calories: 147 | Fat: 12g | Protein: 8g | Carbs: 2g | Fiber: 0g | **Net Carbs: 2g**

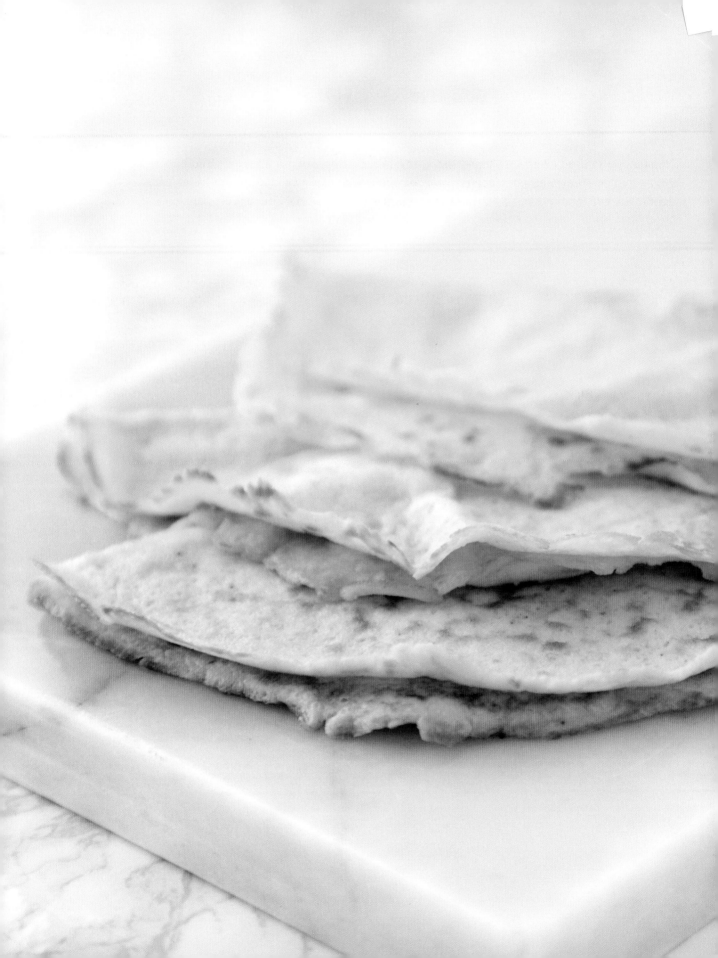

dairy-free egg-free nut-free vegetarian

Cream Cheese Noodles

These noodles are baked instead of fried, which prevents them from browning and keeps the flavor neutral, like real pasta. They work best in creamy sauces. Cutting them into wide noodles rather than a thin spaghetti keeps them from falling apart. You can also custom-cut the sheets for lasagna or even roll them to make stuffed manicotti.

Yield: **4 cups** ◆ Serving Size: **1 cup** ◆ Prep Time: **5 minutes** ◆ Cook Time: **10 minutes**

4 large eggs

3 ounces cream cheese (⅓ cup), softened

⅛ teaspoon kosher salt

⅛ teaspoon ground black pepper

⅛ teaspoon garlic powder

1. Preheat the oven to 325°F. Line a 15 by 10-inch sheet pan with parchment paper or foil.

2. Place all of the ingredients in a small blender and blend for 30 seconds, or until smooth. Let the batter rest for 5 minutes.

3. Pour the batter into the lined pan. Bake for 10 minutes, or until the center doesn't jiggle when you shake the pan. Remove from the oven and let cool in the pan for 5 minutes.

4. Lift the sheet of "pasta" out of the pan with the parchment or foil attached and place it on a cutting board. Gently roll up the pasta, removing the parchment or foil as you roll.

5. Use a sharp knife to slice the pasta into ⅛-inch-wide noodles. Gently unroll and set aside until ready to serve.

6. Store in an airtight container in the refrigerator for up to 5 days or in the freezer for up to 3 months. To reheat the noodles, thaw if frozen, then place in a baking dish and heat in a preheated 325°F oven for 5 minutes. Alternatively, you can microwave them on high, uncovered, for 15 seconds.

Calories: 147 | Fat: 12g | Protein: 8g | Carbs: 2g | Fiber: 0g | **Net Carbs: 2g**

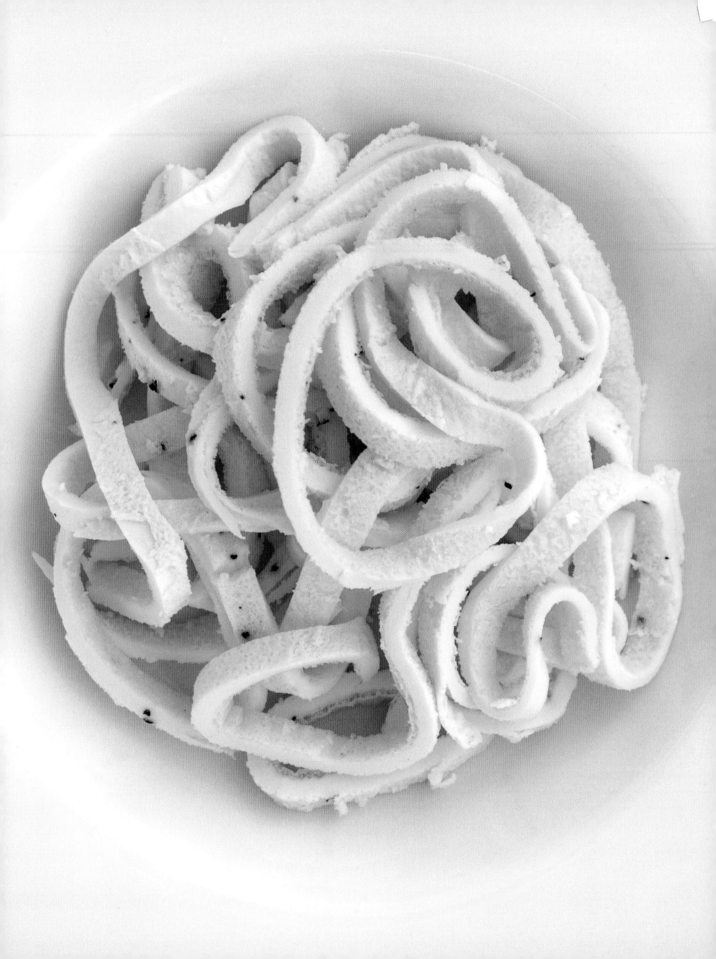

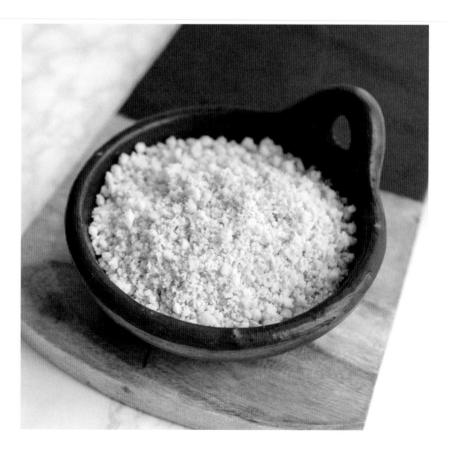

Keto Breadcrumbs

These keto breadcrumbs are prebaked and can be used to top casseroles for added texture and flavor. They also add a nice buttery crunch to seafood dishes, like my Baked Mahi Mahi in Garlic Parsley Butter (page 236).

Yield: **2 cups** ◆ Serving Size: **2 tablespoons** ◆ Prep Time: **5 minutes** ◆ Cook Time: **8 minutes**

6 tablespoons butter, melted

2 cups superfine blanched almond flour

1 Preheat the oven to 350°F. Place the butter and flour in a medium-sized bowl and stir with a fork until pea-sized lumps form.

2 Crumble the dough with your fingers into a 15 by 10-inch sheet pan and spread lightly to form a thin layer. Bake for 8 minutes, or until light golden-brown. Let cool for 30 minutes.

3 Store in an airtight container in the refrigerator for up to 5 days or in the freezer for up to 6 months.

Calories: 118 | Fat: 7g | Protein: 3g | Carbs: 3g | Fiber: 1.5g | **Net Carbs: 1.5g**

Basic Breading

dairy-free egg-free nut-free vegetarian

This basic breading works as a replacement for panko or other breadcrumbs that you might use to coat something before baking or frying. It is just as crispy and flavorful; you'll never miss the carbs!

Yield: ¾ cup • Serving Size: 2 tablespoons • Prep Time: 5 minutes

½ cup superfine blanched almond flour

¼ cup grated Parmesan cheese

½ teaspoon kosher salt

½ teaspoon dried parsley

½ teaspoon garlic powder

½ teaspoon paprika

⅛ teaspoon ground black pepper

Place all of the ingredients in a small bowl and mix well. Store in an airtight container in the refrigerator for up to 5 days or in the freezer for up to 6 months.

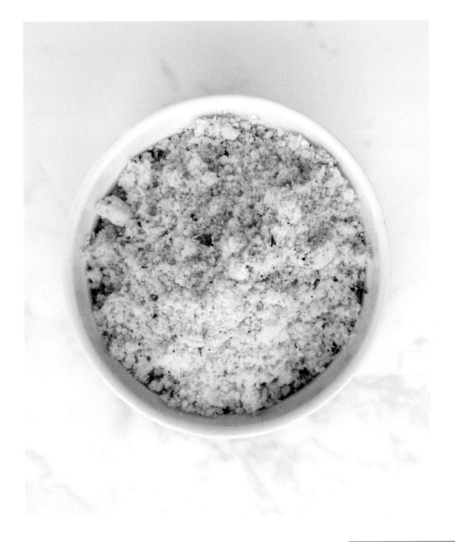

Calories: 69 | Fat: 6g | Protein: 4g | Carbs: 2.5g | Fiber: 1g | **Net Carbs: 1.5g**

Cajun Seasoning

My family loves the flavor and heat that Cajun seasoning delivers, so we use it often. It's fantastic on seafood and chicken or mixed into mayonnaise or sauces for an extra kick!

Yield: **⅓ cup** • Serving Size: **1 teaspoon** • Prep Time: **5 minutes**

1 tablespoon garlic powder

1 tablespoon kosher salt

1 tablespoon paprika

2 teaspoons cayenne pepper

2 teaspoons dried oregano leaves

2 teaspoons dried thyme leaves

2 teaspoons onion powder

1 teaspoon ground black pepper

Place all of the ingredients in a small bowl and mix well. Store in an airtight container for up to 6 months.

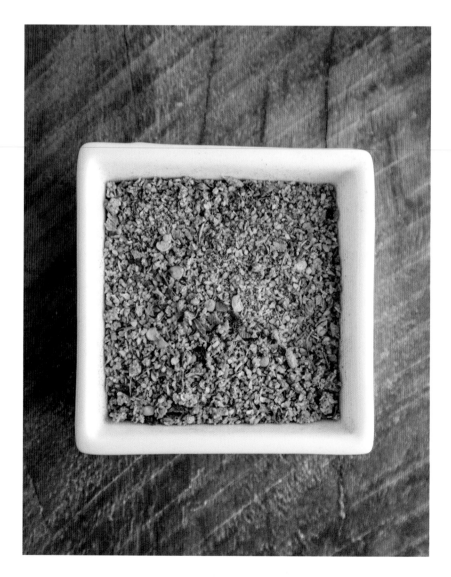

Calories: 5 | Fat: 0g | Protein: 0g | Carbs: 1g | Fiber: 0g | **Net Carbs: 1g**

Chicken Seasoning

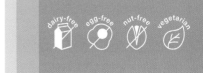

There are tons of chicken seasonings for sale in the spice aisle, but when you make your own at home, you can avoid fillers, MSG, and non-caking agents that might add carbs. I think the flavor is better, too, but maybe that's just me. This is a great all-around seasoning for baked or grilled chicken.

Yield: ¾ cup • Serving Size: 1 teaspoon • Prep Time: 5 minutes

2 tablespoons dried parsley

2 tablespoons kosher salt

2 tablespoons onion powder

2 tablespoons smoked paprika

1 tablespoon dried rosemary leaves

1 tablespoon dried thyme leaves

1 tablespoon garlic powder

2 teaspoons ground black pepper

Place all of the ingredients in a small bowl and mix well. Store in an airtight container for up to 6 months.

Calories: 4 | Fat: 0g | Protein: 0g | Carbs: 1.5g | Fiber: 0.5g | **Net Carbs: 1g**

dairy-free egg-free nut-free vegetarian

Blackening Seasoning

One of my favorite ways to enjoy fresh fish is blackened. Since we ate a lot of fresh fish while living in Belize, I started making my own blackening seasoning, and it's so good that I'll never go back to store-bought! This seasoning is also great on shrimp and chicken. Be sure to use it in a well-ventilated area, and don't breathe in the steam or smoke while your seasoned food cooks or you'll suffer a painful coughing fit from all of the spices.

Yield: **1 cup** ◆ Serving Size: **1 teaspoon** ◆ Prep Time: **5 minutes**

3 tablespoons cayenne pepper

3 tablespoons chili powder

3 tablespoons paprika

2 tablespoons ground black pepper

1 tablespoon chipotle powder

1 tablespoon dried oregano leaves

1 tablespoon dried thyme leaves

1 tablespoon garlic powder

1 tablespoon onion powder

Place all of the ingredients in a small bowl and mix well. Store in an airtight container for up to 6 months.

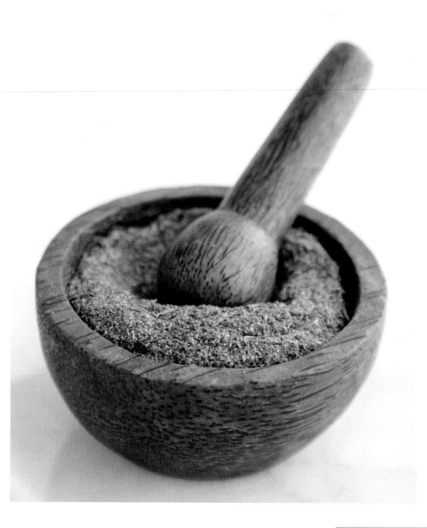

Calories: 7 | Fat: 0g | Protein: 0g | Carbs: 1.5g | Fiber: 0.5g | **Net Carbs: 1g**

Jerk Seasoning

dairy-free · egg-free · nut-free · vegetarian

I love spicy food, and this jerk seasoning delivers not only heat but also amazing flavor to any grilled or roasted fish, chicken, or pork. If you're into sweet-and-spicy combos, then you can't go wrong with any protein cooked with this jerk seasoning and paired with my Sweet Chili Sauce (page 105).

Yield: ⅓ cup • Serving Size: 1 teaspoon • Prep Time: 5 minutes

1 tablespoon cayenne pepper

1 tablespoon granulated erythritol

2 teaspoons dried parsley

2 teaspoons garlic powder

2 teaspoons kosher salt

2 teaspoons onion powder

1 teaspoon dried thyme leaves

1 teaspoon ground allspice

1 teaspoon smoked paprika

½ teaspoon ginger powder

½ teaspoon ground cinnamon

½ teaspoon ground nutmeg

½ teaspoon ground black pepper

Place all of the ingredients in a small bowl and mix well. Store in an airtight container for up to 6 months.

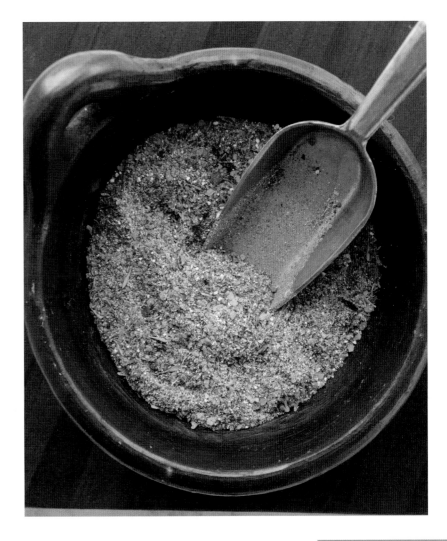

Calories: 5 | Fat: 0g | Protein: 0g | Carbs: 1.5g | Fiber: 0.5g | Erythritol: 1g | **Net Carbs: 1g**

Beef Seasoning

Whether you're seasoning a roast, some steaks for the grill, or even ground meat for burgers, this well-rounded mix will bring out the best flavor in your meat.

Yield: **½ cup** ◆ Serving Size: **1 teaspoon** ◆ Prep Time: **5 minutes**

2 tablespoons kosher salt

1 tablespoon garlic powder

1 tablespoon ground black pepper

1 tablespoon onion powder

1 tablespoon smoked paprika

1 teaspoon dried thyme leaves

1 teaspoon ground coriander

1 teaspoon ground cumin

Place all of the ingredients in a small bowl and mix well. Store in an airtight container for up to 6 months.

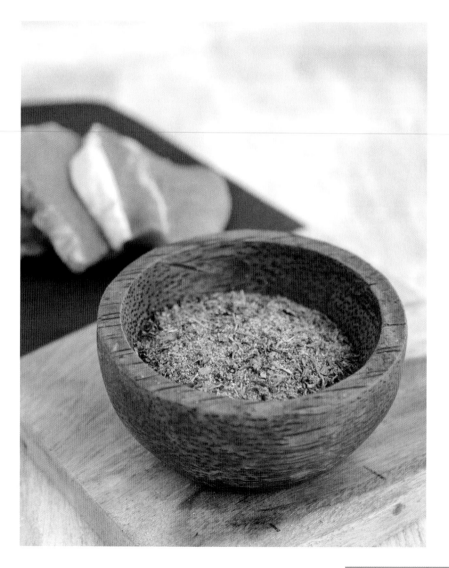

Calories: 4 | Fat: 0g | Protein: 0g | Carbs: 1.5g | Fiber: 0.5g | **Net Carbs: 1g**

Fish and Seafood Seasoning

dairy-free • egg-free • nut-free • vegetarian

I love this seasoning on grilled or oven-roasted fish or shrimp. This specific combination of dried herbs and lemon zest imparts a bright zing that complements pretty much any type of seafood without overpowering its delicate flavor.

Yield: **½ cup** • Serving Size: **1 teaspoon** • Prep Time: **5 minutes**

3 tablespoons dried parsley

1 tablespoon dried chives

1 tablespoon dried dill weed

1 tablespoon grated lemon zest

2 teaspoons celery salt

1 teaspoon dried marjoram leaves

1 teaspoon garlic powder

1 teaspoon ground coriander

1 teaspoon kosher salt

1 teaspoon onion powder

1 teaspoon paprika

½ teaspoon ground white pepper

Place all of the ingredients in a small bowl and mix well. Store in an airtight container for up to 6 months.

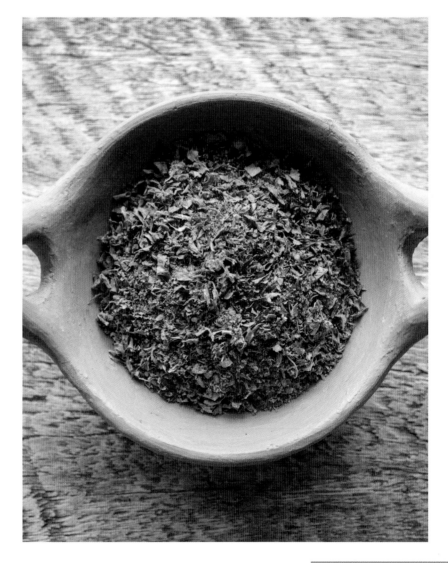

Calories: 2 | Fat: 0g | Protein: 0g | Carbs: 1.5g | Fiber: 0.5g | **Net Carbs: 1g**

dairy-free egg-free nut-free vegetarian

Easy Chicken Bone Broth

Rich and hearty, this bone broth makes a great addition to soups and sauces but also tastes wonderful with some added sea salt as a tonic. When we were living in New York, I loved wrapping my hands around a mug of salted bone broth on chilly winter evenings while watching a movie. It's especially soothing and comforting if you're fighting a cold or the flu, when nothing else seems appealing.

Yield: **12 cups** • Serving Size: **1 cup** • Prep Time: **5 minutes** • Cook Time: **8 hours in a slow cooker**

1 cooked chicken carcass (most of the meat removed), and any pan drippings

1 (1-inch) knob fresh ginger, peeled and sliced

1 small onion, peeled and quartered

1 cup chopped celery tops with leaves

2 cloves garlic, peeled

2 tablespoons apple cider vinegar

4 quarts filtered water

1 Combine all of the ingredients in a 6-quart or larger slow cooker. Cook on high for 8 hours (or longer).

2 Let cool for 1 hour. Then strain the solids from the broth and place in the refrigerator to chill overnight.

3 Skim the solidified fat from the top of the broth. Portion into containers as needed and store in the refrigerator for up to 1 week or in the freezer for up to 3 months.

Variation:
Easy Beef Bone Broth. You can easily use this same basic method to make beef bone broth. Simply replace the chicken carcass and drippings with about 4 pounds of beef bones and cook as directed above. For the best flavor, use short ribs, oxtail, or marrow bones if you can get them.

Alternative Method:
Place all of the ingredients in a 6-quart or larger Instant Pot and seal according to the manufacturer's instructions. Turn the pot on and set it to manual, high pressure, for 1 hour. When finished cooking, release the pressure according to the manufacturer's instructions. Then follow Steps 2 and 3 above to cool, strain, and store the broth.

Calories: 38 | Fat: 2g | Protein: 3g | Carbs: 1.5g | Fiber: 0g | **Net Carbs: 1.5g**

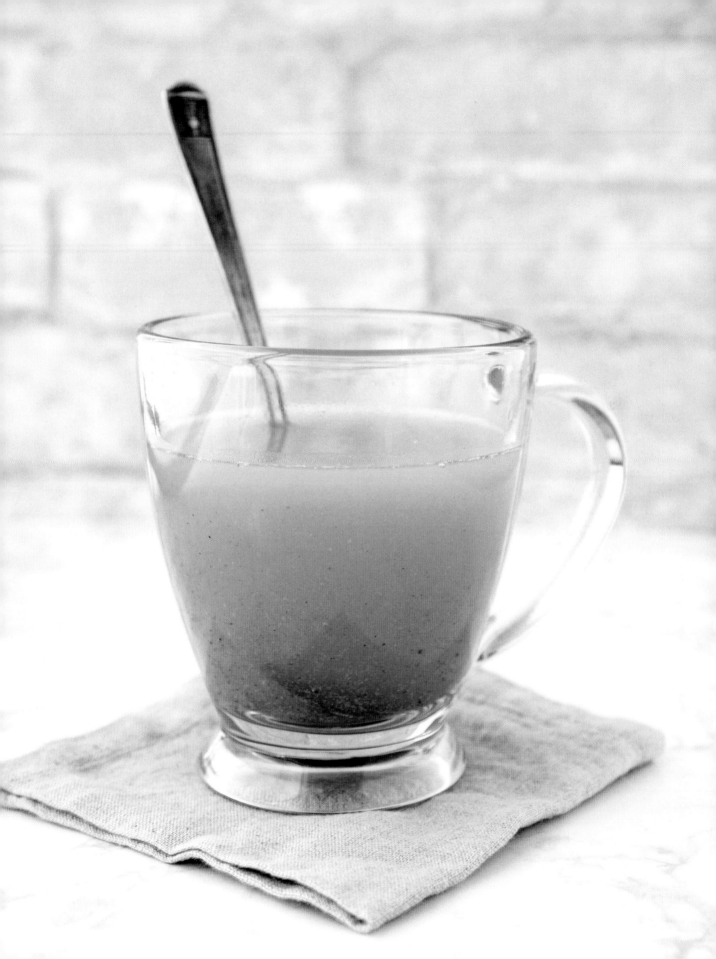

Simple Syrup—
Basic and Flavored

dairy-free *egg-free* *nut-free* *vegetarian*

Simple syrups made with erythritol, especially flavored ones, can be a keto game changer! As the name suggests, these syrups are very easy to make; it takes just minutes, and the syrups will keep for up to a month.

Yield: **2 cups** • Serving Size: **2 tablespoons** • Prep Time: **2 minutes** • Cook Time: **3 minutes**

2 cups filtered water

1 cup granulated erythritol

⅛ teaspoon xanthan gum

1 To make basic simple syrup, combine all of the ingredients in a small saucepan. Cook over medium heat for 3 minutes, stirring occasionally, until all of the sweetener has dissolved. Let cool to room temperature.

2 Pour the syrup into a clean jar with an airtight lid and store in the refrigerator for up to 1 month.

Variations:

Lemon-, Lime-, Orange-, or Grapefruit-Infused Simple Syrup. Add 2 tablespoons grated lemon, lime, orange, or grapefruit zest to the saucepan in Step 1, as described above. Complete Step 1, then let cool and steep at room temperature for 24 hours. Strain out and discard the solids, then continue with Step 2.

Herb-Infused Simple Syrup. Add ¼ cup fresh mint, basil, thyme, or lavender leaves to the saucepan in Step 1, as described above. Complete Step 1, then let cool and steep at room temperature for 24 hours. Strain out and discard the solids, then continue with Step 2.

Coffee-Infused Simple Syrup. Add 2 tablespoons whole roasted coffee beans to the saucepan in Step 1, as described above. Complete Step 1, then let cool and steep at room temperature for 24 hours. Strain out and discard the solids, then continue with Step 2.

Ginger-Infused Simple Syrup. Add ¼ cup peeled and grated fresh ginger to the saucepan in Step 1, as described above. Complete Step 1, then let cool and steep for 24 hours at room temperature. Strain out and discard the solids, then continue with Step 2.

Chili-Infused Simple Syrup. Add 2 tablespoons minced fresh chili peppers to the saucepan in Step 1, as described above. Complete Step 1, then let cool and steep for 24 hours at room temperature. Strain out and discard the solids, then continue with Step 2.

Calories: 0 | Fat: 0g | Protein: 0g | Carbs: 0g | Fiber: 0g | Erythritol: 12g | **Net Carbs: 0g**

Pro Tips for Using Simple Syrups:

Replacing traditional sugar with carb-free erythritol puts simple syrup back on the table, or back in the cocktail shaker, and makes keto cocktail hour possible. I use my basic simple syrup as well as citrus-flavored simple syrup to make the cocktail recipes in this book (see pages 306 to 320), but these syrups aren't limited to cocktails. They also bring lots of flavor to dressings, sauces, coffee, and even desserts without adding carbs. Here are some ideas for their use.

Basic Simple Syrup. Anytime you want to add sweetness to a beverage (like iced tea or lemonade), a sauce, or even a dessert or smoothie without worrying about your sweetener not dissolving and leaving a gritty texture, basic simple syrup is the perfect addition. Because it has no flavor, only sweetness, it can even be used for savory applications—for example, Asian dishes that have that sweet-and-salty thing going on.

Lemon-, Lime-, Orange-, or Grapefruit-Infused Simple Syrup. In addition to cocktails (see pages 306 to 310 and 316 to 318), citrusy simple syrups add a punch of citrus flavor to desserts, sauces, and even smoothies. I love a splash of orange-infused simple syrup in my espresso in the morning!

Herb-Infused Simple Syrup. I love to flavor filtered water or seltzer water with a few slices of lemon and add a splash of mint-, basil-, thyme-, or even lavender-infused simple syrup to break up the monotony. Herb-infused simple syrups will also take your keto cocktails to the next level. They even work great mixed with a little vinegar and avocado oil for a fresh and vibrant keto salad dressing!

Coffee-Infused Simple Syrup. If you love coffee-flavored everything like I do, then you'll love using coffee-infused simple syrup to flavor beverages, ice creams, frostings, baked goods, and even homemade caramel sauce. This syrup is also a great way to sweeten iced coffee and get an extra punch of coffee flavor.

Ginger-Infused Simple Syrup. My favorite way to use ginger-infused simple syrup is to flavor hot or iced green tea. It also makes a fantastic Moscow Mule when paired with vodka, lime juice, and club soda!

Chili-Infused Simple Syrup. This spicy simple syrup is great if you like your cocktails with a kick! It's also fantastic in Thai and other Asian recipes that call for a balance of spicy and sweet flavors.

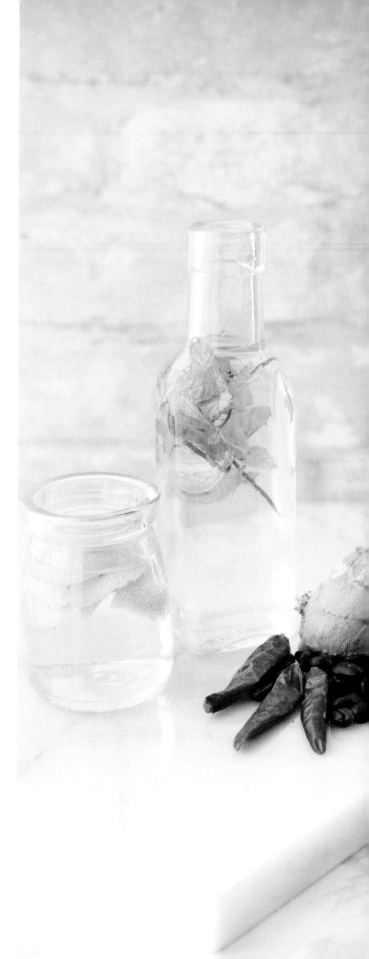

dairy-free egg-free nut-free vegetarian

Creamy Basil-Parmesan Vinaigrette

Bright and fresh, this is the perfect summer salad dressing and a great way to use up all that basil in your garden! It also makes a delicious sauce over grilled chicken.

Yield: **¾ cup** • Serving Size: **2 tablespoons** • Prep Time: **5 minutes**

¼ cup fresh basil leaves

¼ cup sugar-free mayonnaise

2 tablespoons extra-virgin olive oil

2 tablespoons full-fat sour cream

1 tablespoon apple cider vinegar

1 tablespoon lemon juice

1 tablespoon granulated erythritol

1 tablespoon grated Parmesan cheese

½ teaspoon kosher salt

¼ teaspoon ground black pepper

Place all of the ingredients in a small blender and blend until mostly smooth. Store in an airtight container in the refrigerator for up to 1 week.

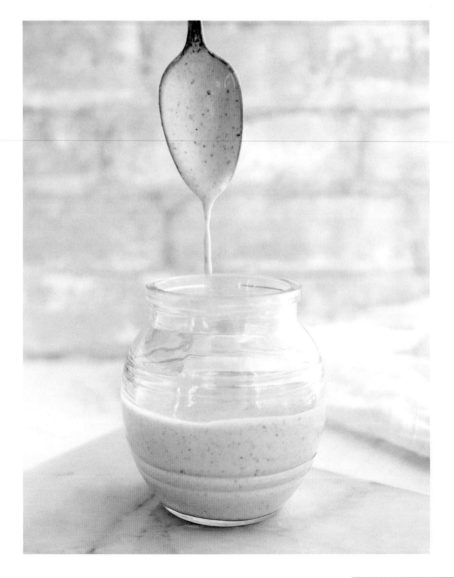

Calories: 123 | Fat: 14g | Protein: 0g | Carbs: 0g | Fiber: 0g | Erythritol: 2g | **Net Carbs: 0g**

Strawberry Basil Vinaigrette

dairy-free · egg-free · nut-free · vegetarian

If you're missing fruit on keto, this dressing is a great way to get a punch of berry flavor without a lot of added carbs!

Yield: **½ cup** • Serving Size: **2 tablespoons** • Prep Time: **5 minutes**

¼ cup chopped fresh strawberries

2 tablespoons avocado oil or other light-tasting oil

1 tablespoon chopped fresh basil

1 tablespoon filtered water

2 teaspoons red wine vinegar

½ teaspoon granulated erythritol

⅛ teaspoon kosher salt

⅛ teaspoon ground black pepper

Place all of the ingredients in a small blender and blend until mostly smooth. Store in an airtight container in the refrigerator for up to 1 week.

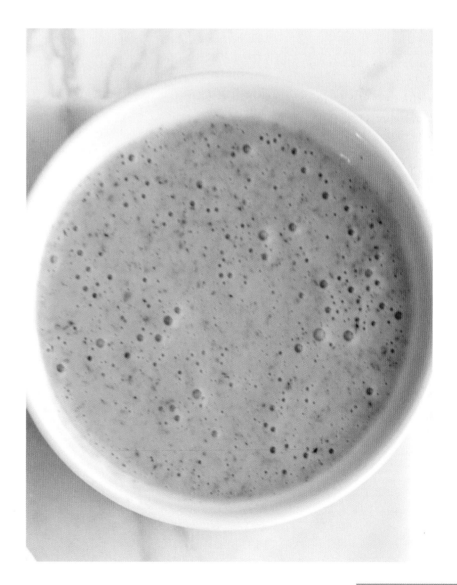

Calories: 65 | Fat: 7g | Protein: 0g | Carbs: 1g | Fiber: 0g | Erythritol: 2g | **Net Carbs: 1g**

dairy-free egg-free nut-free vegetarian

Ginger Scallion Dressing

This Asian-inspired dressing hits all of your favorite flavor notes and will complement not only salad and veggies but also any grilled or fried chicken, fish, or shrimp recipe. It's sweet, it's salty, it's toasty yet bright—we're talking condiment perfection right here!

Yield: **¾ cup** • Serving Size: **2 tablespoons** • Prep Time: **8 minutes**

¼ cup chopped scallions

3 tablespoons avocado oil or other light-tasting oil

2 tablespoons filtered water

2 tablespoons fish sauce (no sugar added)

2 tablespoons granulated erythritol

1 tablespoon lime juice

1 tablespoon white vinegar

1 tablespoon peeled and minced fresh ginger

1 teaspoon toasted sesame oil

Place all of the ingredients in a small blender and blend until mostly smooth. Store in an airtight container in the refrigerator for up to 1 week.

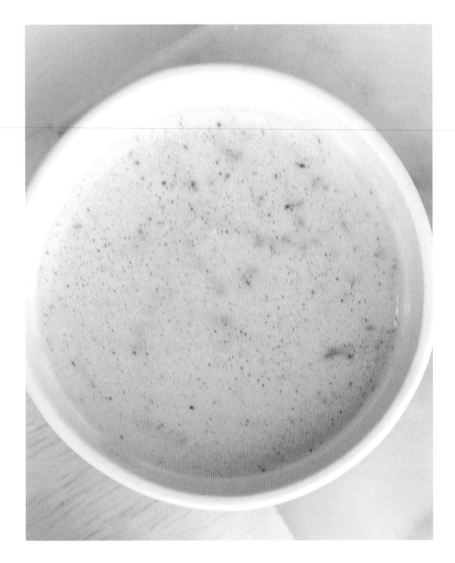

Calories: 75 | Fat: 8g | Protein: 1g | Carbs: 1g | Fiber: 0g | Erythritol: 4g | **Net Carbs: 1g**

Bacon & Tomato Dressing

It's dressing—with bacon in it! If that doesn't sell this recipe to you, then I don't know what will. Smoky and rich, with a hint of sweetness, this is an awesome dressing for Cobb salad, but really any salad leaf would be made better by a drizzle of this tasty elixir.

Yield: ¾ cup ◆ Serving Size: 2 tablespoons ◆ Prep Time: 8 minutes

¼ cup sugar-free mayonnaise

5 cherry tomatoes

3 slices bacon, cooked and chopped

1 clove garlic, peeled

2 tablespoons chopped fresh parsley

½ teaspoon granulated erythritol

¼ teaspoon kosher salt

⅛ teaspoon ground black pepper

Place all of the ingredients in a small blender and blend until mostly smooth. Store in an airtight container in the refrigerator for up to 1 week.

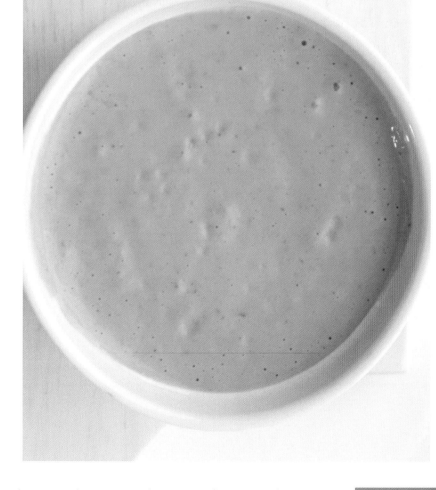

Calories: 93 | Fat: 10g | Protein: 2g | Carbs: 1g | Fiber: 0g | Erythritol: 2g | **Net Carbs: 1g**

Creamy Blue Cheese Dressing

I hated the flavor of blue cheese as a kid, but as an adult I can't get enough of it. I love this dressing on salad, but also with Buffalo wings or even as a dip for raw veggies or pieces of leftover steak.

Yield: **1 cup** • Serving Size: **2 tablespoons** • Prep Time: **5 minutes**

⅓ cup sugar-free mayonnaise

¼ cup crumbled blue cheese

1 ounce cream cheese (2 tablespoons), softened

2 tablespoons heavy whipping cream

1 teaspoon lemon juice

Place all of the ingredients in a small blender and blend for 30 seconds, until creamy and nearly entirely smooth. Store in an airtight container in the refrigerator for up to 1 week.

Pro Tip:

Use a good-quality blue cheese for the best flavor. When I can get it, I prefer Maytag Blue Cheese, but any quality blue cheese, as well as Stilton, Roquefort (made from sheep's milk), or Gorgonzola, will work well in this recipe. Avoid purchasing precrumbled blue cheese, if possible, as it may be coated in starch to prevent sticking and therefore may contain more carbs.

Variation:

Chunky Blue Cheese Dressing. If you prefer your blue cheese dressing chunky and with an extra kick of blue cheese flavor, crumble an additional ¼ cup of blue cheese into the dressing after blending.

Calories: 100 | Fat: 10g | Protein: 1g | Carbs: 0.5g | Fiber: 0g | **Net Carbs: 0.5g**

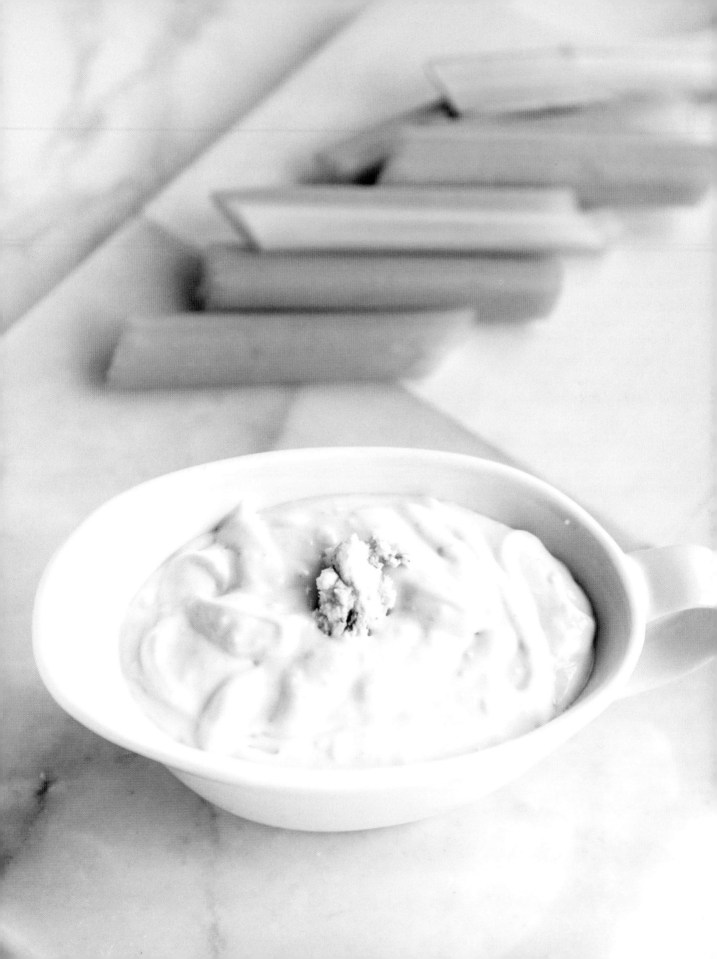

dairy-free · egg-free · nut-free · vegetarian

Creamy Lemon Caper Dressing

This luscious and tangy dressing is not only great on salad but also lends itself well as a sauce for grilled chicken or fish. Toss it with some chilled cooked cauliflower florets and it makes a fun summer salad for any picnic or barbecue.

Yield: **¾ cup** ◆ Serving Size: **2 tablespoons** ◆ Prep Time: **5 minutes**

½ cup sugar-free mayonnaise

2 tablespoons extra-virgin olive oil

1 tablespoon capers, drained

1 tablespoon lemon juice

1 tablespoon white vinegar

1 teaspoon grated lemon zest

½ teaspoon dried dill weed

Place all of the ingredients in a small blender and blend for 30 seconds, until creamy and nearly entirely smooth. Store in an airtight container in the refrigerator for up to 1 week.

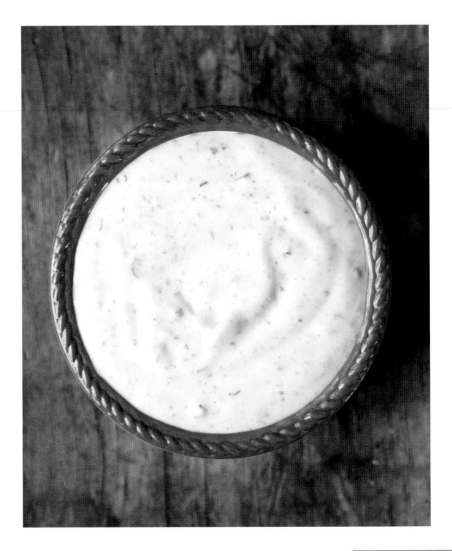

Calories: 107 | Fat: 13g | Protein: 0g | Carbs: 0g | Fiber: 0g | **Net Carbs: 0g**

Tangy Feta & Dill Dressing

dairy-free · egg-free · nut-free · vegetarian

If you're a feta cheese fan, then you're going to L-O-V-E this dressing! It also makes a tasty dip for raw veggies or skewers of grilled chicken, souvlaki-style.

Yield: **1 cup** ◆ Serving Size: **2 tablespoons** ◆ Prep Time: **5 minutes**

¼ cup sugar-free mayonnaise

⅓ cup crumbled feta cheese

2 tablespoons full-fat sour cream

2 tablespoons heavy whipping cream

1 tablespoon chopped fresh dill

1 tablespoon white vinegar

⅛ teaspoon ground black pepper

⅛ teaspoon onion powder

Place all of the ingredients in a small blender and blend for 30 seconds, until creamy and nearly entirely smooth. Store in an airtight container in the refrigerator for up to 1 week.

Pro Tip:
When purchasing feta cheese, avoid the precrumbled variety as it may contain added starches (and therefore carbs) to prevent sticking.

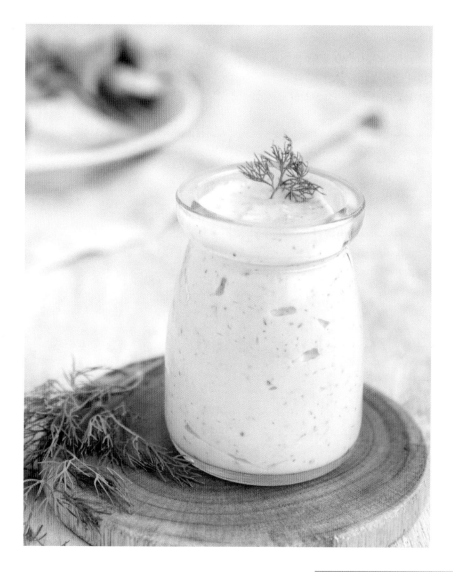

Calories: 76 | Fat: 8g | Protein: 1g | Carbs: 0.5g | Fiber: 0g | **Net Carbs: 0.5g**

dairy-free egg-free nut-free vegetarian

Tahini Lemon Dressing

This easy dressing is the perfect balance of garlic, lemon, and toasty sesame flavors. Tasty on a cabbage salad with chicken and sesame seeds, a no-brainer with my Faux-lafel (page 266) and even as a drizzle over my Tandoori Chicken Meatballs (page 170), there is no end to the applications for this dressing.

Yield: **⅓ cup** • Serving Size: **2 tablespoons** • Prep Time: **5 minutes**

3 tablespoons filtered water

2 tablespoons tahini

1 tablespoon lemon juice

1 teaspoon minced garlic

½ teaspoon kosher salt

Place all of the ingredients in a small blender and blend until smooth. Store in an airtight container in the refrigerator for up to 1 week.

Pro Tip:

When minced garlic is called for, always use fresh and either mince it yourself or press it through a garlic press if you must. Do yourself a favor and avoid the prechopped or preminced garlic in jars that you find in the grocery store. It won't have the same flavor as fresh garlic and is more expensive!

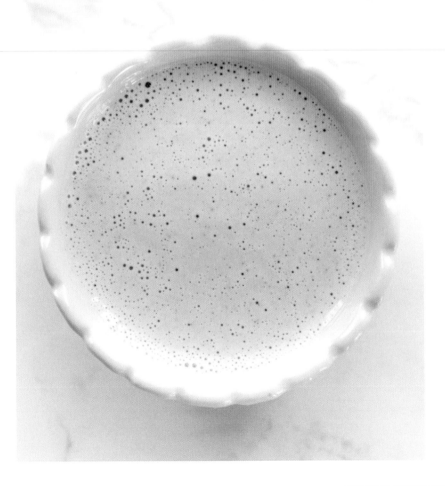

Calories: 63 | Fat: 5g | Protein: 2g | Carbs: 3g | Fiber: 2g | **Net Carbs: 1g**

Raspberry Coulis

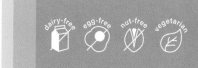

This intensely flavored raspberry sauce is not just for desserts but can be served over Cream Cheese Pancakes (page 138), stirred into your morning kefir (page 118), and blended into smoothies and dressings for a punch of bright raspberry flavor.

Yield: **1½ cups** • Serving Size: **2 tablespoons** • Prep Time: **3 minutes** • Cook Time: **5 minutes**

2 cups fresh or frozen red raspberries

2 tablespoons granulated erythritol

1 Combine the raspberries and sweetener in a small saucepan and cook over medium heat for 5 minutes, or until bubbling.

2 Blend with an immersion blender for 30 seconds or until liquefied, then pour the sauce through a fine-mesh strainer to remove any seed fragments. Let cool before using.

3 Store in an airtight container in the refrigerator for up to 1 week or in the freezer for up to 3 months.

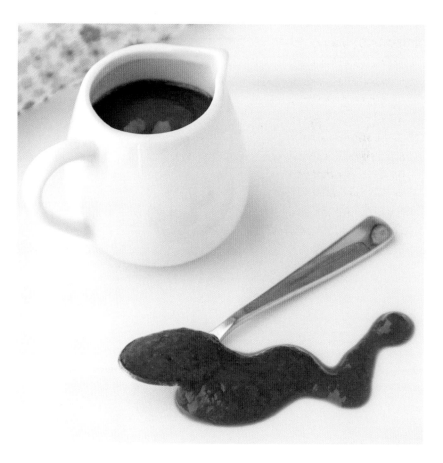

Calories: 12 | Fat: 0g | Protein: 0g | Carbs: 2.8g | Fiber: 1.5g | Erythritol: 2g | **Net Carbs: 1.3g**

Easy Basil Pesto

If I could have only one condiment for the rest of my days, it would be basil pesto. Pungent, fresh, garlicky, and bright, basil pesto adds incredible flavor to poultry, seafood, veggies, and sauces. Let's face it, there is almost nothing it can't make taste better. One of my favorite things is to stir pesto into mayonnaise and spread it on a Cream Cheese Wrap (page 70), then roll it up with roasted red peppers, prosciutto, and provolone cheese inside. It's keto sandwich perfection.

Yield: **¾ cup** ◆ Serving Size: **2 tablespoons** ◆ Prep Time: **5 minutes**

1 cup fresh basil leaves

¼ cup extra-virgin olive oil

¼ cup grated Parmesan cheese

¼ cup pine nuts

1 tablespoon chopped garlic

¼ teaspoon kosher salt

⅛ teaspoon ground black pepper

Put all of the ingredients in a small blender or mini food processor. Pulse until fully combined but not quite smooth. Store in an airtight container in the refrigerator for up to 1 week or in the freezer for up to 3 months.

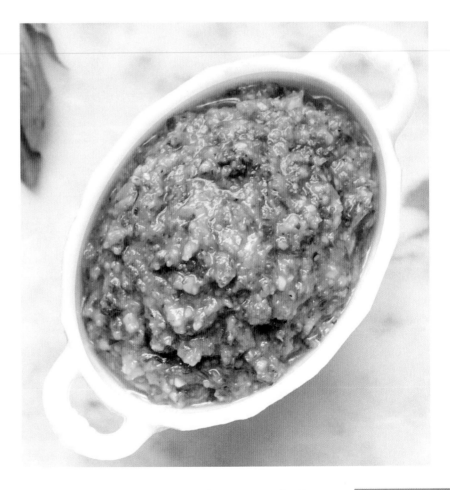

Calories: 139 | Fat: 14g | Protein: 3g | Carbs: 1.5g | Fiber: 0.5g | **Net Carbs: 1g**

Basic Remoulade

dairy-free egg-free nut-free vegetarian

You can never have too many tasty sauce recipes in your repertoire, and this basic remoulade is the perfect accompaniment to grilled, fried, or baked fish, chicken, or shrimp, or even as a zesty dip for veggies.

Yield: **½ cup** • Serving Size: **2 tablespoons** • Prep Time: **5 minutes**

⅓ cup sugar-free mayonnaise

1 tablespoon dill pickle relish

1 teaspoon Cajun Seasoning (page 76)

1 teaspoon capers, drained

1 teaspoon Dijon mustard

1 teaspoon lemon juice

1 teaspoon prepared horseradish

½ teaspoon minced garlic

Place all of the ingredients in a small bowl and mix well. Serve immediately or store in an airtight container in the refrigerator for up to 5 days.

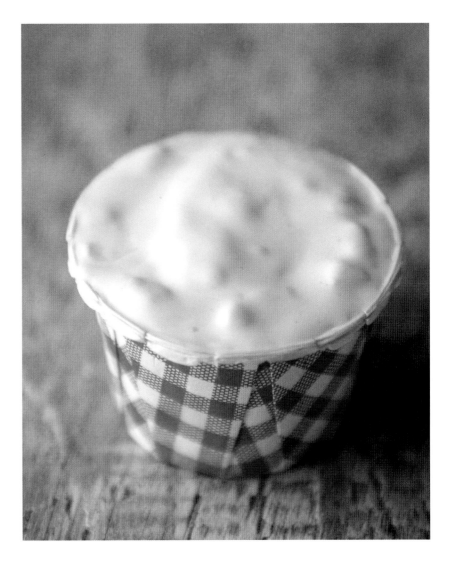

Calories: 160 | Fat: 19g | Protein: 0g | Carbs: 1g | Fiber: 0g | **Net Carbs: 1g**

dairy-free egg-free nut-free vegetarian

Cucumber Raita

The perfect soothing condiment for spicy Indian foods, this cucumber raita has a tangy yogurt base that keeps you coming back for more. I love this with my Tandoori Chicken Meatballs (page 170), but it also pairs well with the Faux-lafel (page 266) and pretty much any grilled chicken or fish!

Yield: **1 cup** • Serving Size: **2 tablespoons** • Prep Time: **8 minutes**

⅓ cup full-fat Greek yogurt

⅓ cup full-fat sour cream

¼ cup finely chopped cucumbers

1 tablespoon chopped fresh cilantro

1 tablespoon chopped fresh mint

1 teaspoon granulated erythritol

1 teaspoon minced red onions

¼ teaspoon ground cumin

Place all of the ingredients in a small bowl and mix well. Serve immediately or store in an airtight container in the refrigerator for up to 3 days.

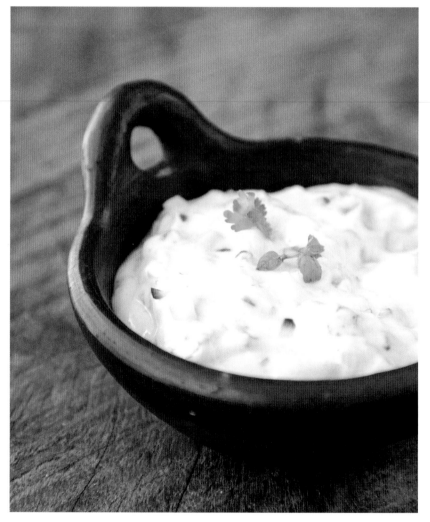

Calories: 29 | Fat: 2g | Protein: 1g | Carbs: 1g | Fiber: 0g | Erythritol: 4g | **Net Carbs: 1g**

Sweet Sriracha Dipping Sauce

dairy-free · egg-free · nut-free · vegetarian

This easy sauce is a tasty alternative to tartar sauce and also for dipping into with baked or fried chicken or fish fingers. We also like this one for dipping chilled cooked shrimp in, cocktail style!

Yield: **¾ cup** ◆ Serving Size: **2 tablespoons** ◆ Prep Time: **5 minutes**

½ cup sugar-free mayonnaise

1½ tablespoons lime juice

1½ tablespoons Sriracha sauce

1 tablespoon granulated erythritol

Place all of the ingredients in a small bowl and stir well until combined. Store in an airtight container in the refrigerator for up to 1 week.

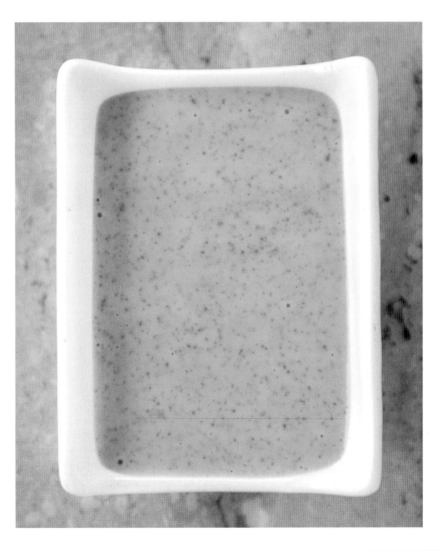

Calories: 138 | Fat: 16g | Protein: 0g | Carbs: 1g | Fiber: 0g | Erythritol: 2g | **Net Carbs: 1g**

Compound Butter

dairy-free · egg-free · nut-free · vegetarian

Compound butter is an easy way to dress up cooked veggies, meats, poultry, or seafood. Here I give you three varieties:

In my catering days, I used classic Hotel Butter all the time for clams casino. Just dab a little of this garlic parsley butter on shucked clams and top them with a slice of raw bacon and some of my Keto Breadcrumbs (page 74), then broil for about 3 minutes.

Flavorful Sun-Dried Tomato & Basil Butter turns plain hot zoodles into side-dish nirvana in seconds. Throw on some grilled chicken and grated Parmesan cheese and people will think you've slaved all day when in reality it took you only minutes to get an amazing and healthy dinner on the table. I won't tell if you don't.

If your love for all things blue cheese can't be contained, Gorgonzola Butter is for you! It takes plain grilled chicken or steak to the next level. It's fantastic on Buffalo chicken or even spread on celery sticks for a quick high-fat snack!

Serving Size: **1 tablespoon** ◆ Prep Time: **10 minutes, plus 1 hour to chill**

Hotel Butter

(makes 1 cup)

1 cup (2 sticks) butter, softened

3 tablespoons chopped fresh parsley

4 teaspoons minced garlic

½ teaspoon kosher salt

¼ teaspoon ground black pepper

Sun-Dried Tomato & Basil Butter

(makes 1¼ cups)

1 cup (2 sticks) butter, softened

2 tablespoons chopped sun-dried tomatoes

½ teaspoon kosher salt

½ teaspoon minced garlic

¼ teaspoon ground black pepper

Gorgonzola Butter

(makes ¾ cup)

½ cup (1 stick) butter, softened

2 ounces Gorgonzola cheese, crumbled

1 tablespoon minced fresh parsley

1 teaspoon minced garlic

1 Place all of the ingredients in a medium-sized bowl and mix thoroughly with a rubber spatula. Place a 12 by 15-inch length of plastic wrap on a cutting board.

2 Spoon the butter mixture into a line approximately 10 inches long in the center of the plastic wrap. Roll up tightly and twist the ends, forming the butter into a log about 10 inches long and 2 inches in diameter. Chill in the refrigerator for 1 hour.

3 Unwrap the butter log and slice into ½-inch-thick rounds. Store in an airtight container in the refrigerator for up to 1 week or in the freezer for up to 3 months.

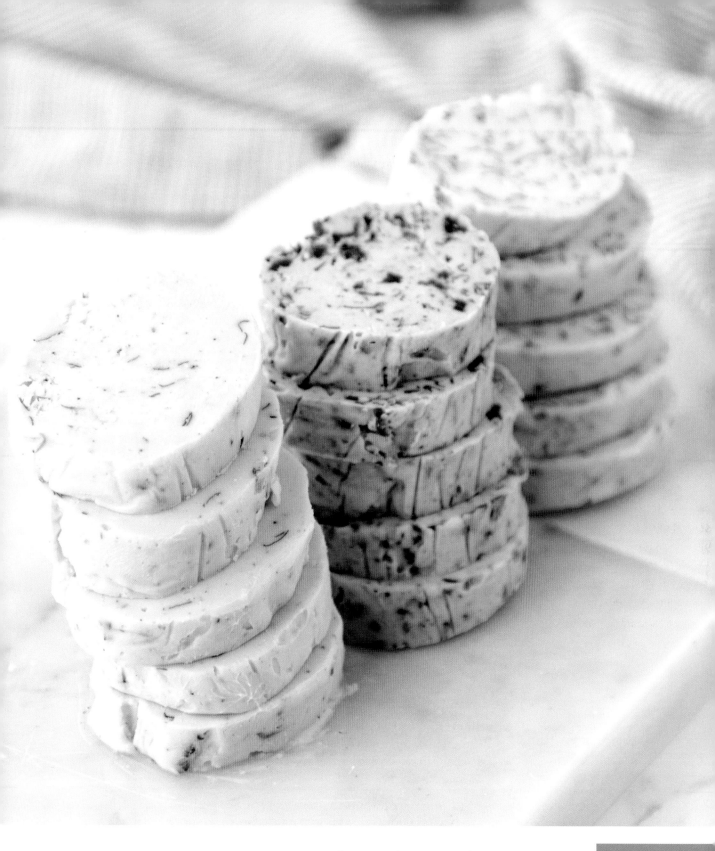

Hotel Butter:	Calories: 102	Fat: 11g	Protein: 0g	Carbs: 0g	Fiber: 0g	**Net Carbs: 0g**
Sun-Dried Tomato & Basil Butter:	Calories: 82	Fat: 9g	Protein: 0g	Carbs: 0g	Fiber: 0g	**Net Carbs: 0g**
Gorgonzola Butter:	Calories: 91	Fat: 10g	Protein: 1g	Carbs: 0g	Fiber: 0g	**Net Carbs: 0g**

Keto Ketchup

This quintessential condiment is usually loaded with sugar—a no-no on keto. My version is keto-friendly and well worth the bit of time it takes to make. It tastes *waaaayyy* better than store-bought, too!

Yield: **2 cups** ◆ Serving Size: **1 tablespoon** ◆ Prep Time: **5 minutes** ◆ Cook Time: **1 hour**

1 (28-ounce) can tomato puree

⅓ cup granulated erythritol

¼ teaspoon cayenne pepper

½ cup white vinegar

1½ teaspoons dehydrated onions

½ teaspoon celery salt

½ teaspoon whole cloves

1 (1-inch) piece of cinnamon stick, broken

1 Combine the tomato puree, sweetener, and cayenne pepper in a medium-sized saucepan and bring to a boil over medium heat, then reduce the heat to low. Simmer until it reduces by half, about 30 minutes, stirring occasionally.

2 Meanwhile, in another small saucepan, combine the vinegar, onions, celery salt, cloves, and cinnamon stick pieces. Bring to a boil, then remove from the heat. Strain out the solids.

3 Add the flavored vinegar to the tomato mixture. Simmer for another 20 minutes, or until the ketchup reaches the desired consistency. Remove from the heat and let cool.

4 Blend the cooled ketchup with an immersion blender or in a small blender until smooth. Store in a clean jar with an airtight lid for up to 1 month in the refrigerator.

Pro Tip:

Turn this into cocktail sauce with a few tablespoons of prepared horseradish, or make it into Thousand Island dressing with chopped pickles and some mayonnaise.

Calories: 16 | Fat: 0g | Protein: 0g | Carbs: 4g | Fiber: 1g | Erythritol: 2g | **Net Carbs: 3g**

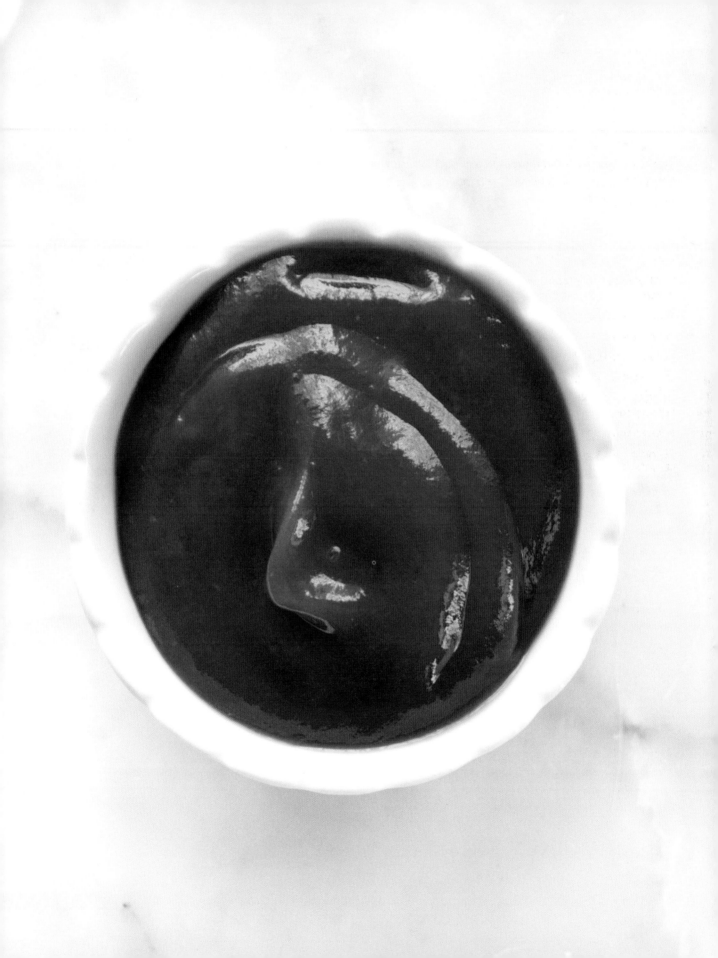

dairy-free egg-free nut-free vegetarian

Easy Keto BBQ Sauce

I'm not always a fan of BBQ sauce, since I actually enjoy the flavor and texture of dry-rubbed ribs and chicken. When I am feeling saucy, though, this tangy potion never disappoints!

Yield: **¾ cup** • Serving Size: **2 tablespoons** • Prep Time: **8 minutes**

½ cup reduced-sugar ketchup, store-bought or homemade (page 102)

2 tablespoons apple cider vinegar

2 tablespoons granulated erythritol

1 tablespoon filtered water

1½ teaspoons ground allspice

1½ teaspoons ground mustard powder

1 teaspoon blackstrap molasses (optional; see note)

½ teaspoon liquid smoke

½ teaspoon onion powder

½ teaspoon Worcestershire sauce

¼ teaspoon ground cloves

¼ teaspoon xanthan gum (optional, to thicken)

Place all of the ingredients in a medium-sized bowl and whisk together. Store in an airtight container in the refrigerator for up to 2 weeks.

> **Note:**
> *While molasses does contain some sugar and you can omit it if that bothers you, the small amount called for in this recipe adds a punch of authentic flavor and texture that I believe is well worth the negligible amount of carbs it adds per serving.*

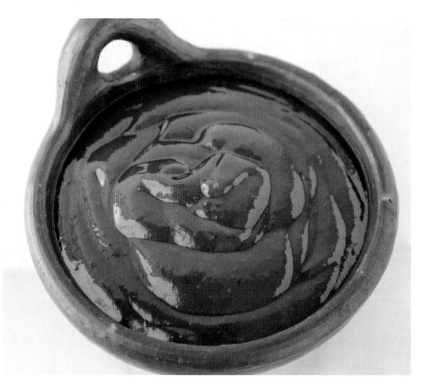

Calories: 15 | Fat: 0g | Protein: 0g | Carbs: 3g | Fiber: 0g | Erythritol: 4g | **Net Carbs: 3g**

Sweet Chili Sauce

dairy-free egg-free nut-free vegetarian

One of my favorite dipping sauces for fried fish or chicken fingers, this sweet and spicy concoction is also fantastic slathered on meatballs or cooked Polish sausage slices for a quick appetizer.

Yield: 1¼ cups • Serving Size: 2 tablespoons • Prep Time: 5 minutes

1 cup sugar-free orange marmalade

1 tablespoon filtered water

1 tablespoon fish sauce (no sugar added)

1 tablespoon lime juice

1 teaspoon granulated erythritol

1 teaspoon red pepper flakes

1 teaspoon toasted sesame oil

Place all of the ingredients in a small bowl and mix well. Store in an airtight container in the refrigerator for up to 2 weeks.

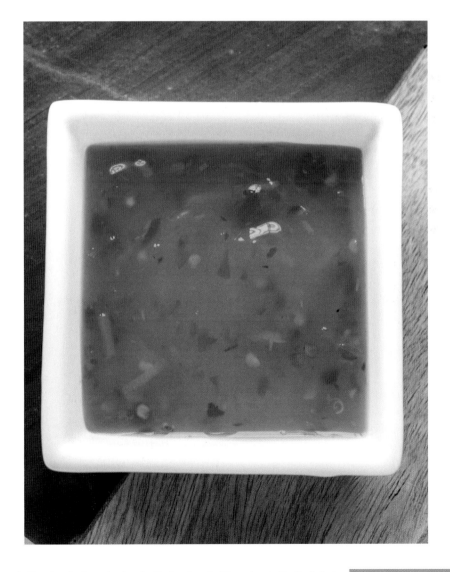

Calories: 22 | Fat: 0g | Protein: 0g | Carbs: 6g | Fiber: 1g | Erythritol: 4g | **Net Carbs: 5g**

Easy No-Cook Marinara

dairy-free *egg-free* *nut-free* *vegetarian*

Store-bought tomato sauces are usually loaded with sugar and preservatives. This incredibly easy and flavorful marinara sauce can be made at home in just five minutes and without the added carbs!

Yield: **4 cups** ◆ Serving Size: **½ cup** ◆ Prep Time: **5 minutes**

1 (28-ounce) can peeled whole San Marzano tomatoes

¼ cup extra-virgin olive oil

2 tablespoons red wine vinegar

1 teaspoon dried basil leaves

1 teaspoon dried oregano leaves

1 teaspoon dried parsley leaves

1 teaspoon garlic powder

1 teaspoon kosher salt

1 teaspoon onion powder

½ teaspoon red pepper flakes

¼ teaspoon ground black pepper

Pro Tip:
If freezing, store this in multiple small containers of 1 cup each so that you don't have to defrost the entire batch when you just need one or two servings for a recipe.

1 Place the tomatoes and olive oil in a blender and blend for 30 seconds, or until the desired consistency is reached. If you prefer a chunkier sauce, pulse instead of blending for about 15 seconds. Stir in the remaining ingredients.

2 Store in an airtight container for up to 1 week in the refrigerator or 6 months in the freezer.

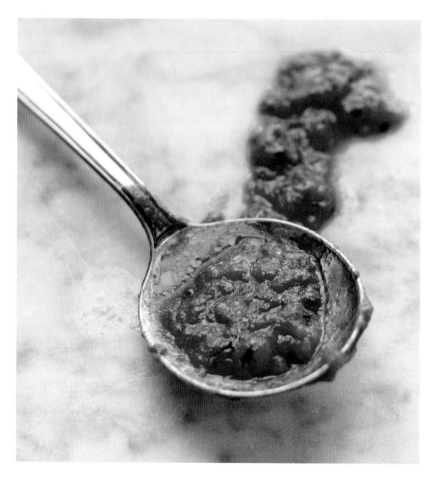

Calories: 84 | Fat: 7g | Protein: 1g | Carbs: 5g | Fiber: 2g | **Net Carbs: 3g**

5-Minute Alfredo Sauce

dairy-free egg-free nut-free vegetarian

If you try only one sauce from this book, make it this one! Made in your microwave in just one minute, this creamy and decadent cheese sauce requires no skill in the kitchen. You can serve it over regular pasta for the rest of the family and over zoodles or cream cheese noodles for you. Pair it with grilled chicken or shrimp and you'll be getting requests for this one over and over again. Pinky promise.

Yield: **1½ cups** ◆ Serving Size: **¼ cup** ◆ Prep Time: **5 minutes** ◆ Cook Time: **1 minute**

½ cup mascarpone cheese (4 ounces)

¼ cup grated Parmesan cheese

¼ cup (½ stick) butter

½ cup heavy whipping cream

½ teaspoon kosher salt

¼ teaspoon ground black pepper

1 Place the mascarpone, Parmesan, and butter in a medium-sized microwave-safe bowl. Microwave on high for 30 seconds, then stir.

2 Microwave on high for 30 seconds more. Add the cream, salt, and pepper to the bowl. Whisk together until smooth. Serve immediately.

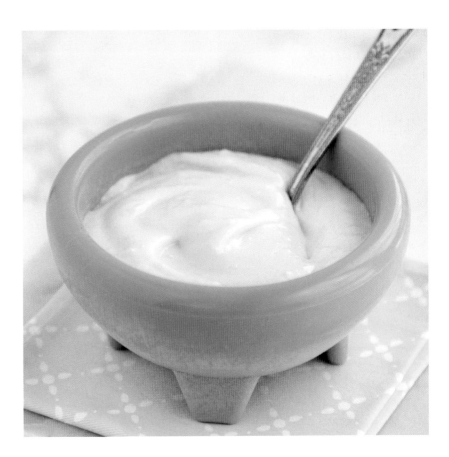

Calories: 237 | Fat: 24g | Protein: 3g | Carbs: 1g | Fiber: 0g | **Net Carbs: 1g**

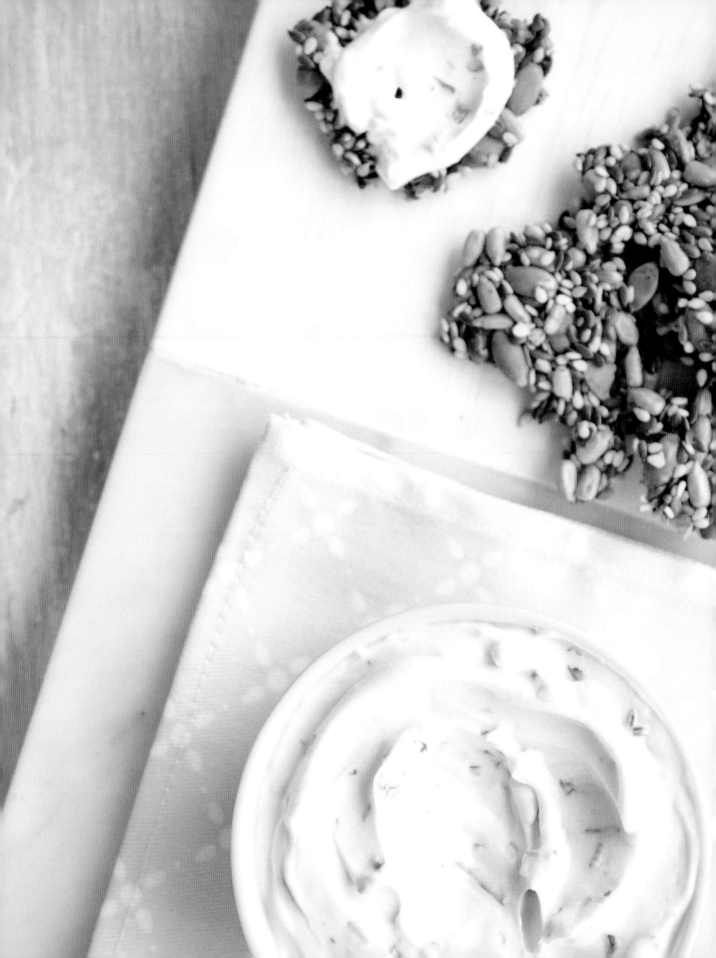

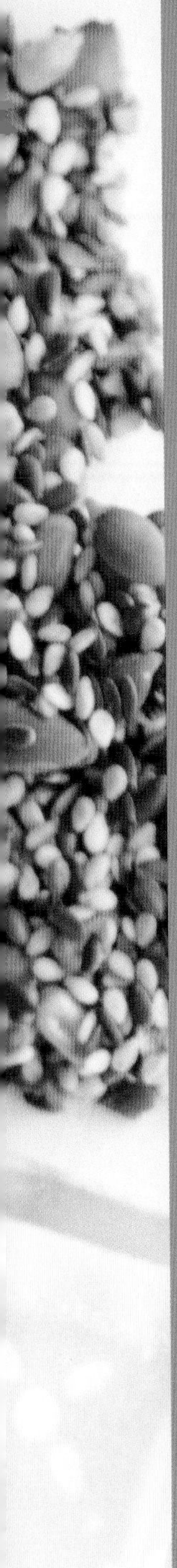

fermented foods

Spicy Sauerkraut / 110

Easy Lacto-Fermented Half-Sour Pickles / 112

Quick Cucumber Pickles / 114

Cultured Red Onion Relish / 116

Homemade Dairy Kefir / 118

Herbed Kefir Cheese / 120

Basic Kombucha / 122

dairy-free · egg-free · nut-free · vegetarian

Spicy Sauerkraut

Sauerkraut is a fantastic keto food because it's loaded with fiber, vitamin C, iron, and, most importantly, lots of beneficial bacteria to promote good gut health and a strong immune system. When I have a stomach bug or feel a cold coming on, I drink a tablespoon of the liquid from my sauerkraut three times a day, and it knocks out the bug in no time! I love this spicy version on salads or even with my eggs in the morning.

Yield: **7 cups drained** ◆ Serving Size: **½ cup** ◆ Prep Time: **10 minutes, plus 6 days to ferment**

½ teaspoon powdered starter culture for vegetables

2 cups plus about 1 quart filtered water, divided

8 cups shredded white cabbage (1 medium head)

1 tablespoon lemon zest

1 tablespoon lemon juice

2 tablespoons kosher salt

1 jalapeño pepper, sliced crosswise and seeded

1 Mix together the starter culture and 2 cups of the water in a medium-sized bowl and set aside.

2 Place the cabbage, lemon zest, lemon juice, salt, and jalapeño slices in a large bowl and mix well. Pack the cabbage into either 1 gallon-sized jar or 2 quart-sized jars, leaving 2 inches of space between the cabbage and the rim of the jar.

3 Add the starter culture mixture to the large jar or divide it evenly between the two smaller jars, and then fill the jar(s) with the remaining water until the cabbage is just covered.

4 Seal the jar(s) and leave on the counter, out of direct sunlight, for 6 days. Each day, open the jar(s) and push any floating cabbage below the surface of the liquid, then reseal.

5 After 6 days, the sauerkraut is ready to serve. Store in the refrigerator for up to 9 months.

Note:
While sauerkraut can be made without the use of a starter culture, this recipe calls for it because it assumes that most of you are new to the fermenting-foods process. The starter culture makes this recipe pretty much foolproof and gives consistent results every time.

Calories: 10 | Fat: 0g | Protein: 1g | Carbs: 2.5g | Fiber: 1g | **Net Carbs: 1.5g**

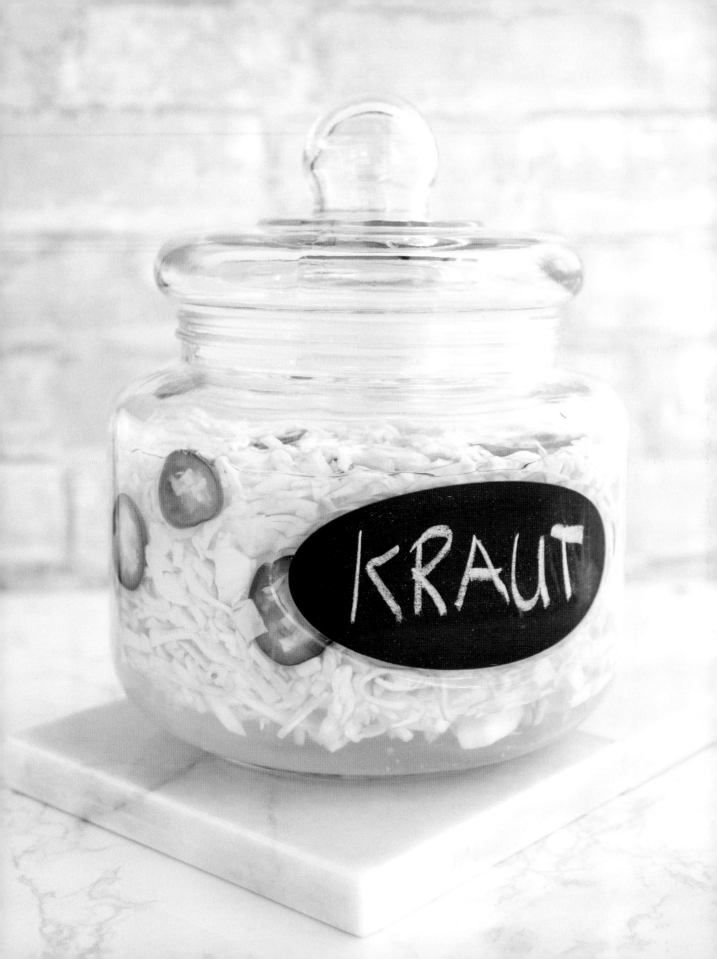

Easy Lacto-Fermented Half-Sour Pickles

dairy-free egg-free nut-free vegetarian

Despite what the name suggests, lacto-fermentation has nothing to do with milk. Rather, it occurs when fruits and vegetables are submerged in brine and fermented by the beneficial bacteria *Lactobacillus*, which are naturally found on their surface. These bacteria convert sugars into lactic acid, which inhibits harmful bacteria, behaves as a natural preservative, and gives fermented foods like sauerkraut and pickles their trademark sour flavor.

Yield: **1 quart** • Serving Size: **½ cup** • Prep Time: **10 minutes, plus 3 days to ferment**

3 cups filtered water

4 teaspoons fine sea salt (see note)

1 teaspoon red pepper flakes

1 pound cucumbers (3 to 4 medium)

5 cloves garlic, peeled

5 sprigs fresh dill

3 bay leaves

1 Place the water, salt, and red pepper flakes in a medium-sized bowl. Whisk until the salt is dissolved and set aside.

2 Rinse the cucumbers and trim off the ends. Cut them in half lengthwise, then into spears about 1 inch wide.

3 Pack a sterilized 1-quart jar with the cucumber spears, garlic, dill, and bay leaves. Pour the brine into the jar until the spears are just covered, leaving 2 inches of space between the liquid and the rim of the jar.

4 Seal the jar and leave it on the counter, out of direct sunlight, for 3 days. Each day, open the jar and push the spears down to make sure they stay submerged in the brine, then reseal.

5 After the third day, the pickles are ready to serve. Store in the refrigerator for up to 3 months.

Note:

While most of my recipes call for kosher salt, I use sea salt when lacto-fermenting vegetables because it doesn't contain anticaking agents, which can inhibit the natural fermentation process. Himalayan pink salt is a good choice if you can find it.

Calories: 8 | Fat: 0g | Protein: 0g | Carbs: 2g | Fiber: 1g | **Net Carbs: 1g**

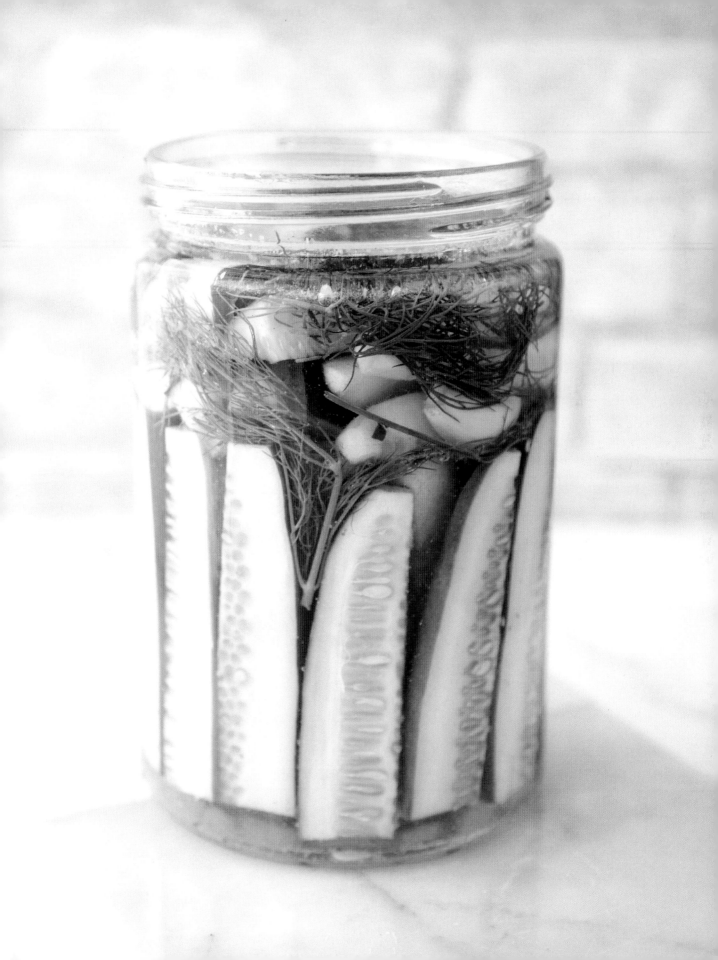

Quick Cucumber Pickles

These quick pickles aren't fermented, so they don't have the health benefits of the other recipes in this chapter, but they are very delicious and make a great condiment or addition to salads!

Yield: **1 quart** ◆ Serving Size: **½ cup** ◆ Prep Time: **5 minutes** ◆ Cook Time: **3 minutes**

1 cup white vinegar

1 cup filtered water

¼ cup granulated erythritol

1 tablespoon kosher salt

1 tablespoon coriander seeds

4 cups thinly sliced cucumbers

1 cup thinly sliced red onions

2 cloves garlic, peeled

2 sprigs fresh cilantro

1   Combine the vinegar, water, sweetener, salt, and coriander seeds in a small saucepan over medium heat. Cook for 3 minutes, or until the sweetener is fully dissolved. Remove from the heat and let cool for 5 minutes.

2   Pack the cucumbers, onions, garlic cloves, and cilantro into a 1-quart jar. Pour the liquid over the vegetables until they are fully submerged.

3   Seal the jar and store in the refrigerator for up to 1 month.

Calories: 11 | Fat: 0g | Protein: 0g | Carbs: 2.5g | Fiber: 0.5g | Erythritol: 5g | **Net Carbs: 2g**

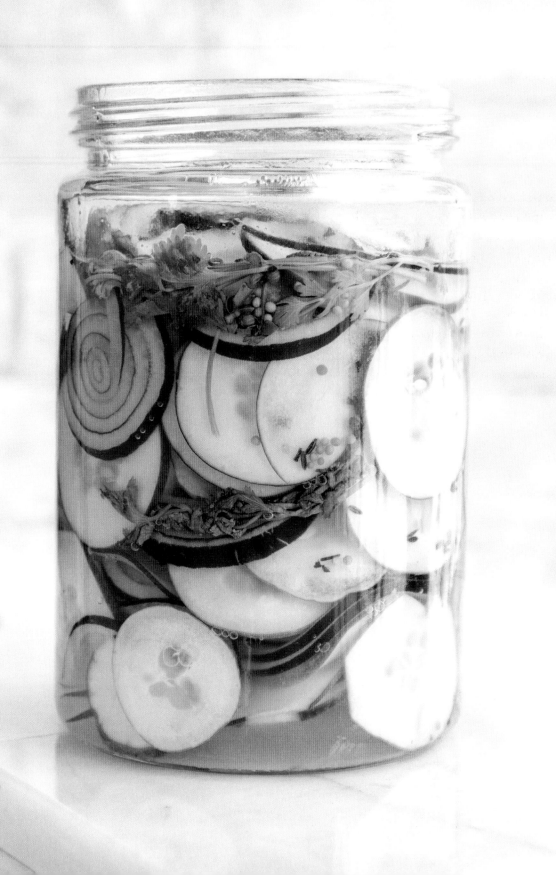

dairy-free   egg-free   nut-free   vegetarian

Cultured Red Onion Relish

This cultured relish is sweet and tart, with a homey spiciness from the cloves and allspice berries. Loaded with gut-friendly bacteria, it makes a healthy addition to salads or a nice little condiment to dress up burgers or grilled chicken or pork.

Yield: **3 cups drained** ◆ Serving Size: **¼ cup** ◆ Prep Time: **10 minutes, plus 4 days to ferment**

¼ teaspoon powdered starter culture for vegetables

2½ cups filtered water, divided

1 cup diced red radishes

1 cup diced red onions

1 cup seeded and diced cucumbers

1 tablespoon peeled and minced fresh ginger

1 tablespoon granulated erythritol

1 teaspoon kosher salt

2 sprigs fresh cilantro

3 whole cloves

2 whole allspice berries

1 Mix together the starter culture and ½ cup of the water in a medium-sized bowl and set aside.

2 Place the radishes, onions, cucumbers, ginger, sweetener, and salt in a large bowl and mix well. Stir in the cilantro, cloves, and allspice berries. Pack the vegetable mixture into a 1-quart jar, leaving 3 inches of space between the vegetables and the rim of the jar.

3 Add the starter culture mixture to the jar, then fill the jar with the remaining 2 cups of water until the vegetables are just covered.

4 Seal the jar and leave it on the counter, out of direct sunlight, for 4 days. Each day, open the jar and push any floating vegetables below the surface of the liquid, then reseal.

5 After the fourth day, the relish is ready to serve. Store in the refrigerator for up to 6 months.

Calories: 8 | Fat: 0g | Protein: 0g | Carbs: 1.5g | Fiber: 0.5g | Erythritol: 1g | **Net Carbs: 1g**

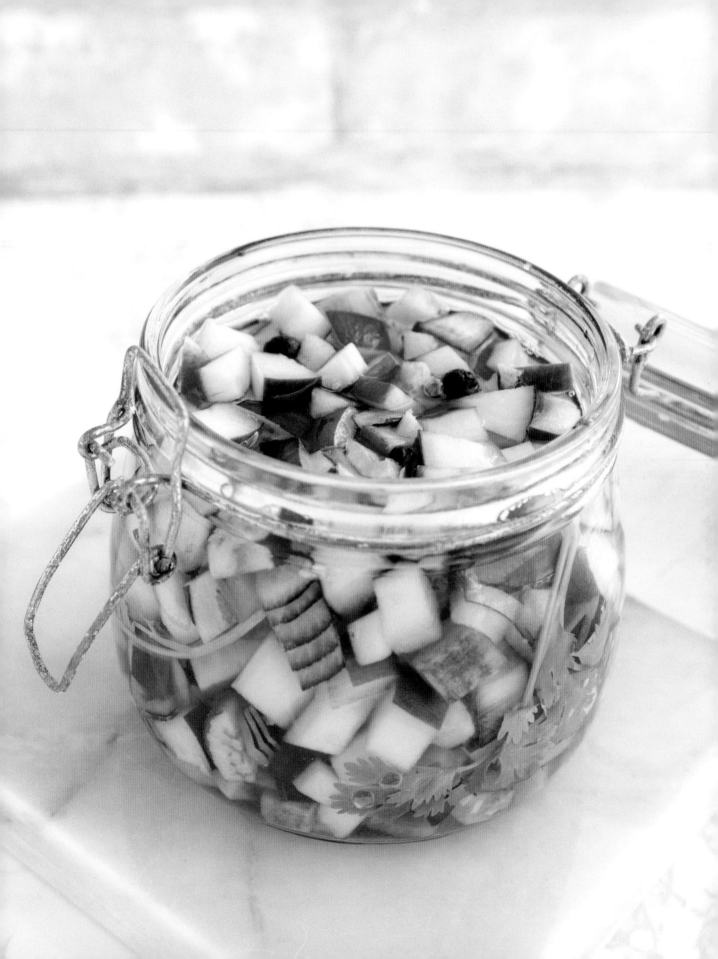

Homemade Dairy Kefir

Kefir is a fermented milk beverage with health benefits similar to yogurt. It's easy to make your own; you simply add a starter culture or kefir grains to milk and let it sit out on the counter for around 24 hours. The culture eats the sugars in the milk, so kefir is lower in carbs than milk. You can make kefir with nut milk, but it's a little trickier to do, so I recommend trying it with dairy milk a few times first until you get the hang of it. There are lots of great resources online for more advanced fermenting when you're ready to take it to the next level. I've added some of my favorites to the Resources section on page 360.

Yield: **4 cups** • Serving Size: **½ cup** • Prep Time: **5 minutes, plus 18 to 24 hours to ferment**

4 cups organic whole milk

1 packet freeze-dried powdered kefir starter culture

1 Pour the milk into a clean quart-sized jar. Add the kefir starter and stir well.

2 Cover the jar with a coffee filter and seal with a rubber band around it. Leave it on the counter, away from direct sunlight, for 18 hours.

3 After 18 hours, uncover the kefir and smell it: if it's sour smelling and has thickened, it's ready to serve; if not, give it a few more hours. After 24 hours, remove the coffee filter and cover it with a lid. Store in the refrigerator for up to 2 weeks.

Note:

You can also make kefir with live, or fresh, kefir grains, which resemble cottage cheese. If you have a source for those, then I recommend trying it out for a wider variety of bacteria in your kefir. They are a little fussier since you have to keep your grains alive in between batches, but the effort is totally worth it. If you're just starting out, though, the method above is foolproof and a great way to get your feet wet in making your own kefir.

Calories: 77 | Fat: 4g | Protein: 4g | Carbs: 4g | Fiber: 0g | **Net Carbs: 4g**

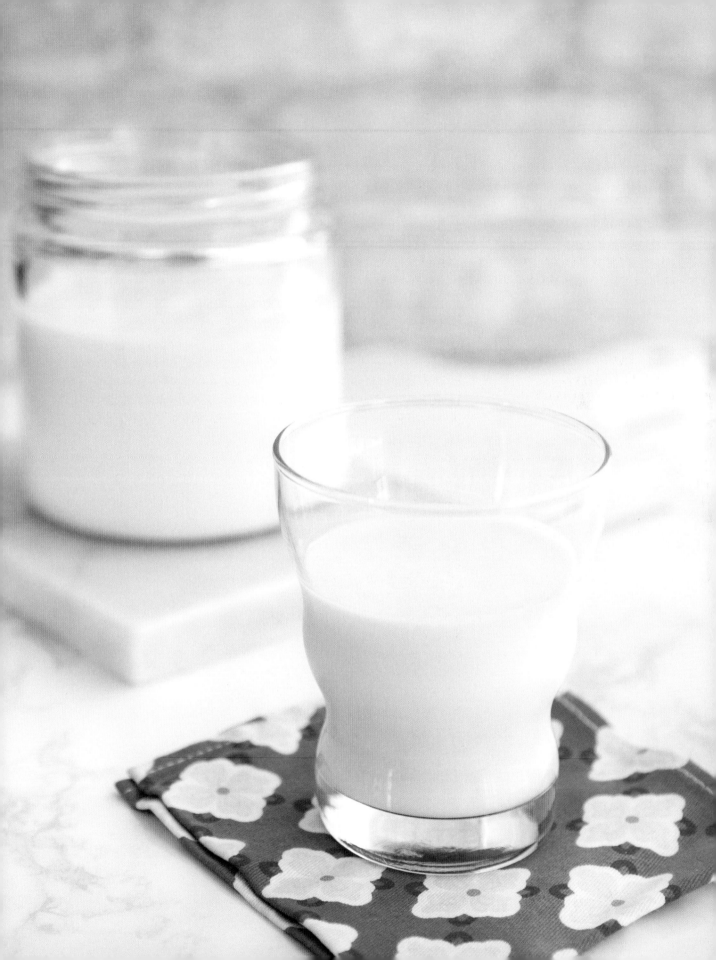

dairy-free · egg-free · nut-free · vegetarian

Herbed Kefir Cheese

Kefir cheese is tangy and smooth, and totally addicting! Whenever I have extra kefir I make this cheese with it, and it never lasts long! We love it with my Keto Seed Crackers (page 300).

Yield: **1 cup**   ◆   Serving Size: **2 tablespoons**   ◆   Prep Time: **5 minutes, plus 12 hours to drain**

2 cups full-fat unsweetened kefir, store-bought or homemade (page 118)

1 ounce cream cheese (2 tablespoons), softened

1 tablespoon chopped fresh parsley

1 teaspoon minced garlic

½ teaspoon fresh thyme leaves

½ teaspoon kosher salt

1   Line a fine-mesh strainer with a large coffee filter. Set the strainer over a bowl and pour the kefir into the filter-lined strainer. Place in the fridge, uncovered, for 12 hours—longer if you want a firmer cheese.

2   When ready to use, discard the whey liquid and place the kefir cheese in a medium-sized bowl. Add the cream cheese and blend with a whisk or fork until smooth. Stir in the parsley, garlic, thyme, and salt until well blended. Chill for at least 1 hour before serving. Store the cheese in the refrigerator for up to 3 weeks.

Calories: 52 | Fat: 3g | Protein: 4g | Carbs: 2g | Fiber: 0g | **Net Carbs: 2g**

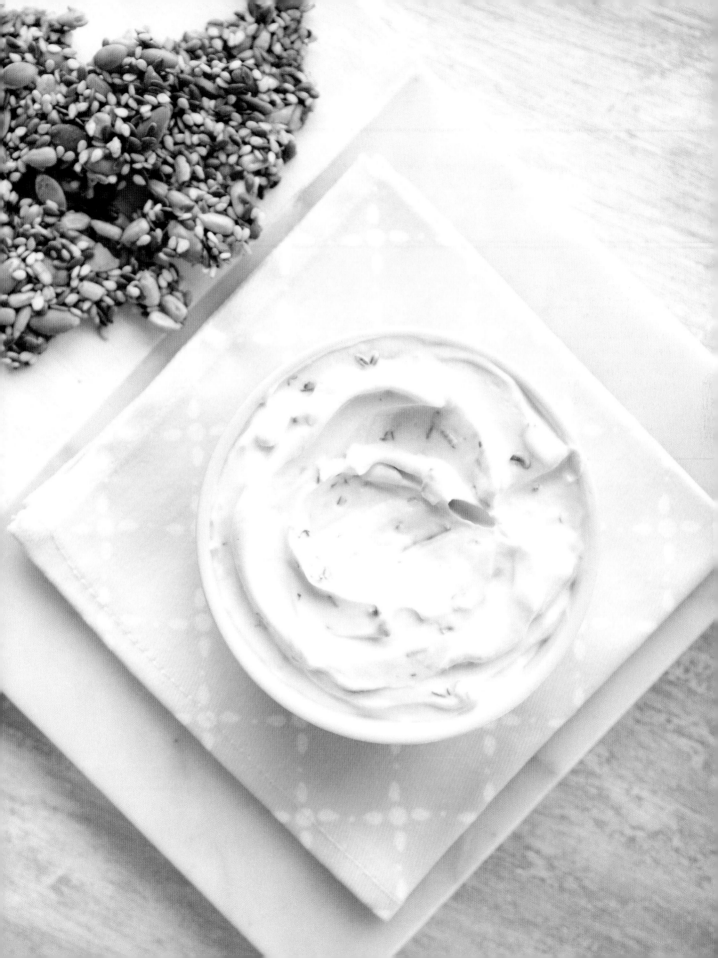

dairy-free · egg-free · nut-free · vegetarian

Basic Kombucha

Kombucha is a fermented tea that contains even more beneficial bacteria than yogurt, and entirely different strains. It's fermented by means of a SCOBY, or Symbiotic Culture of Bacteria and Yeast. If you have a friend who brews "booch," they will likely be happy to give you a SCOBY and one cup of their tea to use as a starter. If not, you can order a kit from Amazon like I did when I first started: it will supply you with a SCOBY and fermented starter tea. Every time you brew a batch, you'll have the SCOBY you started with and a new one that will form on top of your fresh batch. You can keep these SCOBYs thriving in jars of kombucha or give them to friends who want to start brewing. You can do a lot with kombucha, so if you find it tasty and/or interesting, I encourage you to do your own research on its many health benefits, as well as more advanced kombucha-making techniques, such as second fermenting and adding other flavors. I've included some great websites on the subject in the Resources section on page 360. This is just a basic recipe to get you started—I'm excited for you!

Yield: **2½ quarts** ◆ Serving Size: **8 ounces** ◆ Prep Time: **20 minutes, plus 8 to 10 days to ferment**

Cook Time: **5 minutes**

3 quarts filtered water

1 cup white sugar

5 organic black tea bags

1 SCOBY

1 cup fermented starter tea

Special equipment:

1 (1-gallon) glass jug

1   Clean and rinse a 1-gallon glass jug very well before using, or you could end up with mold and have to toss the entire batch.

2   In a large pot, bring the water to a rolling boil. Add the sugar and boil for 5 minutes. Remove from the heat and add the tea bags. Let them steep for 10 minutes, then remove and discard the tea bags.

3   Allow the brewed tea to cool to room temperature. Once cool, pour the tea into the glass jug. Add the SCOBY to the tea (it's okay if it sinks), then pour in the fermented starter tea.

4   Cover the jug with a clean paper towel and secure it around the rim with a large rubber band. Place the jug in a dark but well-ventilated room to ferment. Be aware that kombucha needs relatively warm temperatures (between 65°F and 90°F) for proper fermentation, so don't put it in a cold basement or unheated spare room in the winter.

5   After the eighth day, start tasting a small amount of tea. It should be tart but not sour, and very slightly bubbly. If it's still very sweet, it's not ready, so leave it for another 24 hours and check daily until it reaches the right fermentation level.

Calories: 30 | Fat: 0g | Protein: 0g | Carbs: 5g | Fiber: 0g | **Net Carbs: 5g**

6 Once it reaches proper fermentation, you can remove the SCOBY and at least 1 cup of kombucha to set aside as the starter tea for your next batch. Then pour the remaining booch into jars and store in the refrigerator for up to 3 months. Store the SCOBY and starter tea in a clean jar with a coffee filter secured over the top with a rubber band in a cool, dark place for up to 1 month if you're not making a fresh batch immediately.

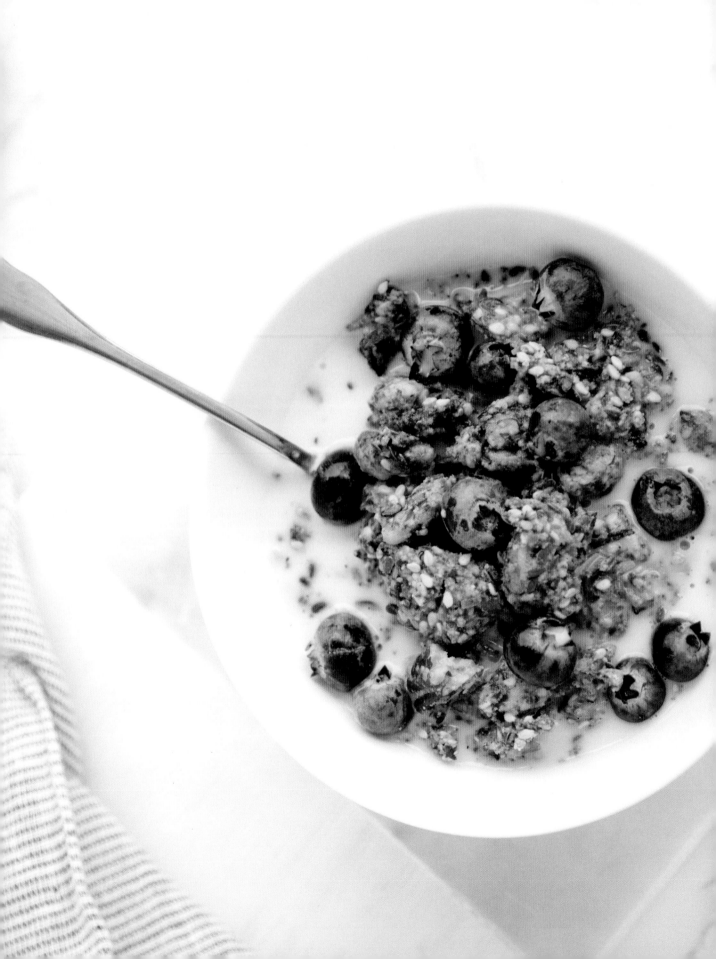

breakfast

Bulletproof Pumpkin Spice Latte / 126

Kefir Strawberry Smoothie / 127

Cinnamon Walnut Streusel Muffins / 128

Spanish Tortilla with Chorizo / 130

Snickerdoodle Crepes / 132

Sausage & Egg-Stuffed Portobello Mushrooms / 134

Savory Chorizo Breakfast Bowl / 136

Cream Cheese Pancakes / 138

Cacao Coconut Granola / 140

Chocolate Hemp Smoothie / 142

Pineapple Ginger Smoothie / 144

Coconut Chai Vanilla Smoothie / 145

Raspberry Chia Smoothie / 146

Moringa Super Green Smoothie / 147

dairy-free egg-free nut-free vegetarian

Bulletproof Pumpkin Spice Latte

Don't you hate it when pumpkin spice lattes are on the menu at all your favorite coffee shops, but you're not indulging because they don't have a sugar-free version? Now you can make a keto-friendly PSL at home, and it won't cost you an arm and a leg.

Yield: **1 serving** ◆ Prep Time: **5 minutes**

6 ounces brewed hot coffee

1 tablespoon coconut oil

1 tablespoon granulated erythritol

1 tablespoon solid-pack pumpkin puree

1 tablespoon unsalted butter

¼ teaspoon pumpkin pie spice

Place all of the ingredients in a small blender and blend until smooth. Pour into a 10-ounce mug and serve immediately.

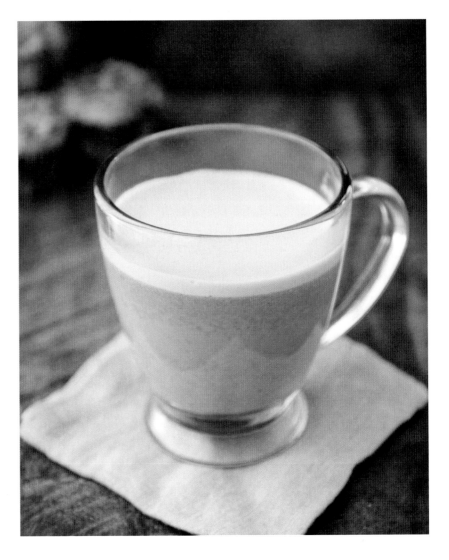

Calories: 226 | Fat: 35g | Protein: 0g | Carbs: 3g | Fiber: 1g | Erythritol: 12g | **Net Carbs: 2g**

Kefir Strawberry Smoothie

dairy-free egg-free nut-free vegetarian

Not only is this smoothie tangy and delicious, but it's loaded with beneficial bacteria to keep your gut and immune system in tip-top shape! Avoid expensive probiotic supplements and add this smoothie to your morning a couple of times a week instead.

Yield: **1 serving** • Prep Time: **5 minutes**

¾ cup unsweetened vanilla-flavored almond milk

¼ cup full-fat unsweetened kefir, store-bought or homemade (page 118)

1 tablespoon granulated erythritol, or more to taste

¼ teaspoon pure vanilla extract

4 medium-sized fresh strawberries, hulled (see tip), plus 1 fresh strawberry for garnish (optional)

3 ice cubes

Place all of the ingredients in a blender and blend until smooth and creamy. Taste and add more sweetener if desired. Pour into a 12-ounce glass and serve immediately. If desired, rest a strawberry on the rim for garnish.

Pro Tip:

You can use frozen strawberries in this recipe—just be sure to purchase a brand that contains only strawberries and no added sweetener. If you use frozen berries, you can omit the ice cubes.

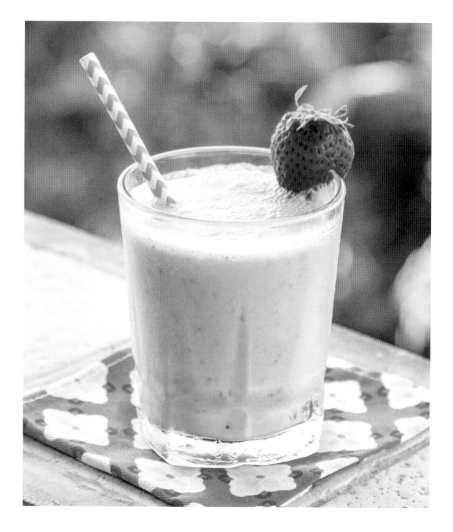

Calories: 73 | Fat: 4g | Protein: 3g | Carbs: 5g | Fiber: 1g | Erythritol: 12g | **Net Carbs: 4g**

Cinnamon Walnut Streusel Muffins

dairy-free · egg-free · nut-free · vegetarian

On hectic mornings, there is nothing easier to grab on the go than a keto-friendly muffin. These Cinnamon Walnut Streusel Muffins go perfectly with a cup of coffee ... or three!

Yield: **12 muffins** ◆ Serving Size: **1 muffin** ◆ Prep Time: **5 minutes** ◆ Cook Time: **22 minutes**

For the muffins:

1 cup unsweetened vanilla-flavored almond milk

½ cup (1 stick) butter, softened

3 large eggs

1 teaspoon pure vanilla extract

1½ cups superfine blanched almond flour

¾ cup granulated erythritol

½ cup coconut flour

2 teaspoons baking powder

1 teaspoon ground cinnamon

¼ teaspoon xanthan gum

Pinch of kosher salt

For the streusel topping:

3 tablespoons butter, melted

¾ cup superfine blanched almond flour

¼ cup chopped raw walnuts

¼ cup granulated erythritol

1 teaspoon ground cinnamon

Pinch of kosher salt

1 Preheat the oven to 375°F. Line a standard-size 12-cup muffin tin with paper or foil liners.

2 Place all of the muffin ingredients in a blender and blend until smooth. Spoon the batter (it will be thick) into the lined muffin cups, filling them about two-thirds full.

3 Place all of the streusel topping ingredients in a small bowl and stir with a fork until a crumbly dough forms. Using your fingers, crumble the streusel into pea-sized pieces over the muffin batter. Bake the muffins for 22 minutes, or until a toothpick inserted in the center of a muffin comes out clean.

4 Remove the muffins from the pan and let cool for at least 10 minutes before serving. Store in an airtight container in the refrigerator for up to 1 week or in the freezer for up to 3 months.

Calories: 272 | Fat: 25g | Protein: 7g | Carbs: 8g | Fiber: 4g | Erythritol: 16g | **Net Carbs: 4g**

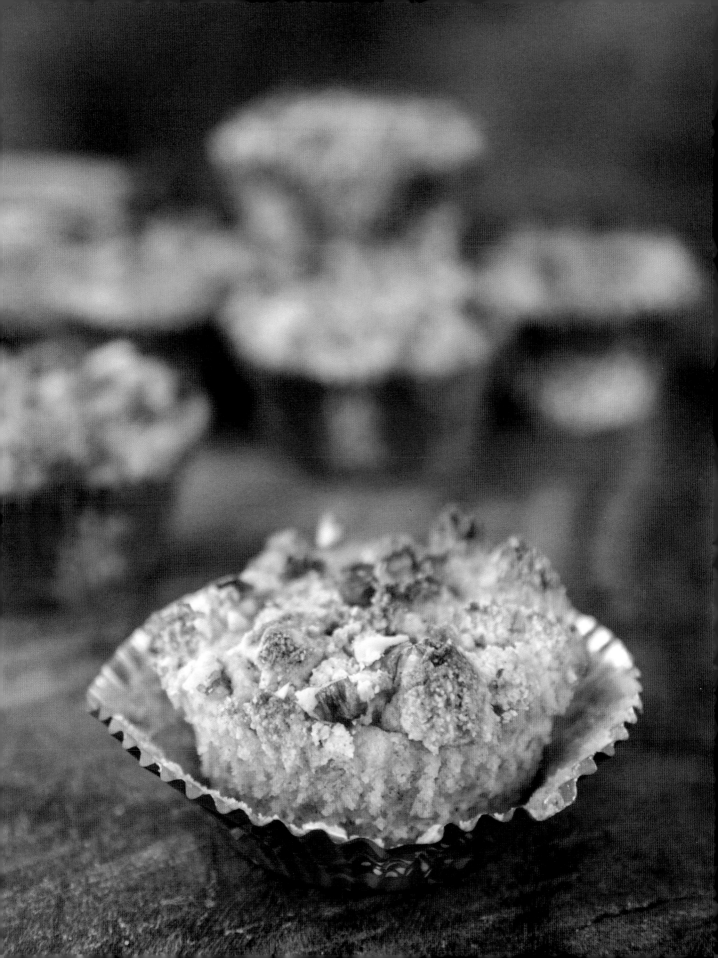

Spanish Tortilla with Chorizo

dairy-free egg-free nut-free vegetarian

A Spanish tortilla is basically a thick omelet, traditionally loaded with potatoes. In this keto version, I have replaced the potatoes with celery root to keep the carbs down. The chorizo and cheese add another layer of flavor and texture, making this a hearty and delicious meal that you can eat at any time of day.

Yield: **1 (10-inch) tortilla** • Serving Size: **¼ tortilla** • Prep Time: **10 minutes** • Cook Time: **18 minutes**

8 ounces Mexican-style fresh (raw) chorizo

2 tablespoons avocado oil or other light-tasting oil

1 cup peeled and thinly sliced celery root (see notes)

½ cup thinly sliced yellow onions

1 teaspoon kosher salt

½ teaspoon ground black pepper

8 large eggs, beaten

½ cup shredded Manchego cheese (see notes)

2 tablespoons chopped fresh cilantro, for garnish (optional)

1 Remove the chorizo from the casing (if applicable) and place in a 10-inch skillet. Cook over medium heat, stirring to break into crumbles, for 5 minutes, or until cooked through. Remove the chorizo from the skillet and set aside.

2 Add the oil, celery root, and onions to the same skillet and cook over medium heat until lightly browned and softened, about 7 minutes. Season with the salt and pepper.

3 Return the cooked chorizo to the skillet and stir to combine. Reduce the heat to low. Add the beaten eggs and stir. Sprinkle with the cheese. Cook on low for 2 minutes, or until the cheese is melting.

4 Stir and bring all of the cooked egg from the sides of the skillet into the center. Stir again, then smooth the mixture back out to the edges with a rubber spatula and cook for 2 minutes, uncovered, until it's beginning to set. Cover the skillet with a lid and cook for another 2 minutes, or until the center is firm.

5 Loosen the edges with a rubber spatula and gently flip over onto a serving dish. Cut into 4 wedges and serve hot. Garnish with chopped cilantro, if desired.

6 Leftovers can be stored in an airtight container in the refrigerator for up to 5 days or in the freezer for up to 3 months. To reheat, thaw if frozen, then place in a baking dish and heat in the oven at 325°F for 8 minutes. Alternatively, you can microwave on high for 30 seconds.

Notes:
If you can't find celery root, sliced radishes or turnips will work just as well.

Manchego is a Spanish cheese that you can usually find in the dairy section of large grocery stores. If you can't get it, sharp cheddar will do just fine.

Serving Suggestion:
While this tortilla is loaded with flavor on its own, you can dress it up with salsa, avocado, sour cream, fresh cilantro, and even more shredded cheese if you like!

Calories: 379 | Fat: 32g | Protein: 22g | Carbs: 5g | Fiber: 1g | **Net Carbs: 4g**

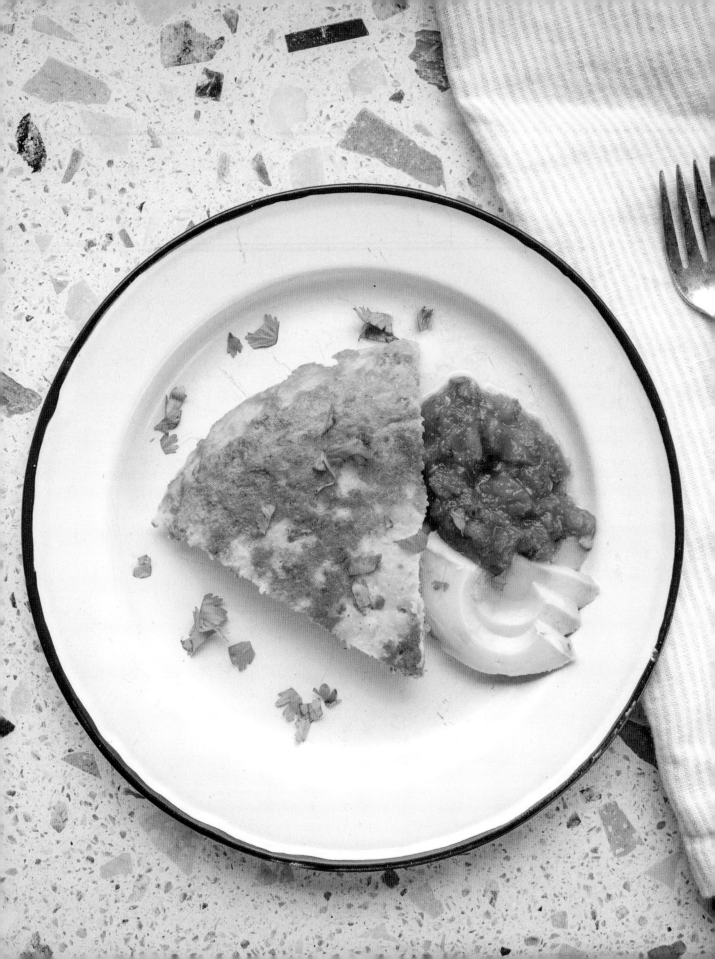

dairy-free egg-free nut-free vegetarian

Snickerdoodle Crepes

I created this recipe for the Egg Fast Diet Plan on my blog, and it quickly became one of the most popular recipes on the website. I'm including it in this book because it's a delicious breakfast that the entire family will love, keto or not.

Yield: **8 crepes** • Serving Size: **2 crepes** • Prep Time: **8 minutes** • Cook Time: **24 minutes**

For the crepes:

6 large eggs

5 ounces cream cheese (½ cup plus 1 tablespoon), softened

1 tablespoon granulated erythritol

1 teaspoon ground cinnamon

2 tablespoons butter, for the pan

For the filling/topping:

⅓ cup granulated erythritol

1 tablespoon ground cinnamon

½ cup (1 stick) butter, softened

1 Make the crepes: Place the eggs, cream cheese, sweetener, and cinnamon in a blender and blend for 30 seconds, or until smooth. Let the batter rest for 5 minutes.

2 Heat a small pat of the butter in a 10-inch nonstick skillet over medium heat until bubbling. Pour about ¼ cup of the batter into the pan and tilt in a circular motion to create a round crepe about 6 inches in diameter. Cook for 2 minutes, or until no longer glossy in the middle. Flip and cook for 1 more minute. Remove the crepe and place on a plate or serving platter. Repeat with the remaining butter and batter to make a total of 8 crepes.

3 Meanwhile, make the filling: Mix the sweetener and cinnamon in a small bowl until combined. Place half of the cinnamon mixture and the softened butter in another small bowl. (Set the other half of the cinnamon mixture aside for the topping.) Stir with a fork until the butter is smooth and the cinnamon mixture is fully incorporated.

4 To serve, spread 1 tablespoon of the filling in the center of each crepe. Roll up each crepe and sprinkle each with 1 teaspoon of the reserved filling.

Calories: 434 | Fat: 42g | Protein: 12g | Carbs: 4.5g | Fiber: 1g | Erythritol: 19g | **Net Carbs: 3.5g**

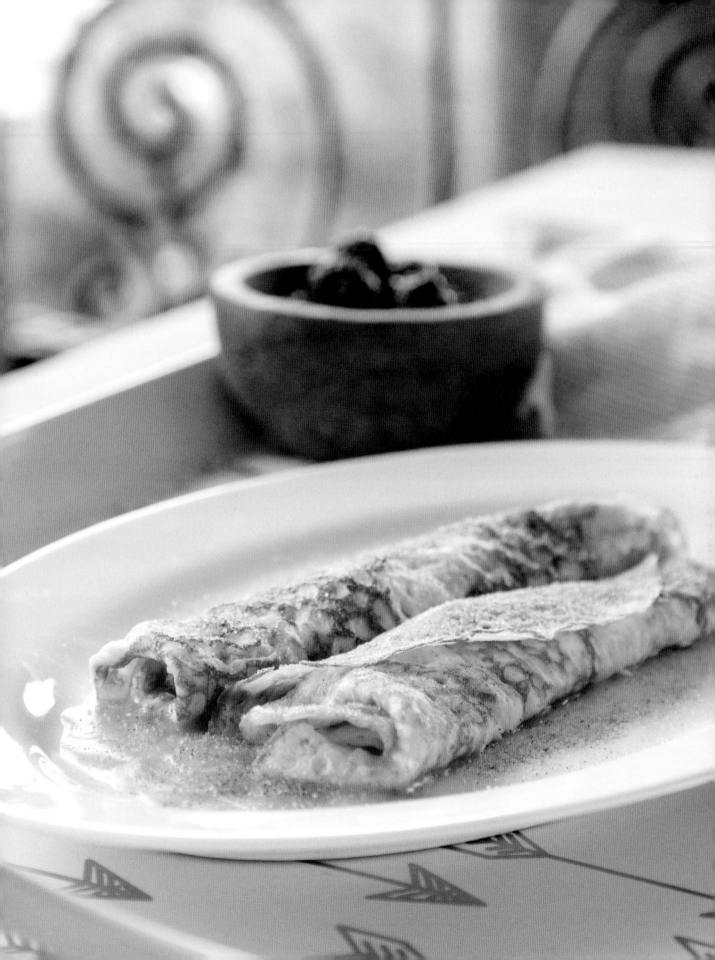

dairy-free egg-free nut-free vegetarian

Sausage & Egg-Stuffed Portobello Mushrooms

This is a fun breakfast when you're looking for something a little different. I love these stuffed mushrooms loaded up with hot sauce, but hollandaise would also be delicious. They are just as tasty chilled or at room temperature, so you can eat them on the go for lunch or add them to your next brunch buffet!

Yield: **4 stuffed mushrooms** ◆ Serving Size: **1 stuffed mushroom** ◆ Prep Time: **8 minutes**

Cook Time: **27 minutes**

4 large portobello mushroom caps

Kosher salt and ground black pepper

1 pound raw country sausage (aka breakfast sausage)

4 medium eggs (see note)

1 tablespoon chopped fresh parsley, for garnish

1 Preheat the oven to 375°F. Remove the stems from the mushroom caps and scrape out the ribs with a spoon. Season the caps with salt and pepper.

2 Divide the sausage into 4 equal portions. Press a portion of the sausage along the bottom and up the sides of each mushroom cap to form a cup for the egg. Place the sausage-stuffed mushrooms on a sheet pan and bake for 15 minutes.

3 Remove the mushroom caps from the oven and blot any liquid from the centers. Crack an egg into each mushroom cap. Return to the oven and bake for 12 more minutes for firm whites and slightly runny yolks. If you prefer hard yolks, increase the cooking time to 15 minutes, or until the eggs are cooked to your liking.

4 Serve hot or at room temperature, garnished with fresh parsley.

5 Store in an airtight container in the refrigerator for up to 3 days. To reheat, microwave on high for 30 seconds.

Note:
While I usually use large eggs in my cooking, I found that a lot of the white overflowed out of the mushroom cap when I tried this recipe with large eggs. Switching to medium eggs resolved the problem. If you must use large eggs, I recommend removing some of the white before adding each egg to a mushroom cap to prevent overflow.

Calories: 465 | Fat: 34g | Protein: 26g | Carbs: 3.5g | Fiber: 1g | **Net Carbs: 2.5g**

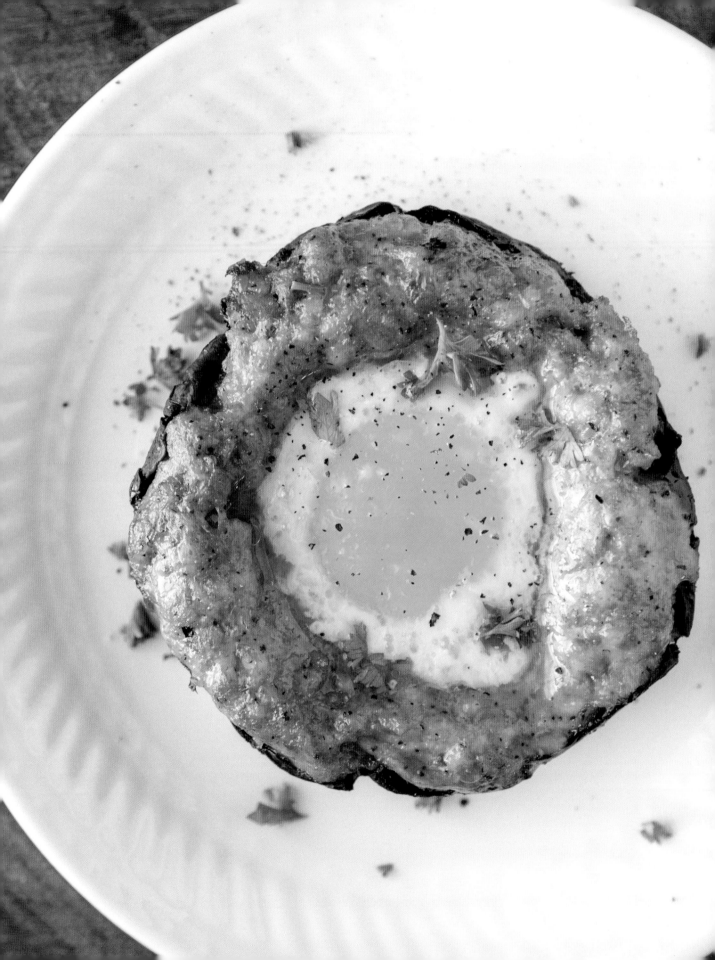

dairy-free egg-free nut-free vegetarian

Savory Chorizo Breakfast Bowl

Who doesn't love a good breakfast bowl? So often breakfast bowls are sweet, but I'm a fan of a savory breakfast, and this one never disappoints! I love the combination of runny egg yolk and spicy chorizo.

Yield: **1 serving** ◆ Prep Time: **8 minutes**

¾ cup Basic Cauliflower Rice (page 250), hot

4 ounces Mexican-style fresh chorizo, cooked

¼ cup shredded cheddar cheese

¼ cup Easy Keto Guacamole (page 293)

2 tablespoons Restaurant-Style Salsa (page 292)

1 large egg, poached (see tip)

1 teaspoon chopped fresh cilantro (optional)

Place the hot cauliflower rice in a serving bowl. Top with the cooked chorizo, shredded cheese, guacamole, salsa, poached egg, and cilantro, if desired. Serve immediately.

Pro Tip:

If poaching eggs stresses you out, you can top this bowl with a fried egg instead. If you're an egg-poaching newbie but game to try it, simply bring a small pot of water to a simmer and add ½ teaspoon of white vinegar (the vinegar helps the egg white firm up quickly). Then break an egg carefully into a small bowl, making sure the yolk stays intact. Swirl a slotted spoon around the water in the pot to create a small whirlpool. (This helps keep the egg white from spreading too much.) Carefully slide the egg from the bowl into the center of the swirling water. Cook for 3 minutes, then remove the egg with the slotted spoon and place the spoon with the egg on it on a paper towel–lined plate. The paper towel will absorb any excess water so your breakfast bowl doesn't become soggy. After 30 seconds, carefully transfer the poached egg from the spoon onto your breakfast bowl.

Calories: 445 | Fat: 32g | Protein: 29g | Carbs: 12g | Fiber: 6g | **Net Carbs: 6g**

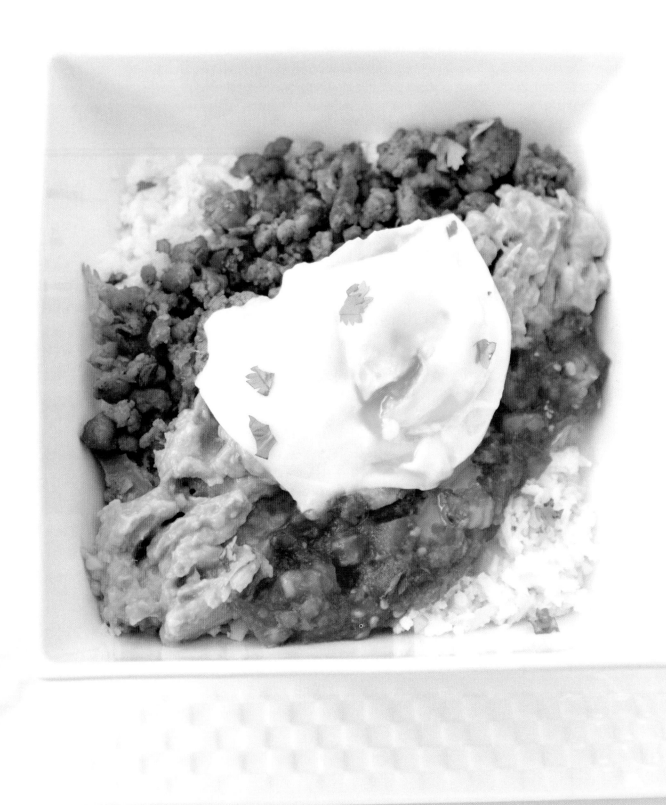

Cream Cheese Pancakes

When I first blended cream cheese and eggs together to make these pancakes for my blog in 2012, I had no idea that the recipe would become so wildly popular! I've since created variations on this batter to make wraps (page 70) and noodles (page 72), but my favorite way to eat it is still in the form of these delicious pancakes, served with butter and lots of sugar-free syrup.

Yield: **4 (6-inch) pancakes** ◆ Serving Size: **1 batch (4 pancakes)** ◆ Prep Time: **5 minutes**

Cook Time: **12 minutes**

2 ounces cream cheese (¼ cup), softened

2 large eggs

1 teaspoon granulated erythritol

½ teaspoon ground cinnamon

1 tablespoon butter, for the pan

1 Place the cream cheese, eggs, sweetener, and cinnamon in a small blender and blend for 30 seconds, or until smooth. Let the batter rest for 2 minutes.

2 Heat the butter in a 10-inch nonstick skillet over medium heat until bubbling. Pour ¼ cup of the batter into the pan and tilt the pan in a circular motion to create a thin pancake about 6 inches in diameter. Cook for 2 minutes, or until the center is no longer glossy. Flip and cook for 1 minute on the other side. Remove and repeat with the rest of the batter, making a total of 4 pancakes.

Make It Easy:

These pancakes are easy to make in double or triple batches when you have time. They can be stored in the refrigerator for up to a week and reheated as necessary. Even better, you can freeze them in individual portions, and they will keep frozen for up to 3 months. To reheat them, place on a plate and cover loosely with a paper towel, microwave on high for 30 seconds, and serve!

Calories: 395 | Fat: 35g | Protein: 17g | Carbs: 3g | Fiber: 0g | Erythritol: 4g | **Net Carbs: 3g**

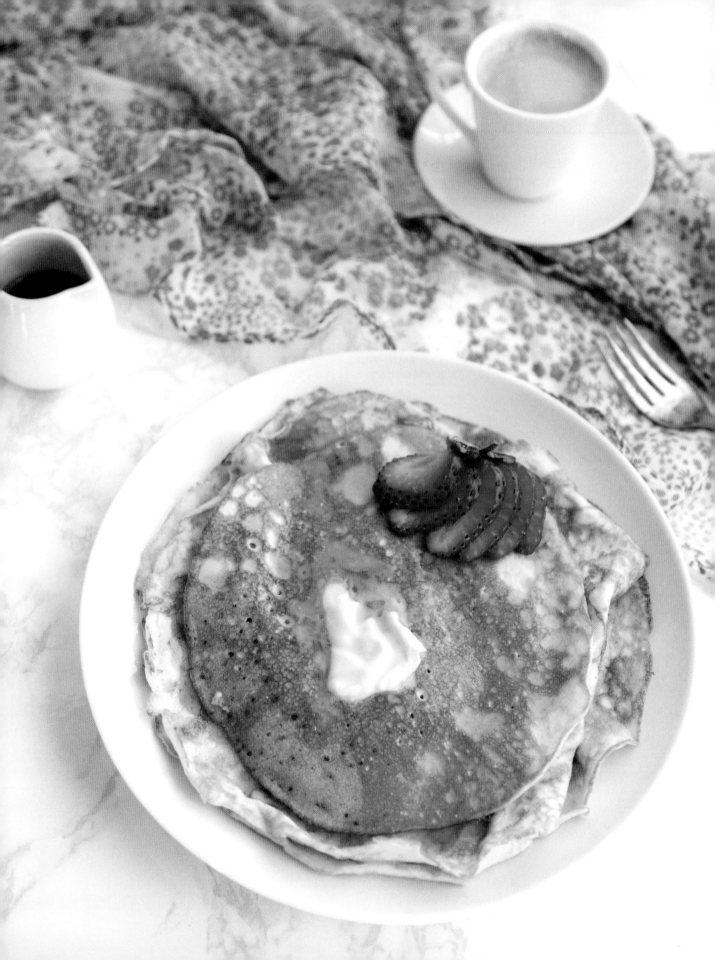

Cacao Coconut Granola

When I went keto years ago, the thing I missed most was cereal in the morning. I just love the sweet crunch of cereal floating in ice-cold milk. I realized recently that a dish I'd made years ago in the dehydrator could be made keto-friendly if I got rid of the maple syrup and dates. Once I got the ratios right, this granola was born, and it perfectly fills the void in my mornings where cereal used to be. Avoid dairy milk because of its high sugar content; serve this granola with unsweetened vanilla-flavored almond milk instead, along with a handful of your favorite fresh berries.

Yield: **3 cups** • Serving Size: **½ cup** • Prep Time: **5 minutes** • Cook Time: **30 minutes**

½ cup chopped raw pecans

½ cup flax seeds

½ cup superfine blanched almond flour

½ cup unsweetened dried coconut

¼ cup chopped cacao nibs

¼ cup chopped raw walnuts

¼ cup sesame seeds

¼ cup sugar-free vanilla-flavored protein powder

3 tablespoons granulated erythritol

1 teaspoon ground cinnamon

⅛ teaspoon kosher salt

⅓ cup coconut oil

1 large egg white, beaten

1 Preheat the oven to 300°F. Line a 15 by 10-inch sheet pan with parchment paper.

2 Place all of the ingredients in a large bowl. Stir well until the mixture is crumbly and holds together in small clumps. Spread out on the parchment-lined pan. Bake for 30 minutes, or until golden brown and fragrant.

3 Let the granola cool completely in the pan before removing. Store in an airtight container in the refrigerator for up to 2 weeks.

Calories: 441 | Fat: 40g | Protein: 15g | Carbs: 14g | Fiber: 10g | Erythritol: 6g | **Net Carbs: 4g**

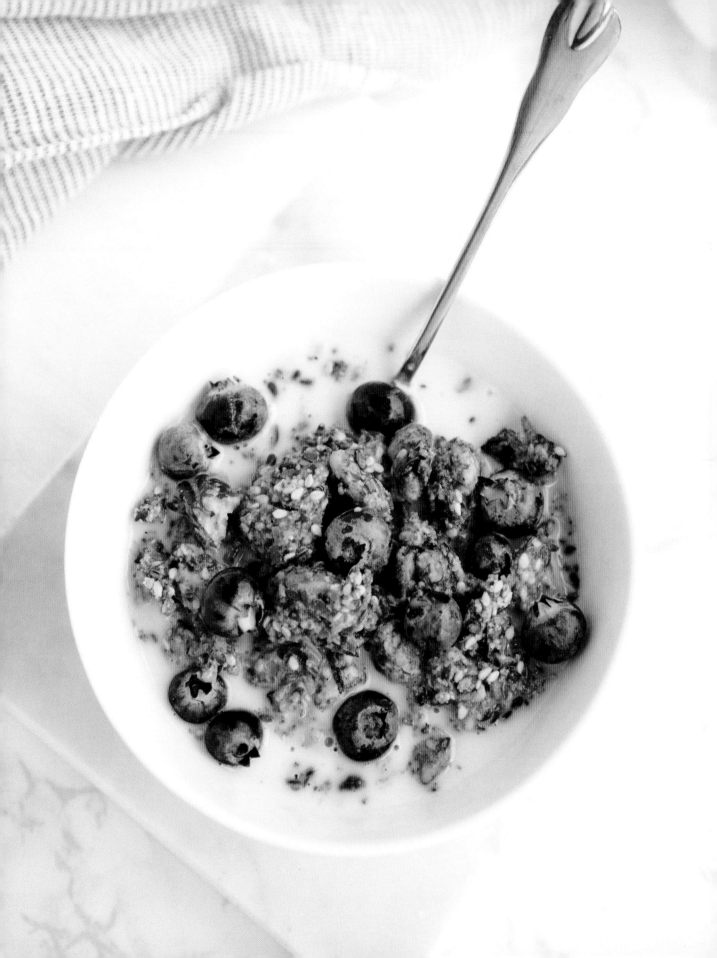

dairy-free · egg-free · nut-free · vegetarian

Chocolate Hemp Smoothie

Chocolate for breakfast? It's how we roll. No need to feel guilty about it, either! Cocoa powder is loaded with antioxidants and phenols that protect your heart, and it's a great source of magnesium and iron. Your family won't believe their ears when you suggest a chocolate shake before school. Just go with it, kids, just go with it.

Yield: **1 serving** ◆ Prep Time: **5 minutes**

1 cup unsweetened vanilla-flavored almond milk

2 tablespoons heavy whipping cream

¼ teaspoon pure vanilla extract

¼ cup unsweetened hemp protein powder

2 tablespoons unsweetened cocoa powder

2 tablespoons granulated erythritol, or more to taste

3 ice cubes

Place all of the ingredients in a blender and blend until smooth and creamy. Taste and add more sweetener, if desired. Pour into a 12-ounce glass and serve immediately.

> **Note:**
> *Hemp protein is highly digestible and is loaded with amino acids, essential fatty acids, fiber, and important nutrients like iron, magnesium, and zinc. To get the best health benefits from hemp protein, always purchase it cold-milled and organic, if possible. While there is no danger of getting high from hemp protein, you can use your favorite unsweetened, unflavored protein powder in this shake if you prefer.*

Calories: 245 | Fat: 17g | Protein: 15g | Carbs: 14g | Fiber: 10g | Erythritol: 24g | **Net Carbs: 4g**

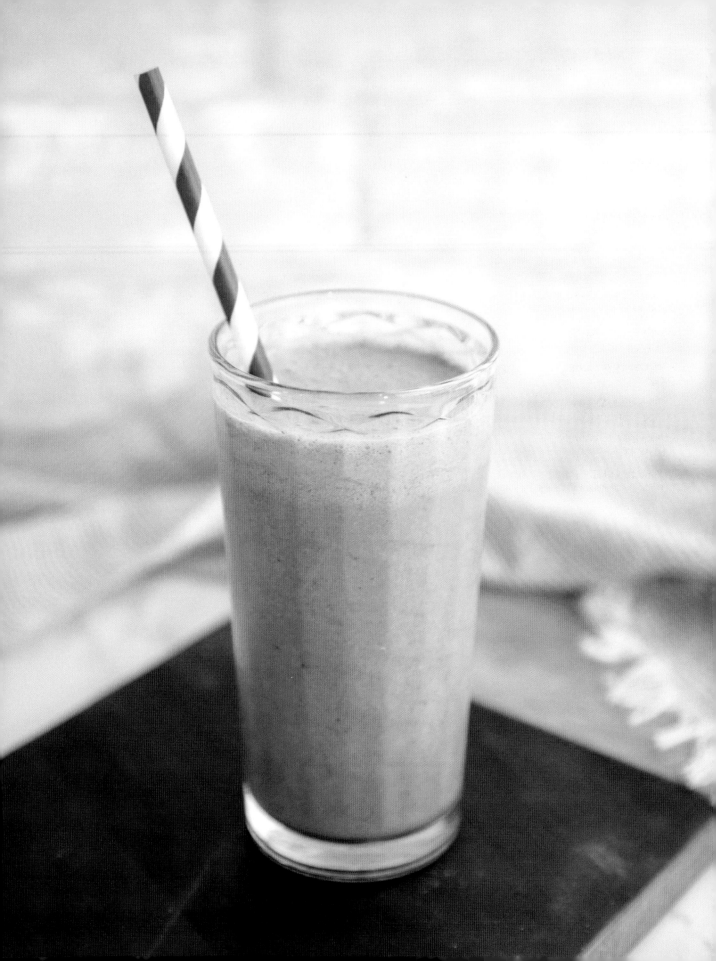

Pineapple Ginger Smoothie

This tasty smoothie has lots of anti-inflammatory benefits from the pineapple, turmeric, and ginger. It's also dairy-free and incredibly refreshing!

Yield: **1 serving** ◆ Prep Time: **8 minutes**

1 cup unsweetened vanilla-flavored almond milk

2 tablespoons full-fat unsweetened coconut milk

¼ cup chopped fresh pineapple

2 tablespoons collagen powder

1 tablespoon granulated erythritol, or more to taste

2 teaspoons chopped fresh turmeric, or 1 teaspoon turmeric powder

1 teaspoon peeled and minced fresh ginger

3 ice cubes

Place all of the ingredients in a blender and blend until smooth and creamy. Taste and add more sweetener, if desired. Pour into a 12-ounce glass and serve immediately.

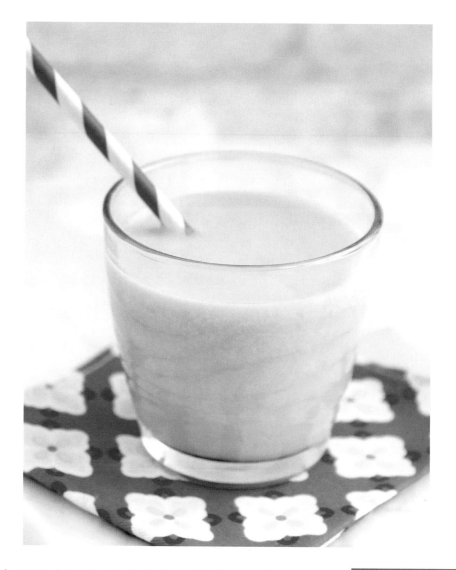

Calories: 149 | Fat: 7g | Protein: 12g | Carbs: 9g | Fiber: 2g | Erythritol: 12g | **Net Carbs: 7g**

Coconut Chai Vanilla Smoothie

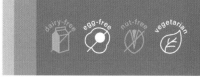

I love iced chai, but commercial brands are loaded with sugar and preservatives. Make this easy and delicious chai smoothie at home, and you'll never go back to store-bought!

Yield: **1 serving** • Prep Time: **5 minutes**

½ cup brewed chai tea, cooled

½ cup unsweetened vanilla-flavored almond milk

2 tablespoons full-fat unsweetened coconut milk

2 tablespoons sugar-free vanilla-flavored protein powder

1 tablespoon granulated erythritol, or more to taste

¼ teaspoon pure vanilla extract

⅛ teaspoon ground cinnamon, plus more for garnish if desired

3 ice cubes

Place all of the ingredients in a blender and blend until smooth and creamy. Taste and add more sweetener, if desired. Pour into a 12-ounce glass and serve immediately. Garnish with a dusting of cinnamon, if desired.

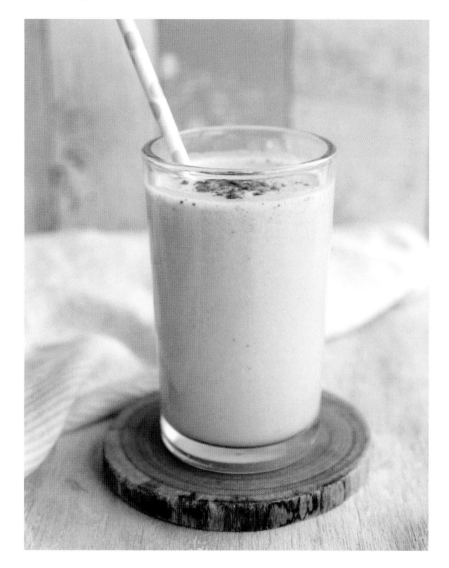

Calories: 170 | Fat: 8g | Protein: 18g | Carbs: 4g | Fiber: 1g | Erythritol: 12g | **Net Carbs: 3g**

Raspberry Chia Smoothie

Chia seeds are naturally rich in healthy omega-3 fatty acids and other important nutrients, making them a healthy addition to any eating plan. Because they are high in fiber and low in carbs, they are also perfectly suited to keto. This tasty smoothie is one of my favorites.

Yield: **1 serving** ◆ Prep Time: **5 minutes**

1 cup unsweetened vanilla-flavored almond milk

⅓ cup fresh raspberries

¼ cup sugar-free vanilla-flavored protein powder

2 tablespoons full-fat unsweetened coconut milk

1 teaspoon chia seeds

3 ice cubes

Pro Tip:
You can use frozen raspberries in this recipe—just be sure to purchase a brand that contains only raspberries and no added sweetener. If you use frozen berries, you can omit the ice cubes.

Place all of the ingredients in a blender and blend until smooth and creamy. Pour into a 12-ounce glass and serve immediately.

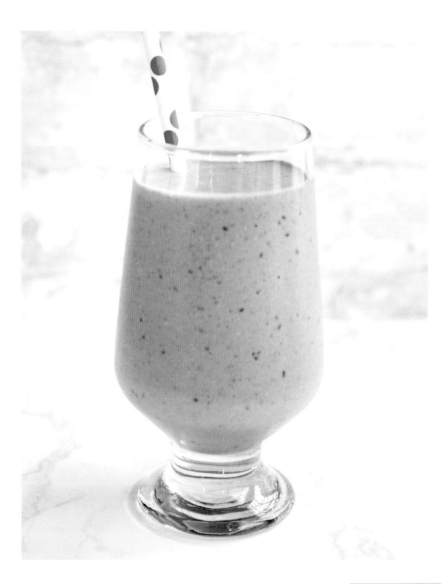

Calories: 222 | Fat: 10g | Protein: 35g | Carbs: 8g | Fiber: 5g | **Net Carbs: 3g**

Moringa Super Green Smoothie

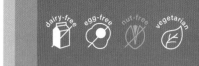

I mentioned some of the health benefits of moringa in the supplements section (see page 39), and this smoothie is a delicious way to get some moringa into your keto diet! Be sure to get unflavored pure moringa powder; it has a mildly grassy flavor.

Yield: **1 serving** • Prep Time: **5 minutes**

1 cup unsweetened vanilla-flavored almond milk

3 tablespoons full-fat unsweetened coconut milk

1 tablespoon pure moringa leaf powder

1 teaspoon granulated erythritol, or more to taste

¼ teaspoon pure vanilla extract

5 ice cubes

Place all of the ingredients in a blender and blend until smooth and creamy. Taste and add more sweetener if desired. Pour into a 12-ounce glass and serve immediately.

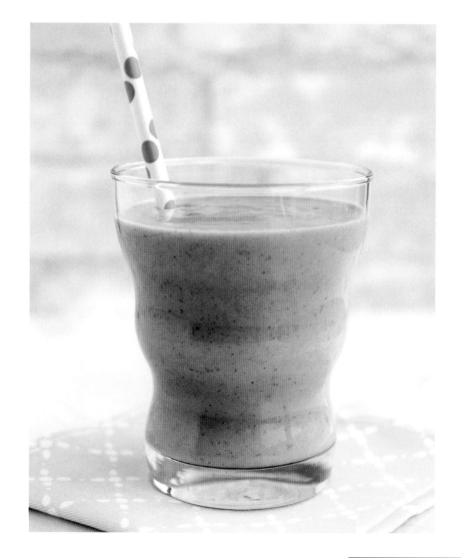

Calories: 115 | Fat: 10g | Protein: 3g | Carbs: 4.5g | Fiber: 1g | Erythritol: 4g | **Net Carbs: 3.5g**

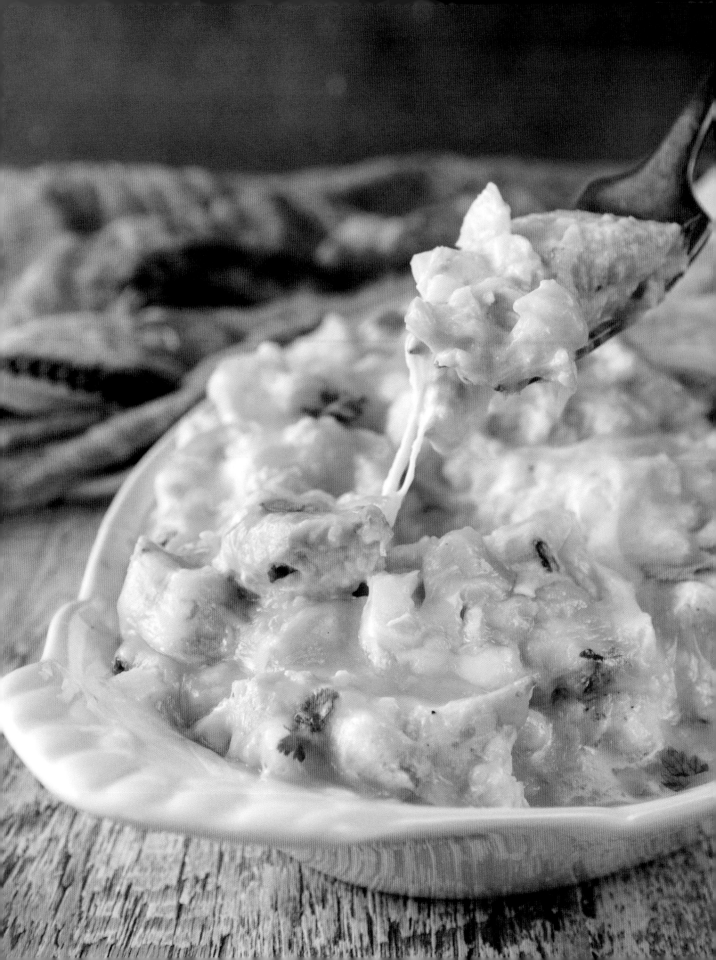

chicken

Chicken Tetrazzini / 150

Pecan-Crusted Chicken Fingers / 152

Chicken Parmesan / 154

Green Chicken Enchilada Cauliflower Casserole / 156

Easy Salsa Chicken / 158

Chicken in Coconut Broth / 160

Green Chicken Curry / 162

Chicken Cacciatore / 164

Cheesy Broccoli–Stuffed Chicken / 166

Chicken Larb / 168

Tandoori Chicken Meatballs / 170

Jerk Chicken / 172

Chicken Tetrazzini

This recipe is a throwback to when I was a kid, but classics are classics for a reason, am I right? Tender pieces of chicken and mushrooms, a few peas thrown in for nostalgia's sake, all swimming in a sherry cream sauce, and with a butter crumb topping? Why are you still here and not making your shopping list? Go already!

Yield: 6 servings ◆ Serving Size: **1 cup tetrazzini and 1 cup zoodles** ◆ Prep Time: **12 minutes**

Cook Time: **35 minutes**

5 tablespoons butter, divided

1 tablespoon extra-virgin olive oil

2 cups sliced white or cremini mushrooms

½ cup chopped yellow onions

1 tablespoon minced garlic

2 teaspoons fresh thyme leaves

⅓ cup dry sherry

3 cups shredded cooked chicken (see tips)

1 cup chicken broth, store-bought or homemade (page 82)

¾ cup heavy whipping cream

¼ teaspoon xanthan gum

⅛ teaspoon ground nutmeg

½ cup fresh or frozen peas

⅓ cup grated Parmesan cheese

¼ cup Keto Breadcrumbs (page 74) (optional, but recommended for texture)

6 cups raw or lightly cooked spiral-sliced zucchini (about 3 medium zucchini)

2 tablespoons chopped fresh parsley, for garnish (optional)

1 Heat 2 tablespoons of the butter and the olive oil in a large sauté pan over medium heat. Add the mushrooms and cook, stirring occasionally, until golden brown, about 8 minutes. Add the onions, garlic, and thyme and cook for 3 more minutes.

2 Stir in the sherry and cook for 2 minutes, scraping any bits off the bottom of the pan. Add the chicken to the pan and stir to coat with the sauce. Spoon the chicken and mushroom mixture into a bowl and return the pan to the stove.

3 Melt the remaining 3 tablespoons of butter in the same pan over medium heat, then whisk in the chicken broth, cream, xanthan gum, and nutmeg. Cook over medium-low heat for 8 minutes, whisking occasionally, until the sauce has reduced and thickened slightly and coats the back of a spoon.

4 Preheat the oven to 450°F.

5 Return the chicken and mushroom mixture to the pan with the thickened sauce, then add the peas and stir until well coated. Transfer to a 13 by 9-inch baking dish and top with the grated Parmesan and breadcrumbs, if using. Bake for 10 minutes, or until the top is golden and the sauce is bubbling.

6 Serve hot over raw or lightly cooked zoodles, garnished with chopped parsley, if desired.

Make It Easy:
Whenever you find yourself with leftover chicken or turkey, freeze it in 1-cup portions for use in recipes like this one—then just thaw it and you're ready to go. No leftovers? Simply pick up a rotisserie chicken on your way home and you're in business!

Calories: 420 | Fat: 26g | Protein: 28g | Carbs: 10g | Fiber: 3g | **Net Carbs: 7g**

Pro Tips:

To shred cooked chicken, simply pull the meat apart with two forks into bite-sized pieces. Shredding the chicken creates more surface area for the yummy sauce to cling to!

Baking the casserole separately from the zoodles keeps the sauce thick. If you bake them together, the moisture will leach out of the zoodles into the sauce, making it watery. The heat from the hot casserole served over the raw zoodles will be just enough to soften them to a pastalike consistency without making them soggy.

Family-Friendly Tip:

Shredding the chicken is a safe and fun task for the kids. They can also spiral-slice the zucchini (watch those blades, though!) while you prep the rest of the ingredients.

dairy-free egg-free nut-free vegetarian

Pecan-Crusted Chicken Fingers

The flavors in the pecan breading are sophisticated enough to make these chicken fingers a hit at your next cocktail party, yet kid-friendly enough to get by even the pickiest eaters at the family dinner table! Serve with Sweet Sriracha Dipping Sauce (page 99).

Yield: **4 servings** • Prep Time: **8 minutes** • Cook Time: **12 minutes**

For the pecan breading:

1 cup raw pecans, finely chopped

2 tablespoons coconut flour

1 teaspoon kosher salt

¼ teaspoon ground black pepper

½ teaspoon garlic powder

½ teaspoon ginger powder

½ teaspoon ground coriander

1 large egg, beaten

1 tablespoon lime juice

1 teaspoon Worcestershire sauce

2 tablespoons avocado oil or other light-tasting oil, for frying

1 pound chicken tenders or boneless, skinless chicken breasts cut into 1½-inch-wide strips

1. Make the breading: Place the pecans, coconut flour, salt, pepper, garlic powder, ginger powder, and coriander in a medium-sized bowl and stir well.

2. Place the beaten egg, lime juice, and Worcestershire sauce in a separate small bowl and stir well.

3. Heat the oil in a large nonstick skillet for 2 minutes. Line a plate with a couple of paper towels.

4. Dip a chicken tender into the egg mixture, then roll it in the pecan breading until completely coated. Repeat with the rest of the tenders. Fry the coated chicken for 2 to 3 minutes per side, or until golden brown and cooked through.

5. Remove the chicken fingers from the skillet and place on the lined plate for a couple of minutes before serving.

Calories: 389 | Fat: 27g | Protein: 31g | Carbs: 7g | Fiber: 4g | **Net Carbs: 3g**

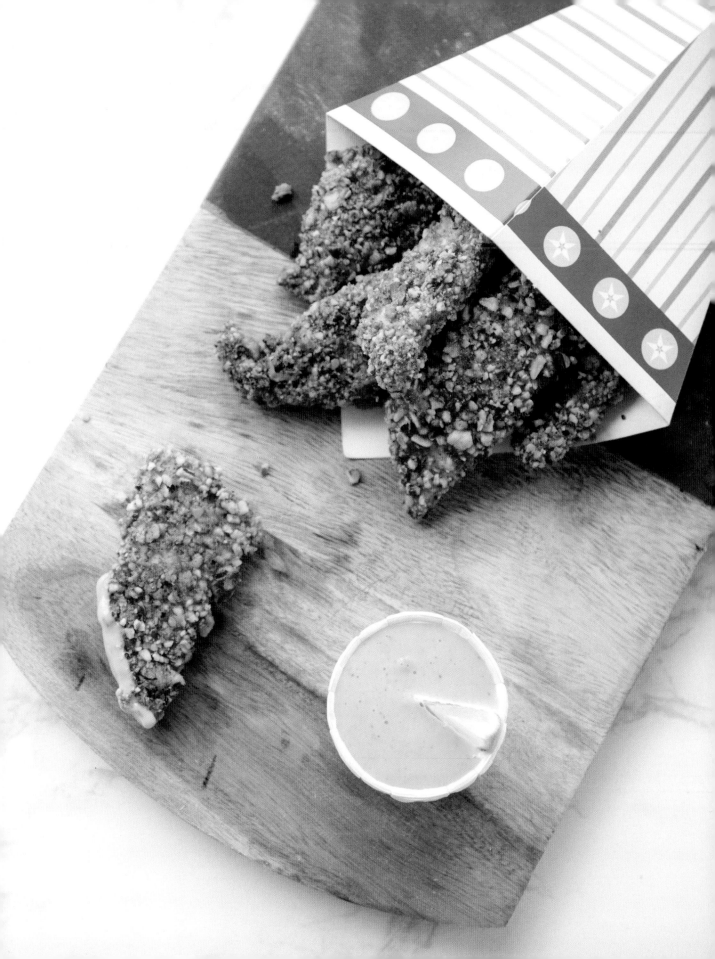

Chicken Parmesan

dairy-free egg-free nut-free vegetarian

Mr. Hungry is half Italian, and chicken Parmesan is one of his favorite meals. For the first ten years of our marriage, he'd order it at every restaurant we went to that had it on the menu. It drove me crazy that he'd never try anything new, since I was the exact opposite and hated ordering the same thing twice. He's since broadened his horizons, but it remains a favorite, and I make this version for him often, to rave reviews every time.

Yield: **4 servings** ◆ Prep Time: **5 minutes** ◆ Cook Time: **28 minutes**

¼ cup extra-virgin olive oil, for frying

1 large egg

1 batch Basic Breading (page 75)

4 (6-ounce) chicken cutlets, pounded to ½-inch thickness

1½ cups marinara sauce, store-bought or homemade (page 106)

4 ounces whole-milk mozzarella cheese, sliced thin

¼ cup julienned fresh basil, for garnish

1 Preheat the oven to 375°F and line a plate with a couple of paper towels.

2 Heat the oil in a large sauté pan over medium heat for 2 minutes. Beat the egg in a small bowl. Place the breading in a medium-sized bowl.

3 Dip the chicken cutlets into the beaten egg, then into the breading until coated on all sides. Place the breaded cutlets in the hot oil and fry until golden brown, about 3 minutes per side.

4 Remove the chicken to the lined plate for a minute or two. Spread ½ cup of the marinara sauce on the bottom of a 2-quart casserole dish.

5 Place the chicken cutlets in the dish and top with the remaining marinara sauce. Place the slices of mozzarella on top of the chicken and bake for 20 minutes, or until golden brown and bubbling. Garnish with fresh basil before serving.

Calories: 509 | Fat: 28g | Protein: 52g | Carbs: 10.5g | Fiber: 6g | **Net Carbs: 4.5g**

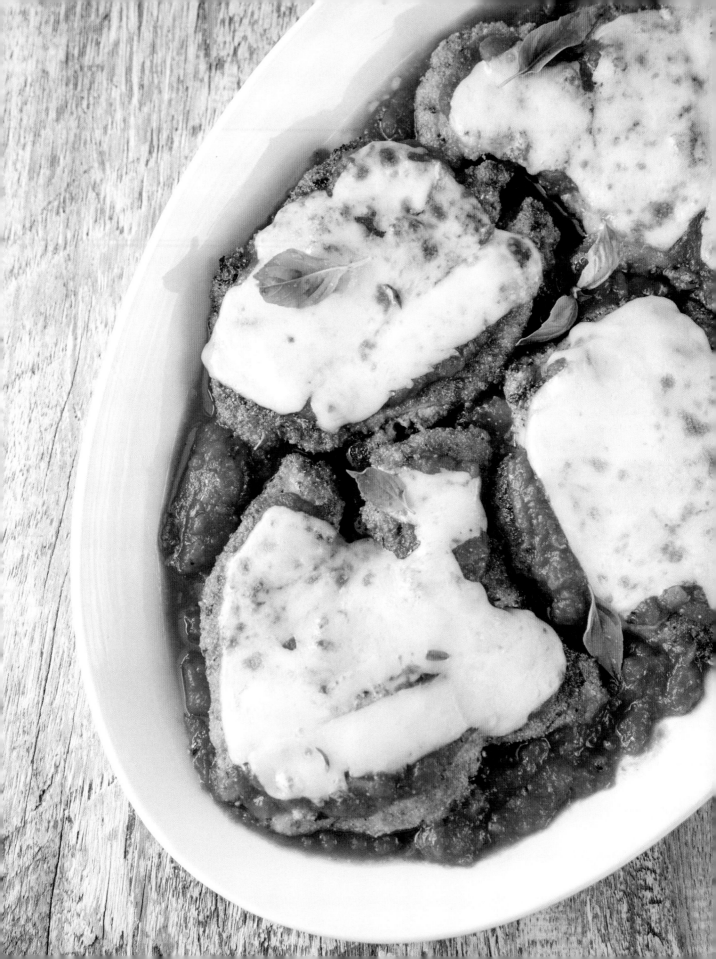

dairy-free   egg-free   nut-free   vegetarian

Green Chicken Enchilada Cauliflower Casserole

This recipe was born out of desperation—I was starving and had only a few ingredients in the house from which to make a tasty keto meal. I threw the following ingredients together and it turned out so good, and took so little effort, that I remade it for my blog. Insanely tasty and comforting to eat, this remains one of the most popular recipes on I Breathe I'm Hungry.

Yield: **6 servings** • Prep Time: **10 minutes** • Cook Time: **33 minutes**

4 cups cauliflower florets

4 ounces cream cheese (½ cup), softened

2 cups shredded cooked chicken breast

1 cup shredded sharp cheddar cheese

½ cup salsa verde

¼ cup full-fat sour cream

1 tablespoon chopped fresh cilantro, plus more for garnish if desired

½ teaspoon kosher salt

⅛ teaspoon ground black pepper

1 Preheat the oven to 375°F.

2 Place the cauliflower in a microwave-safe dish and microwave, uncovered, on high for 12 minutes, or until fork-tender. Add the cream cheese and microwave for 1 more minute, then stir.

3 Add the chicken, cheese, salsa verde, sour cream, cilantro, salt, and pepper and stir well. Transfer the mixture to a 13 by 9-inch baking dish and bake for 20 minutes, or until golden brown and bubbling. Serve hot, garnished with extra cilantro, if desired.

Make It Easy:
This recipe lends itself well to being made ahead for meal prep all week long! Leftovers can be reheated in the microwave on high for 2 minutes.

Calories: 311 | Fat: 18g | Protein: 33g | Carbs: 6.5g | Fiber: 2g | **Net Carbs: 4.5g**

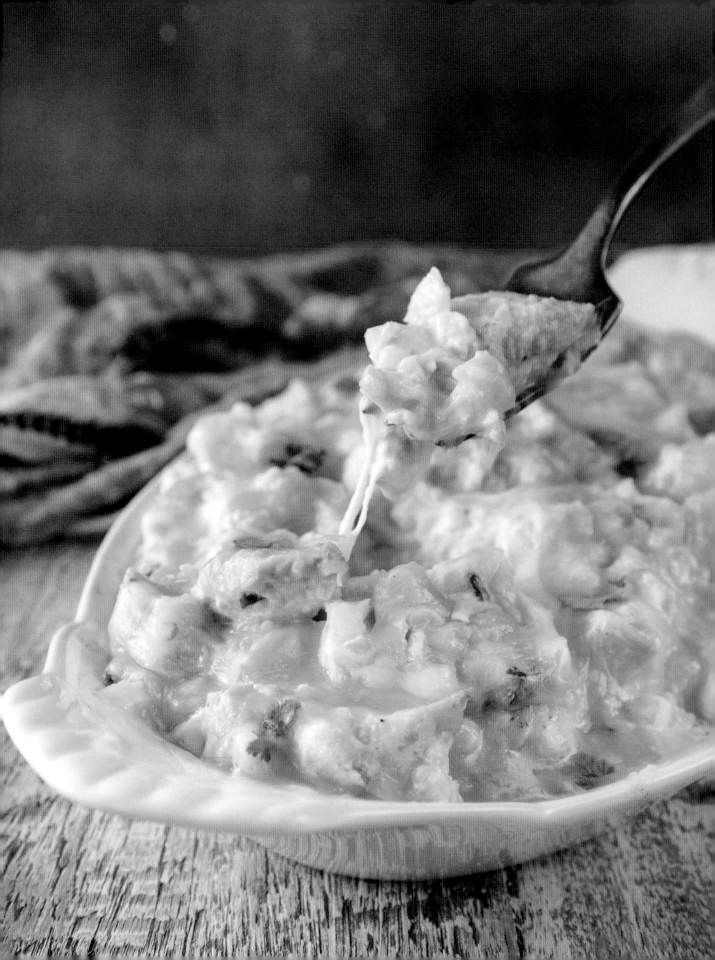

Easy Salsa Chicken

I consider this a Mexican/Creole-themed version of Chicken Parmesan (page 154), since it's breaded chicken cutlets topped with sauce and cheese. My guys like the Italian version, so this was an easy sell, and I make it often. You can make it with regular rice for the rest of the family and cauliflower rice for you!

Yield: **6 servings** • Prep Time: **5 minutes** • Cook Time: **28 minutes**

¼ cup coconut flour

2 tablespoons Creole seasoning

1 large egg

2 tablespoons avocado oil or other light-tasting oil, for frying

6 (6-ounce) chicken cutlets

1 cup Restaurant-Style Salsa (page 292)

1 cup shredded cheddar cheese

For garnish (optional):

Chopped fresh cilantro

Finely diced red onions and/or sliced scallions

Full-fat sour cream

1 Preheat the oven to 375°F and line a plate with a couple of paper towels.

2 Place the coconut flour and Creole seasoning in a small bowl and mix well. Beat the egg in another small bowl. Heat the oil in a large sauté pan over medium heat for 2 minutes.

3 Dip the chicken cutlets into the beaten egg, then into the seasoned coconut flour. Place the breaded cutlets in the hot oil and fry for 3 minutes per side, or until golden brown. Place the chicken on the lined plate for a minute or two.

4 Move the cutlets to a baking dish large enough to comfortably fit all of them. Spoon the salsa over the chicken, then sprinkle the cheese over the top. Bake for 20 minutes, or until the chicken reaches 165°F in the center and the cheese is bubbling. Serve garnished with cilantro, red onions, and/or scallions and plenty of sour cream, if desired.

Calories: 332 | Fat: 14g | Protein: 45g | Carbs: 4.5g | Fiber: 2g | **Net Carbs: 2.5g**

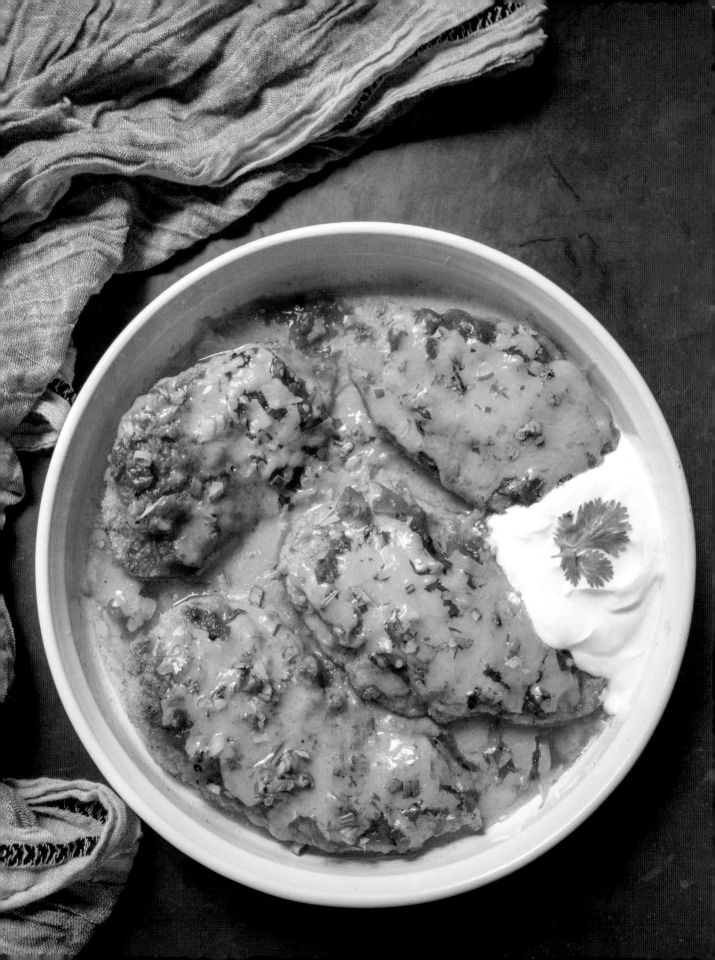

dairy-free egg-free nut-free vegetarian

Chicken in Coconut Broth

This my effort to re-create a dish we had recently in Le Ceiba, Honduras, at a little local joint that some friends had taken us to. They had only a couple of lunch options to choose from, and the coconut stewed chicken sounded the best to me. For the equivalent of about $3 US, it was the best plate of food I ate on the entire trip! The chicken was flavorful and tender, and the creamy coconut sauce was so velvety and rich that I could have eaten it with a spoon, like soup. This version is as close as I can get to what we had, with keto-friendly cauliflower rice replacing the traditional white rice. While it isn't exactly the same, it's still incredibly tasty!

Yield: **6 servings** ◆ Prep Time: **5 minutes** ◆ Cook Time: **40 minutes**

6 whole chicken legs (drumsticks and thighs)

½ teaspoon kosher salt

¼ teaspoon ground white pepper

2 tablespoons coconut oil

1 teaspoon minced garlic

1 teaspoon peeled and minced fresh ginger

1 cup chicken broth, store-bought or homemade (page 82)

1 cup full-fat unsweetened coconut milk

1 tablespoon granulated erythritol

¼ teaspoon xanthan gum

2 tablespoons chopped fresh cilantro, for garnish

3 cups Basic Cauliflower Rice (page 250), for serving (optional)

1 Season the chicken with the salt and pepper. Heat the coconut oil in a large saucepan over medium-high heat. Add the chicken and cook on both sides until golden brown, about 3 minutes per side.

2 Add the garlic and ginger to the pan and cook for 2 minutes, or until fragrant. Pour in the broth, coconut milk, and sweetener. Bring to a boil, then reduce the heat to low. Cover and simmer for 30 minutes, or until the chicken is cooked through.

3 Remove the chicken from the pan and set aside. Whisk the xanthan gum into the sauce and cook on high until the sauce has thickened slightly, about 2 minutes. Taste and season with more salt and pepper, if desired. Return the chicken to the pan and garnish with chopped cilantro before serving. Serve over cauliflower rice if desired.

Calories: 237 | Fat: 15g | Protein: 23g | Carbs: 1g | Fiber: 0g | Erythritol: 2g | **Net Carbs: 1g**

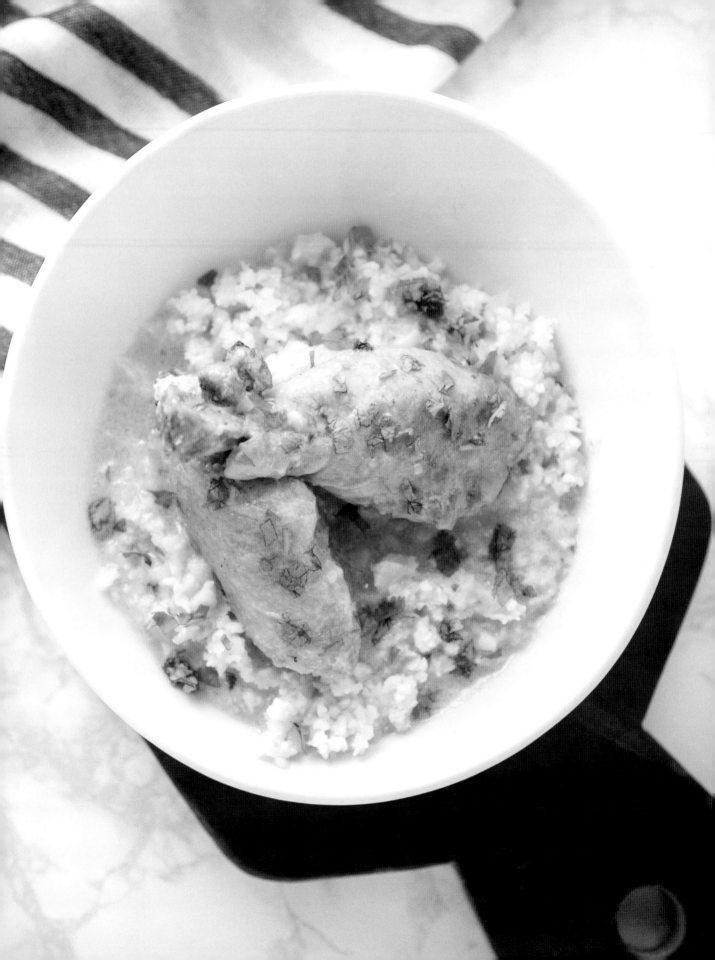

dairy-free egg-free nut-free vegetarian

Green Chicken Curry

Who doesn't love a good curry? Full of flavor and relatively easy to throw together, curry is my favorite dairy-free comfort food. I like it spicy enough to make my nose run, but this version is a tad milder. If you like it spicy, too, add a few slices of fresh habanero pepper like I do and have at it! Serve it over cauliflower rice, if desired.

Yield: **4 servings** • Prep Time: **5 minutes** • Cook Time: **12 minutes**

3 tablespoons green curry paste

1 tablespoon coconut oil

1 (14-ounce) can full-fat unsweetened coconut milk

3 tablespoons granulated erythritol

2 tablespoons fish sauce (no sugar added)

2 cups broccoli florets

1 pound boneless, skinless chicken breasts, cut into thin strips

½ cup sliced yellow bell peppers

½ cup sliced bamboo shoots, drained

1 tablespoon sliced chili peppers

Fresh cilantro leaves, for garnish

1 Combine the curry paste and coconut oil in a large skillet and cook over medium heat for 2 minutes, or until fragrant.

2 Whisk in the coconut milk, sweetener, and fish sauce until smooth. Add the broccoli and simmer over medium-low heat for 5 minutes, being careful not to allow the mixture to boil.

3 Add the chicken, bell peppers, bamboo shoots, and chili peppers. Simmer, stirring occasionally, for another 5 minutes, or until the chicken is cooked through and the broccoli is fork-tender. Garnish with cilantro and serve hot.

Calories: 301 | Fat: 20g | Protein: 29g | Carbs: 8g | Fiber: 4g | Erythritol: 7g | **Net Carbs: 4g**

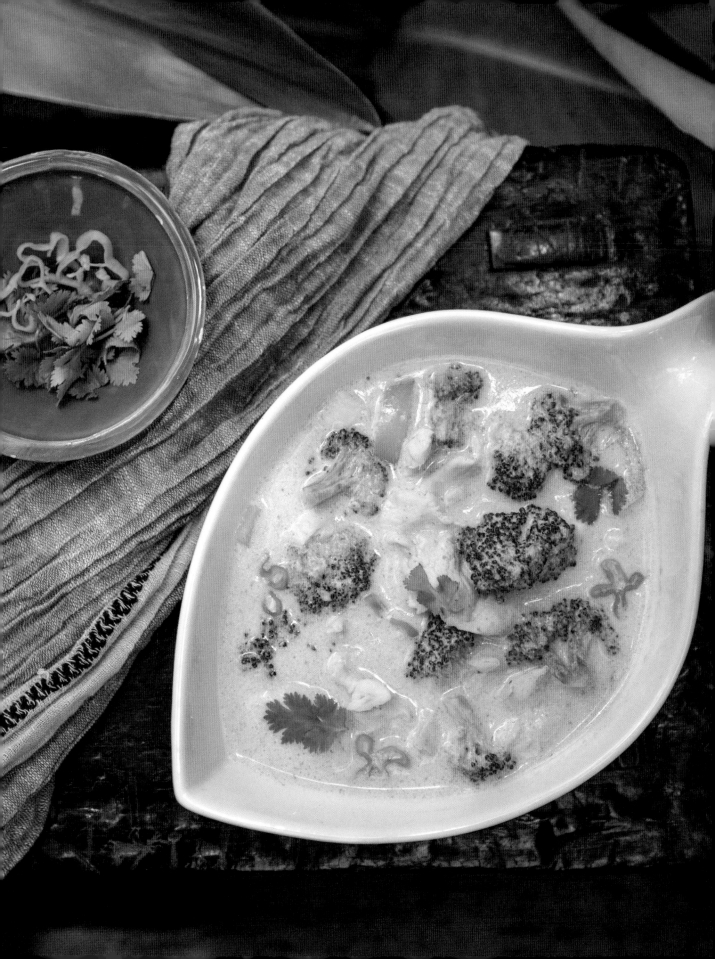

Chicken Cacciatore

My mom made chicken cacciatore for us often when we were kids—mostly because it was economical and there were a lot of us to feed. Her version included potatoes and carrots to stretch it out, but I've gone with a more classic style here that fits keto better. The flavors are familiar and comforting, making this a perfect dish for family meals.

Yield: **8 servings** ◆ Prep Time: **10 minutes** ◆ Cook Time: **45 minutes**

8 bone-in, skin-on chicken thighs

1 teaspoon kosher salt

½ teaspoon ground black pepper

2 tablespoons extra-virgin olive oil

1 cup sliced red bell peppers

1 cup sliced yellow bell peppers

½ cup sliced yellow onions

1 tablespoon minced garlic

½ cup dry white wine

1 (28-ounce) can diced tomatoes

¾ cup chicken broth, store-bought or homemade (page 82)

1 tablespoon capers, drained

1 teaspoon dried oregano leaves

2 tablespoons chopped fresh basil, for garnish

2 tablespoons chopped fresh parsley, for garnish

1 Season the chicken with the salt and pepper. Heat the olive oil in a large sauté pan over medium heat for 2 minutes. Brown the chicken on all sides, about 3 minutes per side. Remove the chicken from the pan and set aside.

2 Place the bell peppers, onions, and garlic in the same pan and cook until the peppers and onions begin to soften, about 5 minutes.

3 Add the wine and cook until reduced by half, about 2 minutes. Add the tomatoes, broth, capers, oregano, and chicken thighs to the pan. Simmer, uncovered, until the chicken is cooked through, about 30 minutes.

4 Remove the chicken to a platter. Increase the heat to high and cook the sauce for about 3 minutes, stirring constantly, until it has reduced and thickened slightly. Taste and season with more salt and pepper, if desired.

5 Pour the sauce over the chicken and garnish with the basil and parsley. Serve immediately.

Family-Friendly Tip:
This dish can be served over regular pasta for your nonketo family members. To keep it keto for you, serve it over zoodles or cauliflower rice.

Calories: 430 | Fat: 26g | Protein: 37g | Carbs: 5.5g | Fiber: 1.5g | **Net Carbs: 4g**

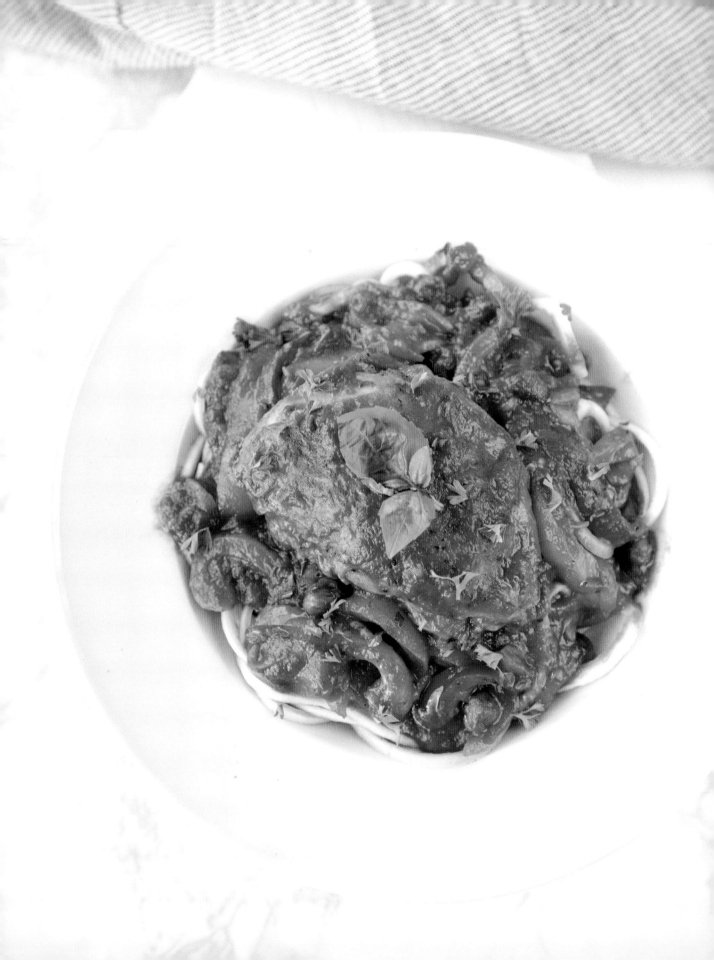

Cheesy Broccoli-Stuffed Chicken

dairy-free *egg-free* *nut-free* *vegetarian*

What better way to get your picky kids to eat broccoli than to smother it in cheese and hide it inside chicken? Even if they're on to you, it will take only one bite to convince them that broccoli *can* be delicious after all!

Yield: **4 servings** ◆ Prep Time: **15 minutes** ◆ Cook Time: **25 minutes**

For the filling:

2 cups chopped cooked broccoli

½ cup mascarpone cheese (4 ounces)

3 tablespoons grated Parmesan cheese

½ teaspoon kosher salt

¼ teaspoon ground black pepper

⅛ teaspoon garlic powder

⅛ teaspoon ground nutmeg

4 (6-ounce) chicken cutlets, pounded to ½-inch thickness

½ cup Keto Breadcrumbs (page 74)

2 tablespoons grated Parmesan cheese

1 teaspoon dried parsley leaves

½ teaspoon kosher salt

¼ teaspoon ground black pepper

⅛ teaspoon garlic powder

1 large egg, beaten

1 Preheat the oven to 375°F. Line a 15 by 10-inch sheet pan with parchment paper.

2 Make the filling: Put the cooked broccoli, mascarpone, Parmesan cheese, salt, pepper, garlic powder, and nutmeg in a medium-sized bowl and mix well.

3 Lay the chicken cutlets on a cutting board and spoon about ½ cup of the filling onto the center of each cutlet. Roll the chicken up around the filling and secure each cutlet with a toothpick.

4 Place the breadcrumbs, Parmesan cheese, parsley, salt, pepper, and garlic powder in a small bowl and mix well. Dip the stuffed cutlets into the beaten egg, then into the seasoned breadcrumbs. Place the breaded cutlets on the lined sheet pan and sprinkle any remaining breadcrumbs over the top of the chicken.

5 Bake for 25 minutes, or until the center of the cutlets reads 165°F on a meat thermometer. Serve immediately.

Calories: 488 | Fat: 25g | Protein: 50g | Carbs: 4g | Fiber: 2g | **Net Carbs: 2g**

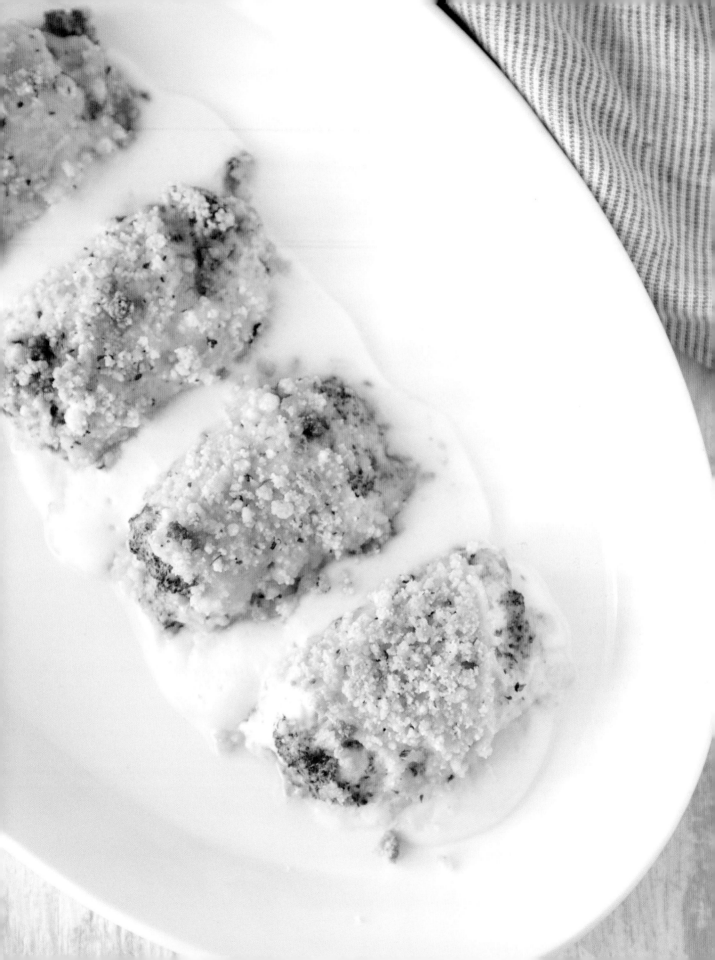

dairy-free egg-free nut-free vegetarian

Chicken Larb

If you've never heard of larb, it's a meat-based salad from Laos that is also popular in Thailand. It's easy to make and incredibly tasty and fragrant. Don't let the unfamiliar name intimidate you; if you can brown meat in a pan and chop some herbs, then you've got this! I promise that once you taste it, you'll be putting it in your regular rotation.

Yield: **4 servings** • Prep Time: **10 minutes** • Cook Time: **8 minutes**

1 tablespoon coconut oil

1 pound ground chicken

½ cup thinly sliced red onions, plus more for garnish if desired

1 tablespoon peeled and minced fresh ginger

1 teaspoon minced garlic

½ teaspoon red pepper flakes

1 tablespoon fish sauce (no sugar added)

1 tablespoon wheat-free soy sauce

1 teaspoon Sriracha sauce, plus more for serving if desired

1 tablespoon lime juice

For serving/garnish:

Leaves from 1 large head or 2 small heads butter and/or leaf lettuce

2 cups Basic Cauliflower Rice (page 250), hot

2 tablespoons chopped fresh basil

2 tablespoons chopped fresh cilantro

2 tablespoons chopped fresh mint

Lime wedges, for serving (optional)

1   Heat the coconut oil in a large sauté pan. Add the chicken, onions, ginger, garlic, and red pepper flakes and cook, stirring occasionally, for 5 minutes, or until fragrant.

2   Add the fish sauce, soy sauce, and Sriracha and cook for 3 more minutes, or until most of the liquid has been absorbed.

3   Remove from the heat and stir in the lime juice. Serve the chicken mixture over the lettuce leaves and cauliflower rice and garnish with the fresh herbs. If desired, top with a few extra slices of onion and serve with lime wedges and Sriracha on the side.

Calories: 200 | Fat: 8g | Protein: 26g | Carbs: 6g | Fiber: 1g | **Net Carbs: 5g**

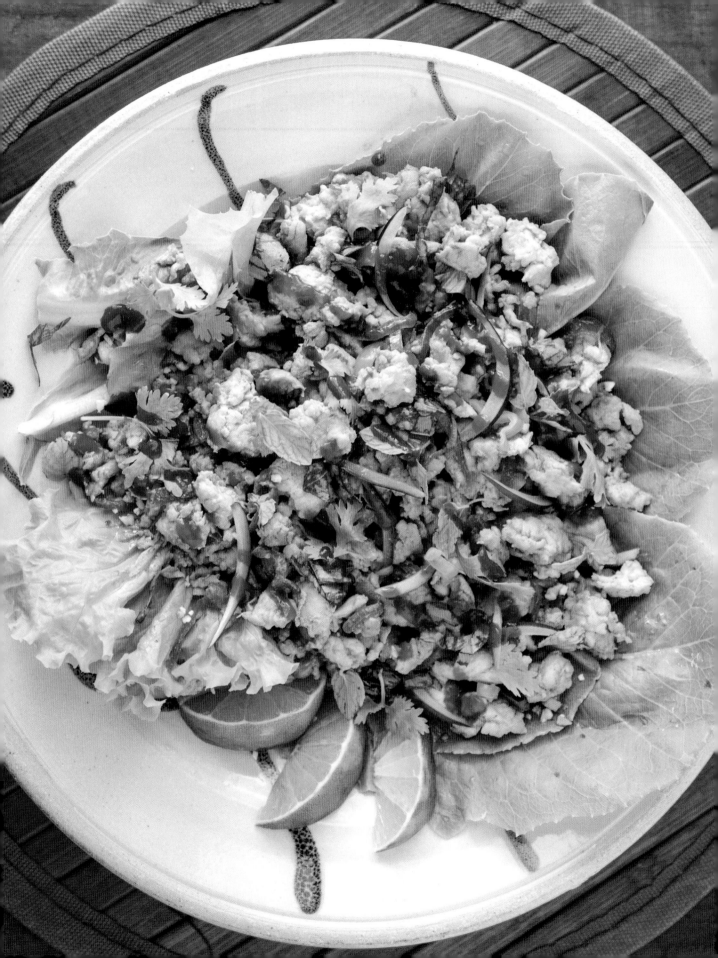

dairy-free · egg-free · nut-free · vegetarian

Tandoori Chicken Meatballs

I've got more than fifty meatball recipes on my blog and a long list of ideas for more in my notes. I'd been kicking this concept around in my head for a while, and when I finally made it, I liked it so much that I decided to add it to this book. Mr. Hungry thinks it's one of my best yet—and he's tried them all, so I believe him! Shown served with Cucumber Raita (page 98).

Yield: 12 meatballs ◆ Serving Size: **3 meatballs** ◆ Prep Time: **10 minutes, plus 1 hour to chill**

Cook Time: **10 minutes**

1 pound ground chicken

2 tablespoons full-fat Greek yogurt

2 tablespoons minced red onions

2 teaspoons lemon juice

1 teaspoon kosher salt

1 teaspoon peeled and minced fresh ginger

1 teaspoon minced garlic

1 teaspoon paprika

½ teaspoon cayenne pepper

½ teaspoon garam masala

½ teaspoon ground cumin

½ teaspoon turmeric powder

1 large egg, beaten

½ cup superfine blanched almond flour

2 tablespoons avocado oil or other light-tasting oil, for the pan

1. Place all of the ingredients, except for the oil, in a medium-sized bowl and mix well. Chill for at least 1 hour or up to 24 hours to allow the flavors to come together.

2. Use your hands to form the chicken mixture into 12 meatballs, each about 2 inches in diameter.

3. Heat the oil in a large sauté pan over medium heat. Place the meatballs in the pan and cook for about 4 minutes per side, until golden brown and cooked through.

4. Meanwhile, turn on the oven to broil-high.

5. Transfer the meatballs to a sheet pan and broil in the oven for 2 to 3 minutes, until slightly charred on the outside.

Calories: 355 | Fat: 27g | Protein: 24g | Carbs: 5g | Fiber: 2g | **Net Carbs: 3g**

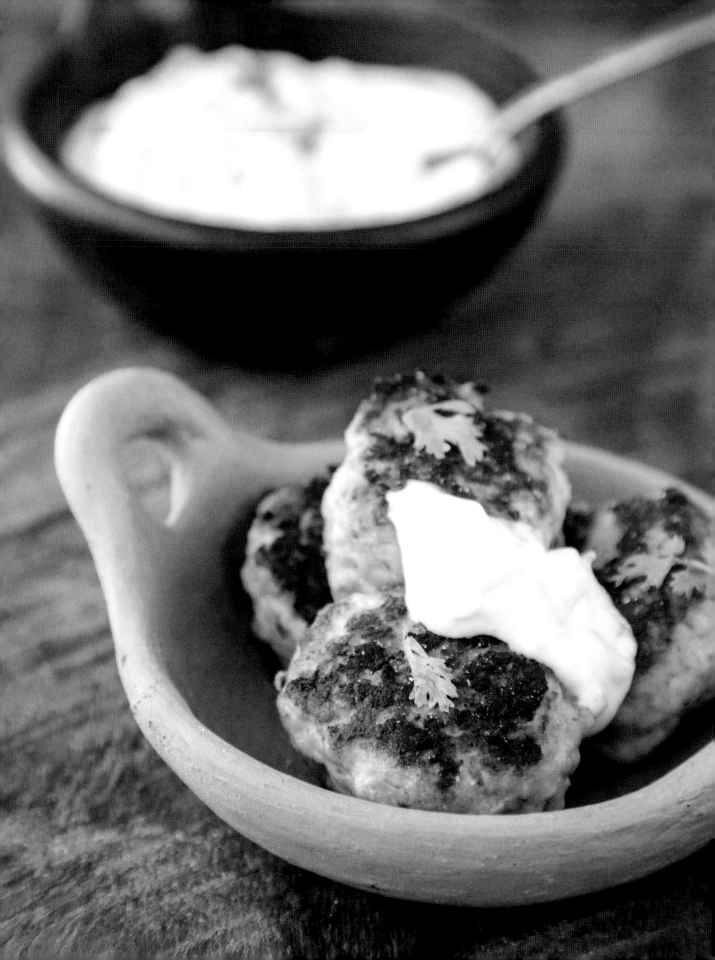

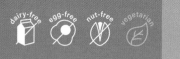

Jerk Chicken

A couple of hundred yards from where we lived in Belize, there is a tiny BBQ shack called Robin's Kitchen, where we'd get jerk chicken on the regular. Robin and his wife, Dulcie, are from Jamaica, and they are legit—which is why their jerk chicken always sells out early. This keto version is as close as I can get to replicating the flavor of theirs; to get the real thing, you'll have to visit them in Belize!

Yield: **6 servings** • Prep Time: **2 minutes** • Cook Time: **30 minutes**

6 whole chicken legs (drumsticks and thighs)

2 tablespoons Jerk Seasoning (page 79)

1½ teaspoons kosher salt

½ cup Easy Keto BBQ Sauce (page 104)

1 Preheat a grill to medium heat.

2 Coat the chicken legs liberally with the jerk seasoning and salt. Grill the chicken for 20 minutes, turning occasionally.

3 Brush the BBQ sauce on the chicken and grill for 5 more minutes per side, or until a meat thermometer inserted in the thickest part of a thigh reads 165°F.

> **Alternative Method:**
> *If you don't feel like firing up the grill, you can bake the seasoned chicken legs at 400°F for 30 minutes. Then baste the chicken with the BBQ sauce and bake for another 10 minutes, or until a meat thermometer inserted in the thickest part of a thigh reads 165°F.*

Calories: 350 | Fat: 20g | Protein: 38g | Carbs: 3g | Fiber: 0.5g | **Net Carbs: 2.5g**

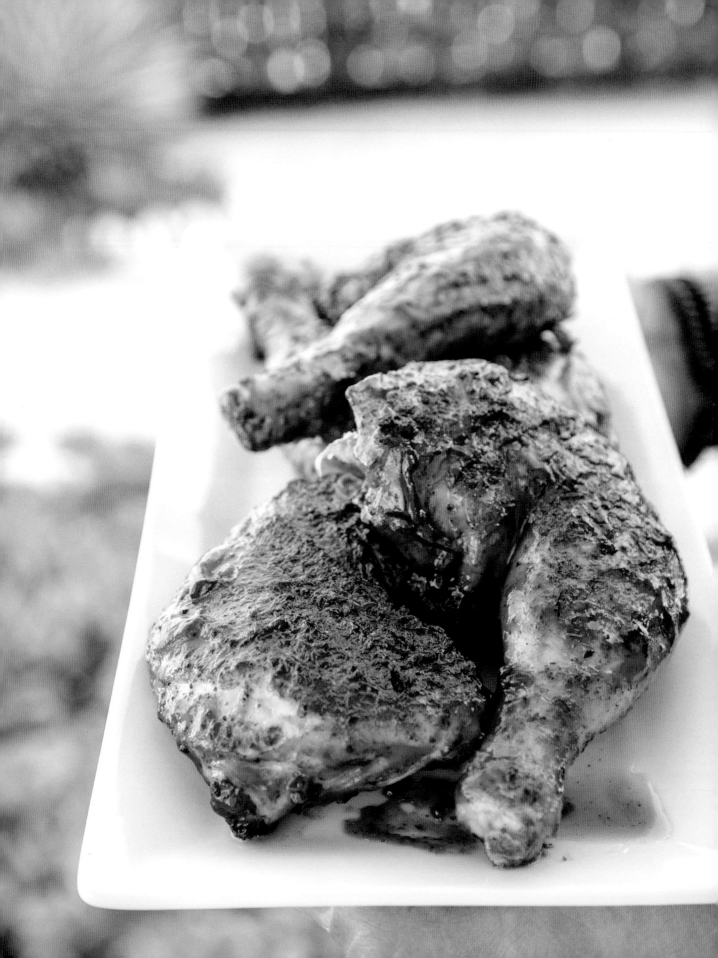

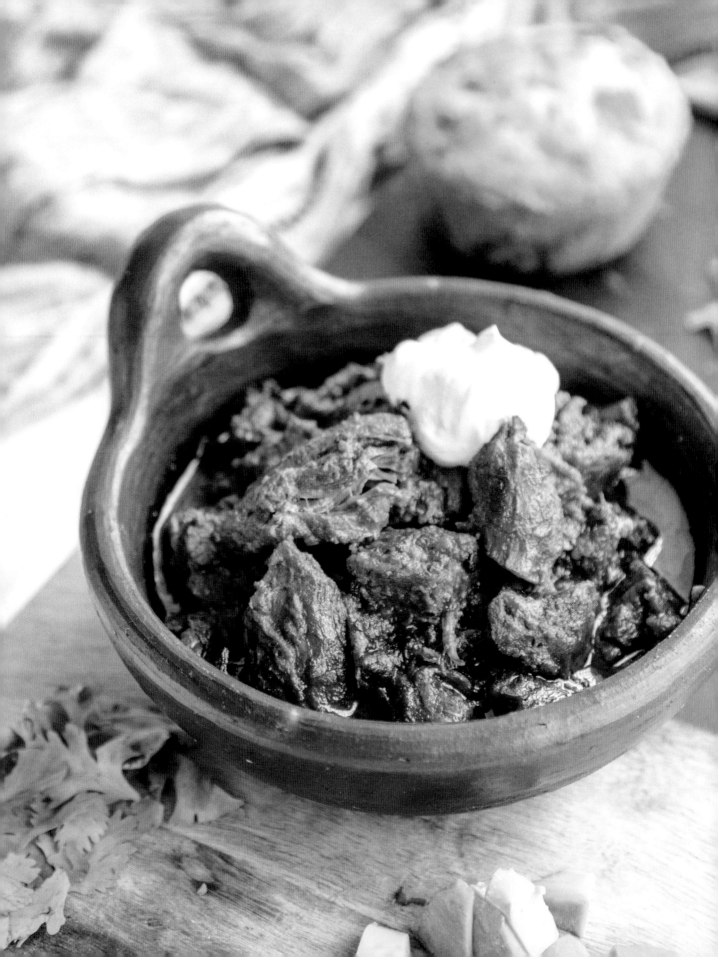

beef

Caprese Burgers / 176

Marinated Skirt Steak / 178

Easy No-Chop Chili / 180

Chili con Carne / 182

Chicken-Fried Steak with Sour Cream Gravy / 184

Pepperoni Pizza Meatloaf / 186

Beef Burrito Bowl / 188

Korean BBQ Beef Wraps / 190

Meatballs alla Parmigiana / 192

Cheesy Beef Stroganoff Casserole / 194

Coffee-Rubbed Rib-Eyes with Balsamic Butter / 196

Caprese Burgers

Who needs a bun when so many flavors and textures are packed into this delicious burger?! This is an easy recipe to customize according to individual preferences. And if your family wants to have their burgers on buns, no extra cooking from you is required!

Yield: **4 burgers** • Serving Size: **1 burger** • Prep Time: **8 minutes** • Cook Time: **8 minutes**

For the burger patties:

1 pound ground beef (80/20)

½ teaspoon kosher salt

½ teaspoon ground black pepper

¼ teaspoon garlic powder

8 red or green lettuce leaves

¼ cup sugar-free mayonnaise

¼ cup Keto Ketchup (page 102)

4 ounces fresh mozzarella, cut into 4 slices

4 slices ripe tomato

¼ cup fresh basil leaves

4 teaspoons sugar-free balsamic glaze (optional; see note)

1 Place the beef, salt, pepper, and garlic powder in a medium-sized bowl and mix well with your hands. Form into 4 burger patties of equal size, about 1½ inches thick.

2 Place the burger patties in a medium-sized nonstick skillet over medium-high heat. Cook for about 4 minutes per side for medium-done burgers. Remove the burgers from the skillet and place on a paper towel–lined plate.

3 To assemble: Place 2 lettuce leaves on another plate and top with 1 tablespoon of mayonnaise and 1 tablespoon of ketchup. Place a burger patty on top of the lettuce, then top with a slice of mozzarella, a slice of tomato, a few basil leaves, and 1 teaspoon of balsamic glaze, if using. Repeat for the rest of the burgers and serve immediately.

Note:

The balsamic glaze adds a few grams of carbs but also brings a lot of flavor, so you decide if it's worth it. You can make your own by reducing balsamic vinegar in a saucepan until thick, or you can purchase it in the condiment aisle of most grocery stores. Try to purchase a brand with no sugar added and use sparingly.

Calories: 420 | Fat: 32g | Protein: 27g | Carbs: 6g | Fiber: 1g | **Net Carbs: 5g**

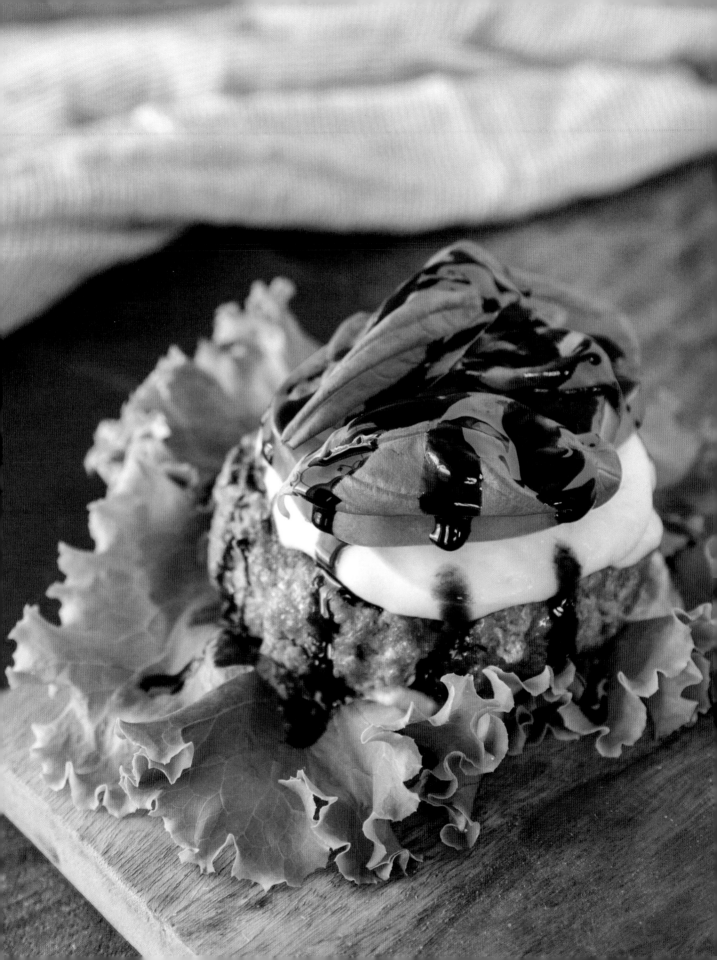

Marinated Skirt Steak

dairy-free egg-free nut-free vegetarian

A properly prepared skirt steak is a thing of beauty, and this tasty marinade ensures that the meat will be tender and flavorful every time! Grilling is recommended for the best flavor, but in a pinch you can pan-sear the steak in a hot cast-iron pan.

Yield: **6 servings** ◆ Serving Size: **4 ounces steak and 1 tablespoon of sauce**

Prep Time: **2 minutes, plus 2 hours to marinate** ◆ Cook Time: **6 minutes**

¼ cup balsamic vinegar (no sugar added)

2 tablespoons extra-virgin olive oil

1 tablespoon fresh chopped parsley

1 teaspoon minced garlic

1 teaspoon kosher salt

¼ teaspoon ground black pepper

2 pounds skirt steak, trimmed of fat

1   In a medium-sized bowl, whisk together the vinegar, olive oil, parsley, garlic, salt, and pepper. Add the skirt steak and flip to ensure that the entire surface is covered in marinade. Cover with plastic wrap and marinate in the refrigerator for at least 2 hours, or up to 24 hours.

2   Take the bowl out of the refrigerator and let the steak and marinade come to room temperature. Meanwhile, preheat a grill to high heat.

3   Remove the steak from the marinade (reserve the marinade) and place on the grill over direct high heat. Grill for 3 minutes per side for medium (recommended) or 5 minutes per side for well-done.

4   Remove the steak from the grill when the desired doneness is reached and let rest for 10 minutes before slicing. Meanwhile, place the reserved marinade in the microwave and cook on high for 3 minutes, or until boiling. Stir and set aside; you will use the boiled marinade as a sauce for the steak.

5   Slice the steak, being sure to cut against the grain for best results. Serve with the sauce.

> **Serving Suggestion:**
> *Serve with Cheesy Cauliflower Puree (page 272) and Sautéed Mushrooms (page 281).*

Calories: 354 | Fat: 25g | Protein: 31g | Carbs: 0g | Fiber: 0g | **Net Carbs: 0g**

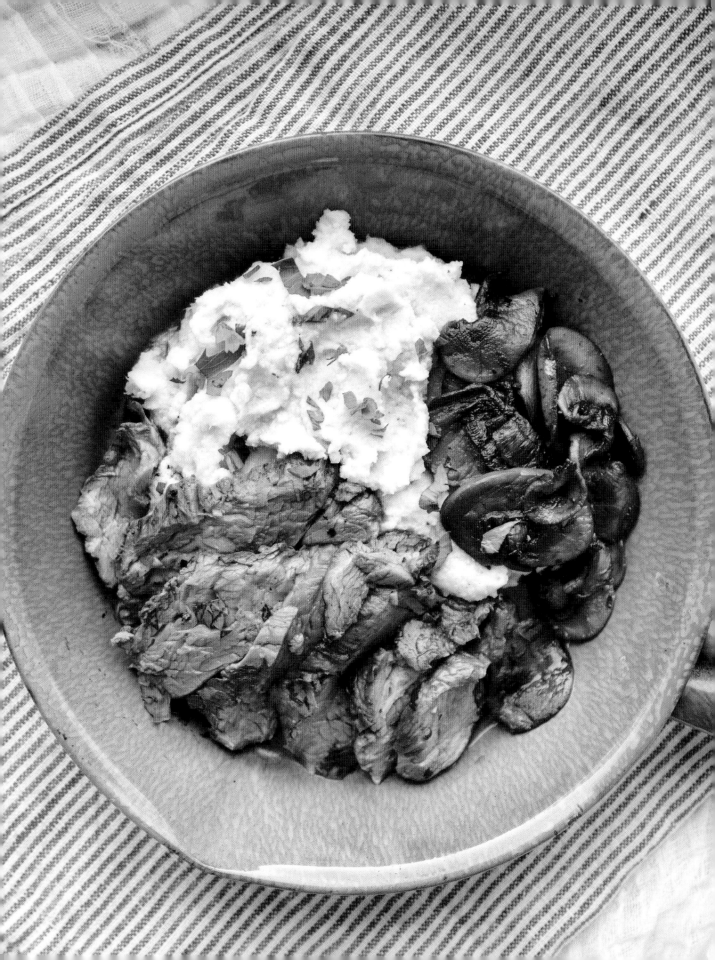

Easy No-Chop Chili

This easy, tasty, family-friendly chili can be whipped up in about ten minutes, making it a perfect weeknight meal. And since it is on the drier side, it has all sorts of uses: you can serve it with tortilla chips for the rest of the family and enjoy it in a lettuce-lined bowl for yourself, taco salad style, or you can use it to make burrito bowls (see page 188) or as an inspiration for a Mexican-themed casserole. If you prefer, you can easily convert it to a souplike chili for a cold winter day (see the variation below).

Yield: **4 servings** • Serving Size: **⅔ cup** • Prep Time: **5 minutes** • Cook Time: **8 minutes**

1 pound ground beef (80/20)

1 teaspoon kosher salt

1 teaspoon ground coriander

1 teaspoon ground cumin

½ teaspoon cayenne pepper

½ teaspoon garlic powder

½ teaspoon onion powder

¼ teaspoon ground black pepper

½ cup Restaurant-Style Salsa (page 292)

For serving (optional):

Lettuce leaves

Diced fresh tomatoes

Sliced avocados

Shredded cheese

Full-fat sour cream

Chopped fresh cilantro

1 Place the ground beef, salt, coriander, cumin, cayenne, garlic powder, onion powder, and pepper in a medium-sized saucepan. Cook over medium heat, stirring occasionally, for about 5 minutes, until the beef is cooked through and crumbly.

2 Add the salsa and stir, then simmer for 5 more minutes, or until the liquid is reduced by half. Serve hot.

3 To serve this as a keto taco salad, as shown in the photograph, line 4 serving bowls with lettuce leaves, top the lettuce with the hot chili, then garnish with diced tomatoes, avocado slices, shredded cheese, sour cream, fresh cilantro, or your other favorite keto-friendly chili toppings!

Variation:
Easy No-Chop Chili Soup. To make this recipe into a chili you can enjoy as a soup, simply add 1 cup of beef broth, store-bought or homemade (page 82), along with the salsa in Step 2 and simmer just long enough to heat through and give you the consistency you are looking for. The Bacon & Cheddar Cornless Muffins on page 302 are the perfect side to make this a hearty and comforting meal the entire family will love!

Calories: 230 | Fat: 9g | Protein: 33g | Carbs: 3g | Fiber: 0.5g | **Net Carbs: 2.5g**

Make It Easy:
This chili freezes well and can be reheated in the microwave, so to keep life easy, you can make a double or triple batch and freeze it in 1-cup portions for whenever you need a quick keto meal in minutes!

dairy-free egg-free nut-free vegetarian

Chili con Carne

This hearty chili boasts tender chunks of beef in a rich, smoky sauce that's loaded with earthy spices like cumin and coriander. You can customize the spice level according to the preference of your tribe by using more or less of the canned chipotles or adding some chopped habanero if you like it super spicy. Great for stormy days or hanging out with friends, this chili is always a crowd-pleaser, and nobody will ever guess that it's "diet food."

Yield: **6 servings** ◆ Serving Size: **1½ cups** ◆ Prep Time: **8 minutes** ◆ Cook Time: **2 hours 15 minutes**

2 pounds boneless beef chuck, trimmed and cut into 1-inch cubes

1 teaspoon kosher salt

½ teaspoon ground black pepper

2 tablespoons avocado oil or other light-tasting oil

½ cup chopped yellow onions

1 tablespoon minced garlic

3 cups beef broth, store-bought or homemade (page 82)

1 tablespoon chili powder

2 teaspoons ground cumin

1 teaspoon cayenne pepper

1 teaspoon dried oregano leaves

1 teaspoon ground coriander

¼ teaspoon ground cinnamon

¼ cup canned chipotles in adobo sauce

1 tablespoon apple cider vinegar

1 tablespoon coconut flour

1 Season the beef with the salt and pepper. Heat the oil in a large heavy-bottomed saucepan (make sure it has a lid) or a 4- or 6-quart Dutch oven over medium-high heat.

2 Add the beef and brown on all sides, about 4 minutes. Remove the meat and set aside.

3 Add the onions and garlic to the pan and cook for 5 minutes, or until browned and translucent. Add the meat back to the pan along with the broth, spices, and chipotles. Simmer, covered, until the meat is tender, about 2 hours.

4 Stir in the vinegar. Remove about ¼ cup of the sauce to a small bowl. Whisk the coconut flour into the bowl of sauce, then add the sauce back to the pot and stir well. Simmer, uncovered, for 5 more minutes, until the sauce has thickened. Taste and season with more salt and pepper, if desired.

Serving Suggestion:

Garnish with your choice of fresh cilantro, sliced or cubed avocado, shredded cheddar cheese, chopped onions, and/or sour cream. Shown with Bacon & Cheddar Cornless Muffins (page 302).

Calories: 363 | Fat: 27g | Protein: 29g | Carbs: 3.5g | Fiber: 1.5g | **Net Carbs: 2g**

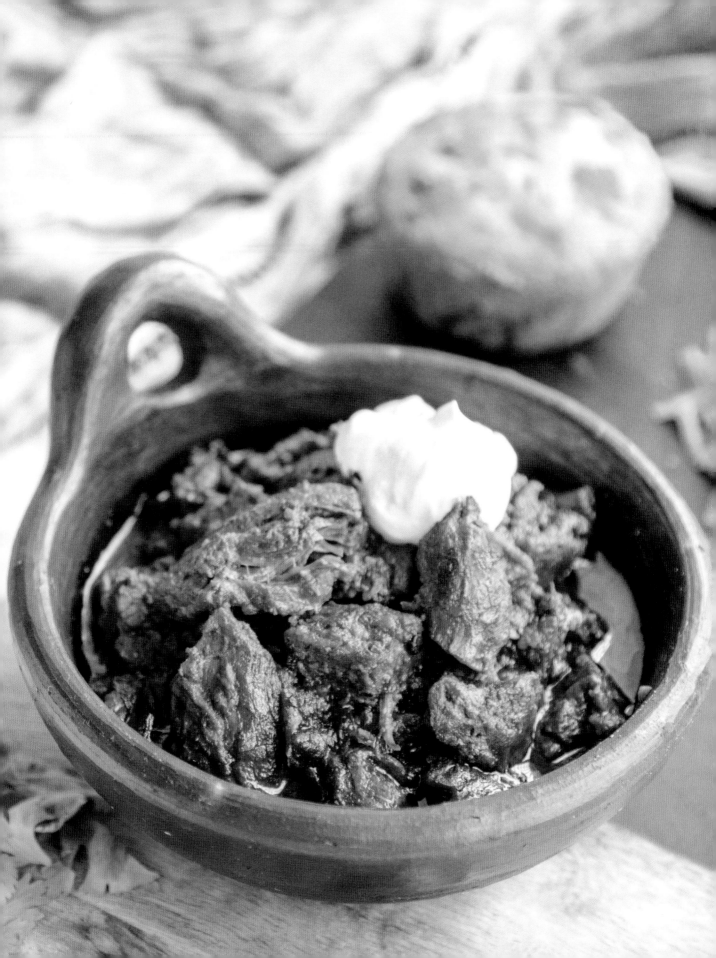

Chicken-Fried Steak with Sour Cream Gravy

dairy-free egg-free nut-free vegetarian

Talk about comfort food! What's not to love about crispy fried steak smothered in rich, creamy gravy? This is one of those quick and easy meals that the entire family will love. Serve it over cauliflower puree to soak up all that luscious gravy. If your family hasn't been won over to cauliflower yet, you can easily serve their steaks with regular mashed potatoes instead.

Yield: 4 steaks • Serving Size: **1 steak and 2 tablespoons gravy** • Prep Time: **5 minutes**

Cook Time: **8 minutes**

4 (6-ounce) cube steaks (see tip)

¼ teaspoon kosher salt

¼ teaspoon ground black pepper

1 large egg, beaten

1 batch Basic Breading (page 75)

2 tablespoons butter

2 tablespoons avocado oil or other light-tasting oil

⅓ cup full-fat sour cream

1 Season the steaks with the salt and pepper. Dip the steaks in the beaten egg and then in the breading, turning to coat the meat on both sides.

2 Heat the butter and oil in a large nonstick sauté pan over medium-high heat until bubbling, about 2 minutes. Add the steaks and cook for about 2 minutes per side, until golden brown. Remove the steaks from the pan and set aside.

3 Whisk the sour cream into the pan juices and cook for 2 minutes, until golden and slightly thickened. Serve the warm gravy over the steaks.

Pro Tip:
Cube steaks are simply thinly cut sirloin steaks that have been tenderized mechanically or with a meat mallet. If you can't find them, you can use any lean cut of beef sliced ½ inch thick and pounded with a meat mallet to tenderize it.

Calories: 517 | Fat: 35g | Protein: 45g | Carbs: 4.5g | Fiber: 1.5g | **Net Carbs: 3g**

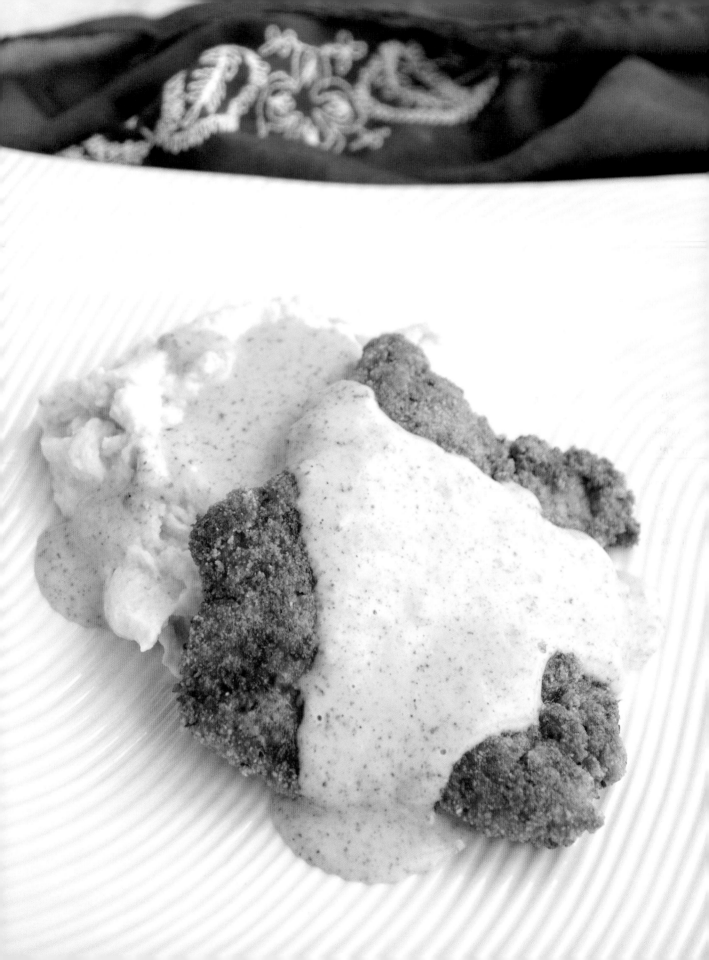

dairy-free egg-free nut-free vegetarian

Pepperoni Pizza Meatloaf

Meatloaf plus pizza equals winning, if you ask me! This is one of those recipes that nobody will guess is keto, and they won't notice that you used almond flour instead of breadcrumbs in the mix. That being said, if someone in your group has a nut allergy, you can replace the almond flour with crushed pork rinds and get a similar result.

Yield: **8 servings** ◆ Prep Time: **10 minutes** ◆ Cook Time: **1 hour**

2 pounds ground beef (80/20)

⅓ cup superfine blanched almond flour

¼ cup grated Parmesan cheese

1 tablespoon dried parsley

1 tablespoon dried onion flakes

1 teaspoon kosher salt

½ teaspoon dried oregano leaves

½ teaspoon garlic powder

½ teaspoon ground black pepper

2 large eggs

1 cup marinara sauce, store-bought or homemade (page 106), plus more for serving if desired

2 cups shredded whole-milk mozzarella cheese

4 ounces thinly sliced pepperoni

Chopped fresh parsley, for garnish (optional)

1 Preheat the oven to 375°F. Line a 9 by 5-inch loaf pan with foil, leaving 2 inches of foil folded over the outside edges of the pan. The extra foil will make it easier to lift the cooked meatloaf out of the pan.

2 Place the ground beef, almond flour, Parmesan cheese, parsley, onion flakes, salt, oregano, garlic powder, pepper, and eggs in a large bowl and mix well by hand until the texture is uniform.

3 Press the meatloaf mixture into the prepared loaf pan and flatten it out. Spoon the marinara evenly over the top and then sprinkle with the mozzarella cheese. Layer the pepperoni slices on top. Bake, uncovered, for 1 hour, or until a meat thermometer inserted in the center reads 160°F.

4 Remove the meatloaf from the oven and let cool for at least 10 minutes in the pan to allow it to firm up before slicing.

5 Carefully remove the meatloaf from the pan using the foil as handles. Place on a cutting board and remove the foil. You can then cut it into slices and serve on individual plates, or, to dress it up a bit, spread some warm marinara sauce on the bottom of a serving platter, then place the loaf on top of the sauce and garnish with fresh parsley, as shown.

Family-Friendly Tip:
This is a fun recipe to get the kids involved in. They can put the mozzarella cheese and pepperoni slices on before cooking. To make it even more kid approved, you can make eight mini meatloaves or even bake them as meatloaf cupcakes. Serve with pasta for nonketo family members and Basic Zucchini Noodles (page 252) or Cheesy Cauliflower Puree (page 272) for you.

Calories: 439 | Fat: 31g | Protein: 33g | Carbs: 3.5g | Fiber: 1g | **Net Carbs: 2.5g**

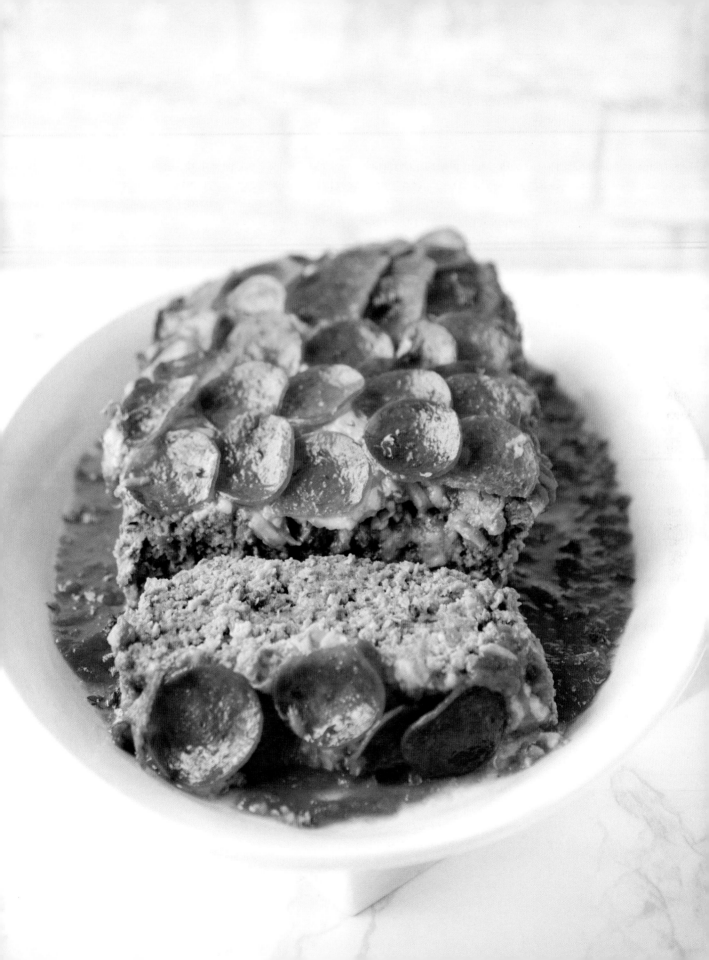

Beef Burrito Bowl

dairy-free · egg-free · nut-free · vegetarian

More a method than a recipe, this burrito bowl can be customized in a variety of ways. If you're feeding a crowd, just lay out the fixings and let everyone build their own bowl! You can provide real rice and tortilla chips for the nonketo peeps, if desired. The burrito bowl comes together almost instantly if you have the components made already, but if not, allow up to half an hour to make the cauliflower rice, chili, guacamole, and salsa.

Yield: **1 serving** ◆ Prep Time: **5 minutes**

½ cup Basic Cauliflower Rice (page 250), hot

⅔ cup Easy No-Chop Chili (page 180), hot

½ cup shredded romaine lettuce

¼ cup shredded cheddar cheese

¼ cup Easy Keto Guacamole (page 293)

¼ cup Restaurant-Style Salsa (page 292)

¼ cup full-fat sour cream

1 tablespoon chopped fresh cilantro, for garnish (optional)

Arrange all of the ingredients in a serving bowl as shown, or place the cauliflower rice in the bowl first, then top the cauliflower rice with the remaining ingredients. Garnish with the cilantro, if desired. Serve immediately.

Calories: 441 | Fat: 26g | Protein: 43g | Carbs: 10g | Fiber: 3g | **Net Carbs: 7g**

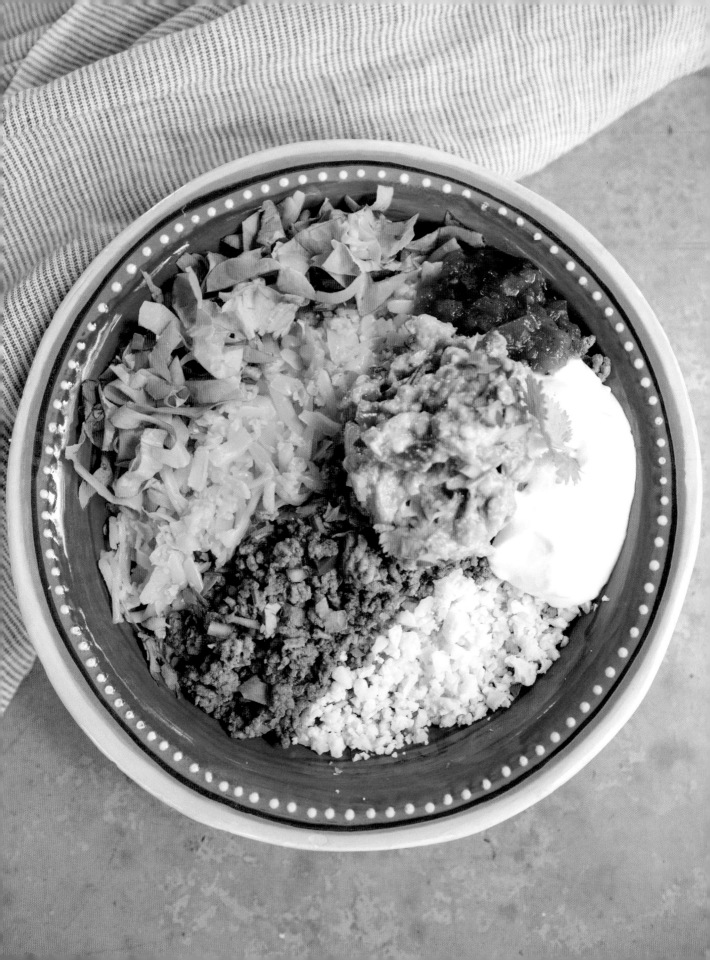

dairy-free egg-free nut-free vegetarian

Korean BBQ Beef Wraps

Loosely based on the bulgogi that we love to order from a Korean restaurant in New York City, this version is easy to make at home because it's cooked in a skillet rather than grilled. To keep it keto-friendly, I have replaced the traditional sticky rice with cauliflower rice and the copious amounts of sugar with erythritol—I promise you won't miss the carbs!

Yield: **4 servings** • Prep Time: **8 minutes, plus 2 hours to marinate** • Cook Time: **8 minutes**

For the BBQ beef:

1 pound boneless beef sirloin, thinly sliced

¼ cup chopped scallions

2 tablespoons granulated erythritol

2 tablespoons peeled and minced fresh ginger

1 tablespoon minced garlic

2 teaspoons cayenne pepper

¼ cup filtered water

¼ cup wheat-free soy sauce

1 tablespoon toasted sesame oil

For serving:

8 large red or green lettuce leaves

1 cup Basic Cauliflower Rice (page 250)

For garnish (optional):

Sliced scallions

Thinly sliced red chili peppers

1 Place the beef, scallions, sweetener, ginger, garlic, cayenne pepper, water, soy sauce, and sesame oil in a medium-sized bowl and stir well to coat. Cover and place in the refrigerator to marinate for 2 hours or overnight.

2 Heat a large skillet over medium-high heat. Add the beef (reserve the marinade) to the skillet and cook for about 3 minutes, or until just cooked through. Remove the meat from the pan and set aside.

3 Return the skillet to the stove and pour the marinade into it. Bring to a boil and simmer for 2 minutes; if you want to thin out the sauce, add 1 or 2 tablespoons of filtered water.

4 Add the cooked meat back to the sauce and stir to coat. To serve each portion, place 2 lettuce leaves on a plate, then add ¼ cup of the cauliflower rice and one-quarter of the BBQ beef. Top with sliced scallions and chili peppers, if desired. Repeat for the remaining servings.

Pro Tip:
Kimchee, a traditional Korean condiment of spicy fermented cabbage that is usually served with bulgogi, would be a great addition to this if you can get it, with the added bonus that it's good for your gut!

Calories: 287 | Fat: 18g | Protein: 26g | Carbs: 5g | Fiber: 1.5g | Erythritol: 6g | **Net Carbs: 3.5g**

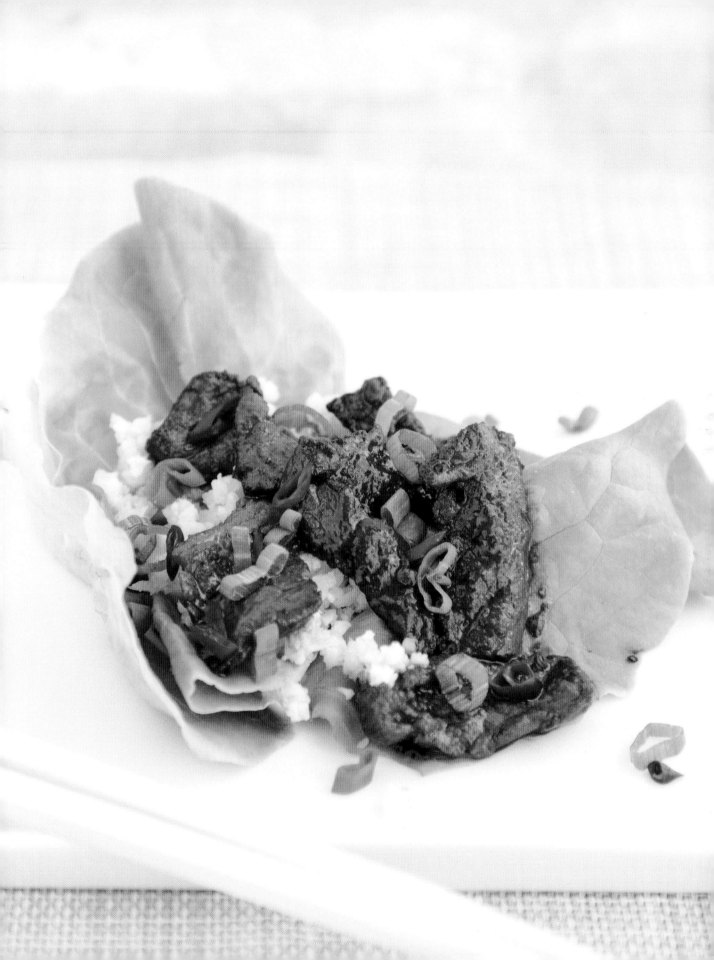

dairy-free · egg-free · nut-free · vegetarian

Meatballs alla Parmigiana

Tender meatballs smothered in marinara sauce and mozzarella cheese—need I say more? This recipe never fails to get rave reviews from even the pickiest eaters. Serve it with zoodles for you and pasta for them and you're good to go with no complaints!

Yield: **4 servings** ◆ Prep Time: **10 minutes** ◆ Cook Time: **40 minutes**

For the meatballs:

1 pound ground beef (80/20)

2 tablespoons chopped fresh parsley, plus more for garnish if desired

⅓ cup grated Parmesan cheese

¼ cup superfine blanched almond flour

1 large egg, beaten

1 teaspoon kosher salt

¼ teaspoon ground black pepper

¼ teaspoon garlic powder

¼ teaspoon onion powder

¼ teaspoon dried oregano leaves

¼ cup warm filtered water

1 cup marinara sauce, store-bought or homemade (page 106)

1 cup shredded whole-milk mozzarella cheese

1 Preheat the oven to 350°F. Line a 15 by 10-inch sheet pan with foil or parchment paper.

2 Put the ground beef, parsley, Parmesan, almond flour, egg, salt, pepper, garlic powder, onion powder, oregano, and water in a medium-sized bowl. Mix thoroughly by hand until fully combined.

3 Form the meat mixture into 12 meatballs about 2 inches in diameter and place them 2 inches apart on the sheet pan. Bake for 20 minutes.

4 Place the meatballs in a casserole dish large enough to fit all of the meatballs. Spoon the marinara evenly over the meatballs, then sprinkle the cheese over the meatballs. Bake for 20 minutes, or until the meatballs are cooked through, the sauce is bubbling, and the cheese is golden. Garnish with chopped fresh parsley, if desired.

Make It Easy:
This recipe freezes well and can be reheated in the microwave. So, to keep life simple, you can make a double or triple batch and freeze it in single servings for whenever you need to get a quick keto meal on the table!

Calories: 430 | Fat: 31g | Protein: 33g | Carbs: 5g | Fiber: 2g | **Net Carbs: 3g**

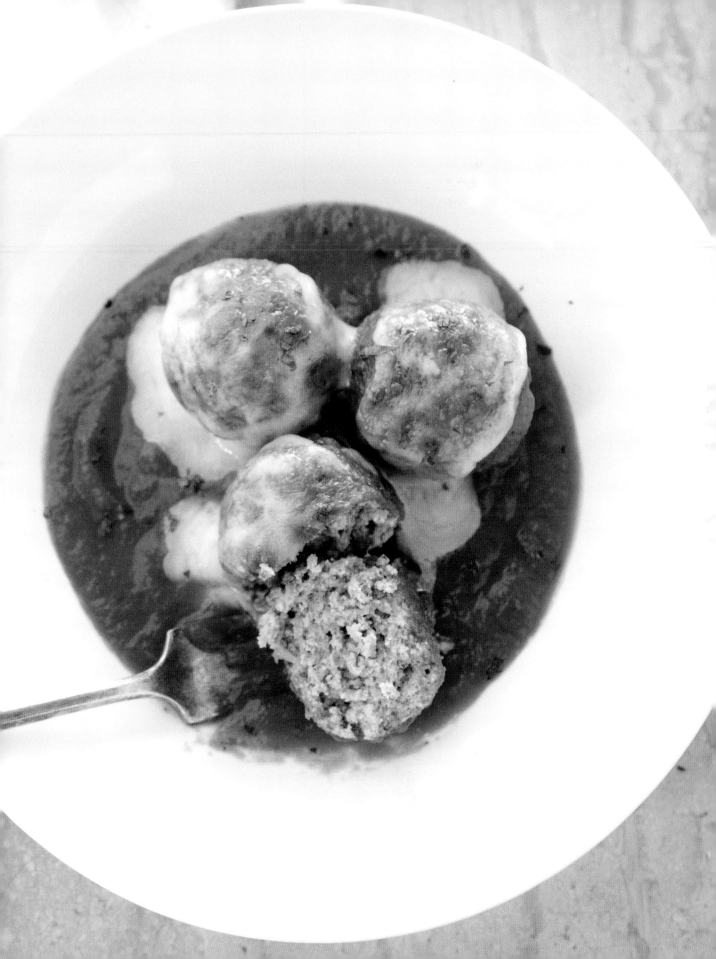

dairy-free egg-free nut-free vegetarian

Cheesy Beef Stroganoff Casserole

This hearty casserole is the ultimate winter comfort food: tender chunks of beef swimming in a creamy, flavorful sauce and topped with a thick and cheesy cauliflower mash. Sigh... dieting is so hard.

Yield: **8 servings** • Prep Time: **8 minutes** • Cook Time: **47 minutes**

2 pounds stew beef, cut into bite-sized pieces

1½ teaspoons kosher salt

½ teaspoon ground black pepper

3 tablespoons butter, divided

2 cups sliced white mushrooms

½ cup sliced yellow onions

1 tablespoon minced garlic

1 cup beef broth, store-bought or homemade (page 82)

1 teaspoon Worcestershire sauce

¾ cup full-fat sour cream

¼ teaspoon xanthan gum

½ teaspoon fresh thyme leaves

1 batch Cheesy Cauliflower Puree (page 272)

2 tablespoons chopped fresh parsley, for garnish (optional)

1   Season the beef with the salt and pepper. Melt 2 tablespoons of the butter in a large sauté pan over high heat. Add the beef and sear for 3 minutes, or until browned, stirring occasionally. Remove the beef to a bowl and set aside.

2   Lower the heat to medium. Add the mushrooms to the pan and cook until golden brown, about 5 minutes. Remove to the bowl with the beef. Add the onions, garlic, and remaining tablespoon of butter to the pan. Cook until the onions are translucent, about 4 minutes. Remove to the bowl with the beef and mushrooms.

3   Add the beef broth and Worcestershire sauce to the pan and whisk up all of the browned bits into the liquid. Whisk in the sour cream and xanthan gum and cook over medium heat until reduced and thickened, about 5 minutes.

4   Add the beef, mushroom, and onion mixture back to the pan and stir to coat. Remove from the heat and stir in the thyme. Taste and season with more salt and pepper, if desired.

5   Preheat the oven to 375°F. Transfer the beef mixture to a 2-quart or 9-inch square casserole dish. Spread the cauliflower puree evenly over the top of the beef mixture. Bake for 30 minutes, or until the top is turning golden and the stroganoff is bubbling at the edges.

6   Remove the casserole from the oven and let cool for 5 minutes. Garnish with fresh parsley, if desired, and serve hot.

Calories: 518 | Fat: 41g | Protein: 27g | Carbs: 10.5g | Fiber: 4g | **Net Carbs: 6.5g**

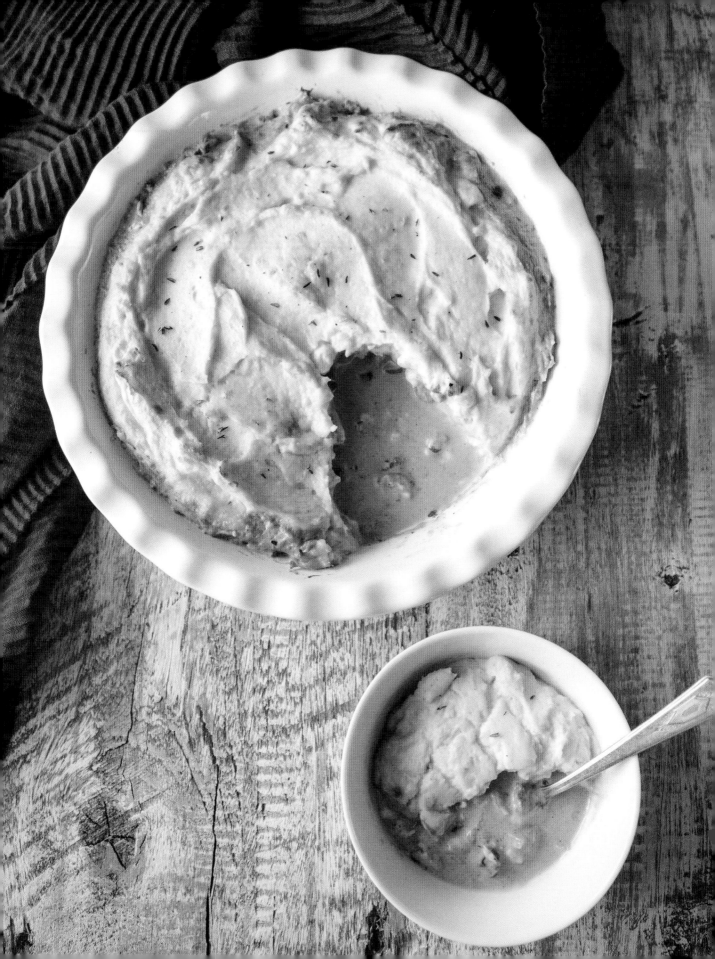

Coffee-Rubbed Rib-Eyes with Balsamic Butter

Hungry Jr. pronounced this "the best steak you've ever made, Mom," and I agree! The complex flavors of the coffee, chili, and cocoa rub combined with the meaty beef and sweet balsamic butter are truly sublime. This ain't your mama's steak! Unless you're Hungry Jr.; then I guess it is.

Yield: **2 servings** ◆ Prep Time: **5 minutes** ◆ Cook Time: **15 minutes**

For the rub:

1 tablespoon ground coffee

1 tablespoon unsweetened cocoa powder

2 teaspoons kosher salt

¼ teaspoon cayenne pepper

2 (8-ounce) bone-in rib-eye steaks, room temperature

For the balsamic butter:

3 tablespoons butter, softened

2 tablespoons balsamic vinegar (no sugar added)

1 teaspoon granulated erythritol

For garnish (optional):

Chopped fresh parsley

1 Preheat a grill to medium heat. Combine the coffee, cocoa powder, salt, and cayenne in a small bowl. Rub the steaks generously with the coffee mixture.

2 Grill the steaks on direct heat for 6 minutes (for medium) to 8 minutes (for medium-well) per side, or until your desired doneness is reached.

3 Remove the steaks from the grill and let rest for 5 minutes. Meanwhile, place the butter, balsamic vinegar, and sweetener in a small bowl and mix with a fork until blended. Serve the steaks with a generous dollop of balsamic butter. Garnish with chopped parsley, if desired.

Calories: 583 | Fat: 45g | Protein: 53g | Carbs: 4g | Fiber: 1g | Erythritol: 2g | **Net Carbs: 3g**

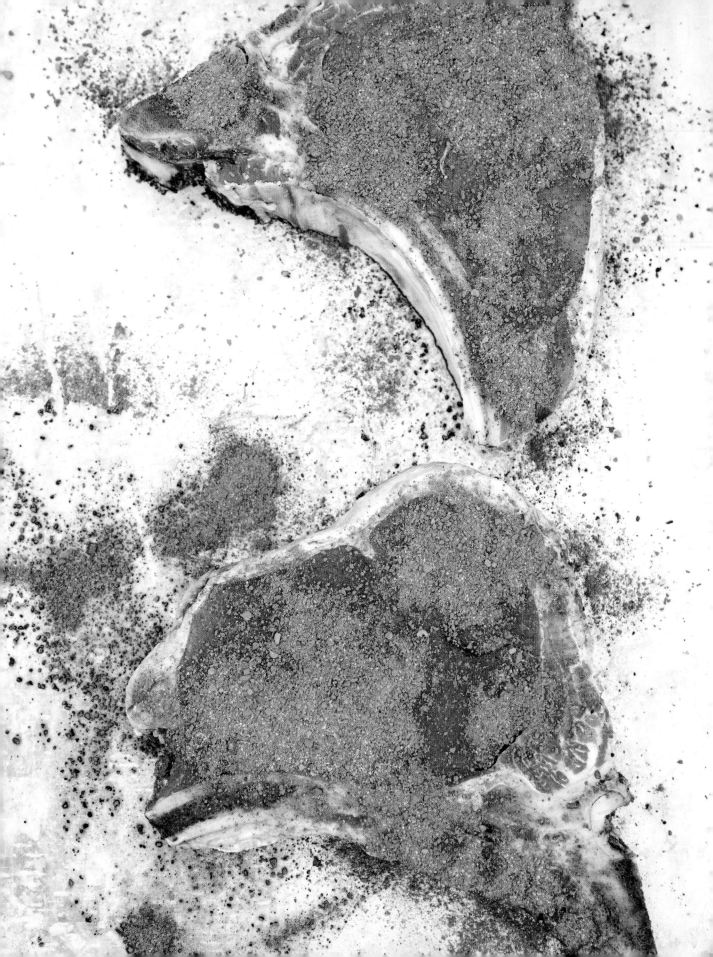

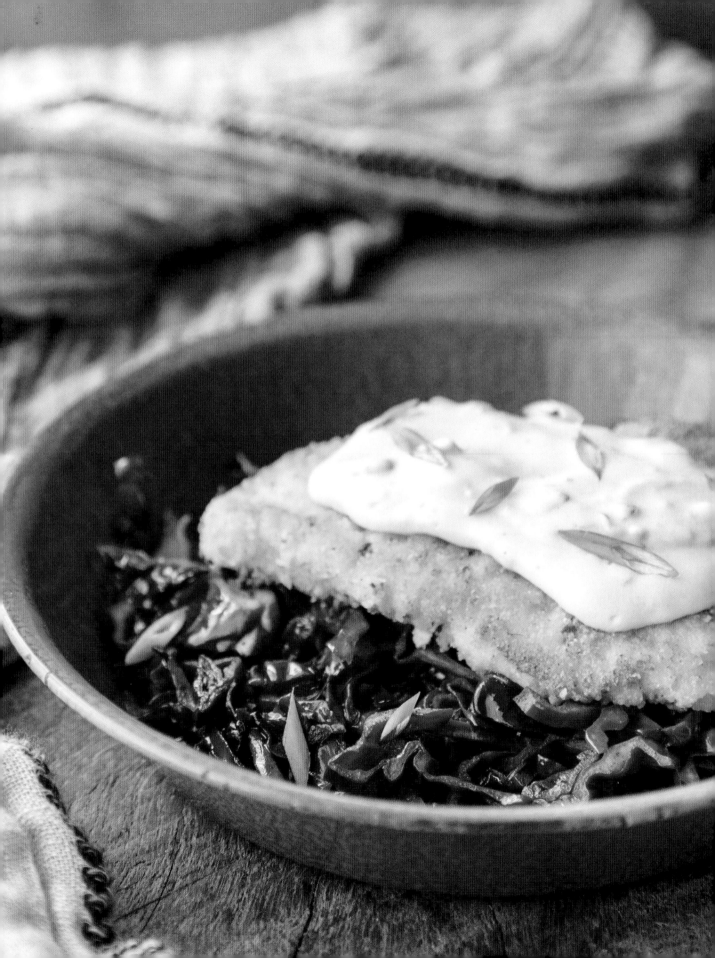

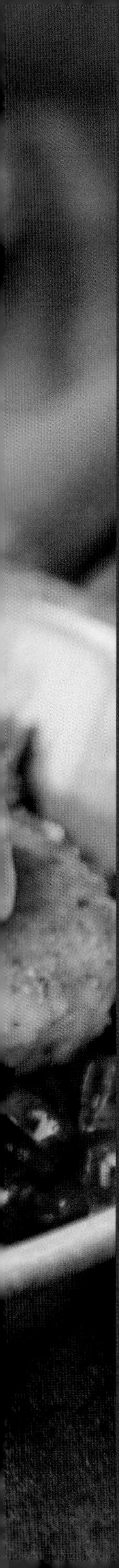

pork

Cajun Pork Chops with Aioli / **200**

Sweet & Spicy Asian Meatballs / **202**

Pork Fried Cauliflower Rice / **204**

Mojo Pork Tenderloin / **206**

Pork Chili Verde / **208**

Easy Sausage & Cauliflower Bake / **210**

Schnitzel with Sour Cream & Scallion Sauce / **212**

Bahn Mi Pork Burgers / **214**

Pork Chops with Dijon Tarragon Sauce / **216**

Easy Jerk Ribs / **218**

dairy-free egg-free nut-free vegetarian

Cajun Pork Chops with Aioli

Dinner doesn't get much easier than these Cajun pork chops. While the chops are delicious on their own, the garlicky aioli really makes them shine. Aioli doesn't typically include parsley, but I love the bright flavor that it adds. Serve them with a simple side salad and you've got dinner on the table in less than twenty minutes!

Yield: **4 servings** ◆ Serving Size: **1 chop and 2 tablespoons aioli** ◆ Prep Time: **5 minutes**

Cook Time: **14 minutes**

1 tablespoon avocado oil or other light-tasting oil

4 (8-ounce) bone-in pork chops

1 tablespoon Cajun Seasoning (page 76)

For the aioli (garlic mayo):

½ cup sugar-free mayonnaise

1 tablespoon chopped fresh parsley

1 teaspoon lemon juice

½ teaspoon minced garlic

1 Heat the oil in a large skillet over medium heat for 2 minutes, or until shimmering. Season the pork chops on both sides with the Cajun seasoning.

2 Place the chops in the hot oil and cook for about 6 minutes per side for medium doneness, or longer if you want them well-done. (When medium-done, a meat thermometer will read 160°F when inserted in the middle of a chop.) Remove from the pan and let rest for 5 minutes.

3 Meanwhile, make the aioli: Place the mayonnaise, parsley, lemon juice, and garlic in a small bowl and mix well.

4 Serve the pork chops with the aioli.

Calories: 579 | Fat: 45g | Protein: 46g | Carbs: 1g | Fiber:0g | **Net Carbs: 1g**

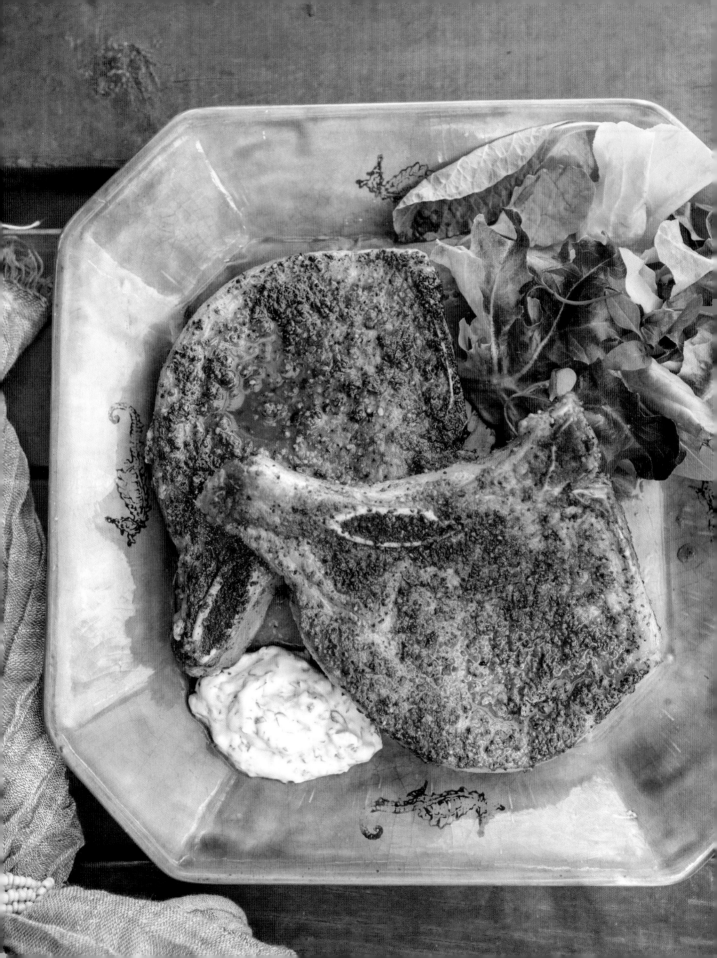

dairy-free egg-free nut-free vegetarian

Sweet & Spicy Asian Meatballs

These addictive little morsels make a fantastic appetizer or cocktail party nosh served with fancy toothpicks. Just as good as a main course, these meatballs can be served with cauliflower rice for you and regular rice for the rest of the family. You can easily double the sauce and throw in some broccoli or zucchini to get your veggies in, too!

Yield: **16 meatballs** ◆ Serving Size: **4 meatballs** ◆ Prep Time: **8 minutes** ◆ Cook Time: **13 minutes**

For the meatballs:

1 pound ground pork

⅓ cup superfine blanched almond flour

2 tablespoons chopped scallions

2 tablespoons chopped water chestnuts

2 tablespoons minced red bell peppers

1 tablespoon wheat-free soy sauce

¼ teaspoon cayenne pepper

½ teaspoon minced garlic

1 large egg, beaten

1 tablespoon avocado oil or other light-tasting oil, for the pan

For the sauce:

½ teaspoon toasted sesame oil

3 tablespoons sugar-free rice wine vinegar

3 tablespoons wheat-free soy sauce

¼ cup filtered water

3 tablespoons granulated erythritol

¼ cup chopped scallions

1 tablespoon red pepper flakes

½ teaspoon xanthan gum

1 Place all of the meatball ingredients in a medium-sized bowl and mix well with your hands. Form into 16 meatballs about 1½ inches in diameter.

2 Heat the avocado oil in a large nonstick skillet over medium heat. Add the meatballs to the hot oil and cook for about 3 minutes per side, or until browned and cooked through. Remove the meatballs from the pan and set aside.

3 Return the skillet to the stove over medium heat. Make the sauce: Pour the sesame oil, vinegar, soy sauce, water, and sweetener into the skillet and whisk until combined. Add the scallions, red pepper flakes, and xanthan gum to the skillet. Simmer, stirring occasionally, for about 5 minutes, until thickened enough to coat a spoon.

4 Add the meatballs to the sauce and cook for 2 more minutes, or until the sauce adheres to the meatballs. Serve hot.

Calories: 391 | Fat: 35g | Protein: 24g | Carbs: 4.5g | Fiber: 1.5g | Erythritol: 9g | **Net Carbs: 3g**

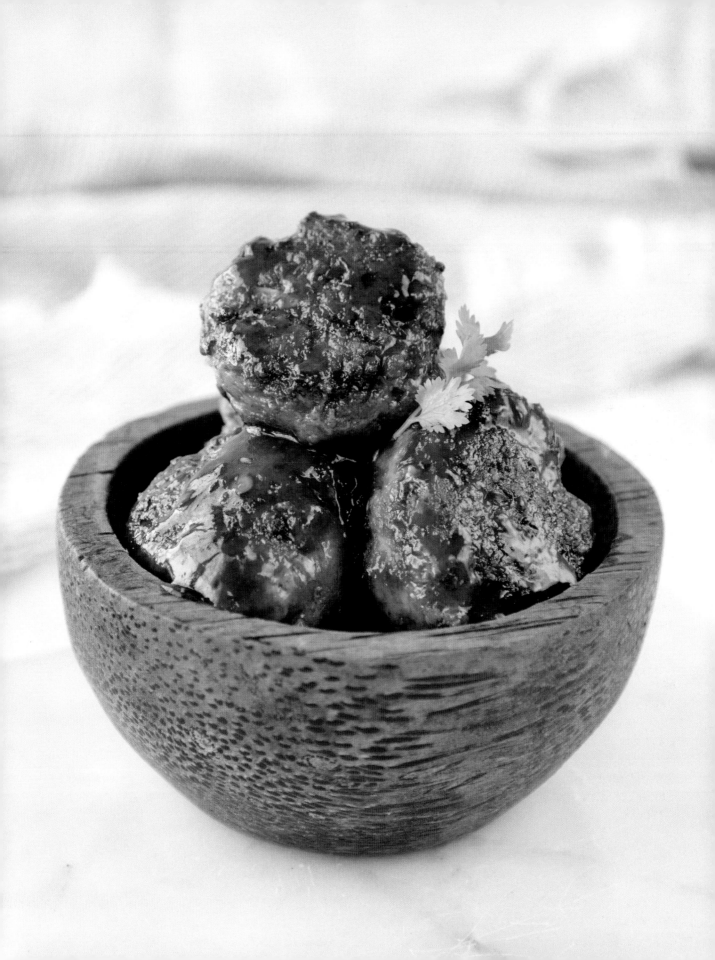

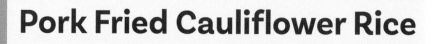

Pork Fried Cauliflower Rice

Pork fried rice is a Chinese takeout staple, and back in the day I could eat it by the pint. This keto version has all the flavor and texture of the original, but without the carbs and MSG that would leave me in a fog for hours afterward!

Yield: **4 servings**   •   Serving Size: **1½ cups**   •   Prep Time: **8 minutes**   •   Cook Time: **15 minutes**

1 pound boneless pork sirloin cutlets

½ teaspoon kosher salt

⅛ teaspoon ground black pepper

1 tablespoon coconut oil

1 teaspoon toasted sesame oil

1 large egg, beaten

3 cups riced cauliflower (see page 250)

1 teaspoon peeled and minced fresh ginger

1 teaspoon minced garlic

¼ cup frozen peas

2 tablespoons wheat-free soy sauce

1 teaspoon Sriracha sauce, plus more for serving if desired

¼ cup sliced scallions

2 tablespoons chopped fresh cilantro

1 teaspoon lime juice

1   Slice the pork cutlets into strips about ½ inch wide. Season with the salt and pepper.

2   Heat the coconut oil and sesame oil in a large skillet over medium-high heat. Put the seasoned pork in the skillet and cook for 3 to 5 minutes, until browned and cooked through. Remove the pork from the skillet and set aside.

3   Return the skillet to the stove and lower the heat to medium. Pour the beaten egg into the skillet and scramble for 2 minutes. Remove the cooked egg from the skillet and set aside.

4   Return the skillet to the stove and increase the heat to medium-high. Spoon the riced cauliflower, ginger, and garlic into the skillet and cook for 2 minutes, or until fragrant and slightly browned. Add the peas and cook for 2 more minutes.

5   Add the cooked pork and scrambled eggs back into the skillet and stir in the soy sauce and Sriracha. Cook, stirring occasionally, for another 3 minutes, or until the cauliflower is tender. Remove the skillet from the heat and stir in the scallions, cilantro, and lime juice. Serve immediately, with extra Sriracha on the side, if desired.

Calories: 218 | Fat: 8g | Protein: 30g | Carbs: 5g | Fiber: 2g | **Net Carbs: 3g**

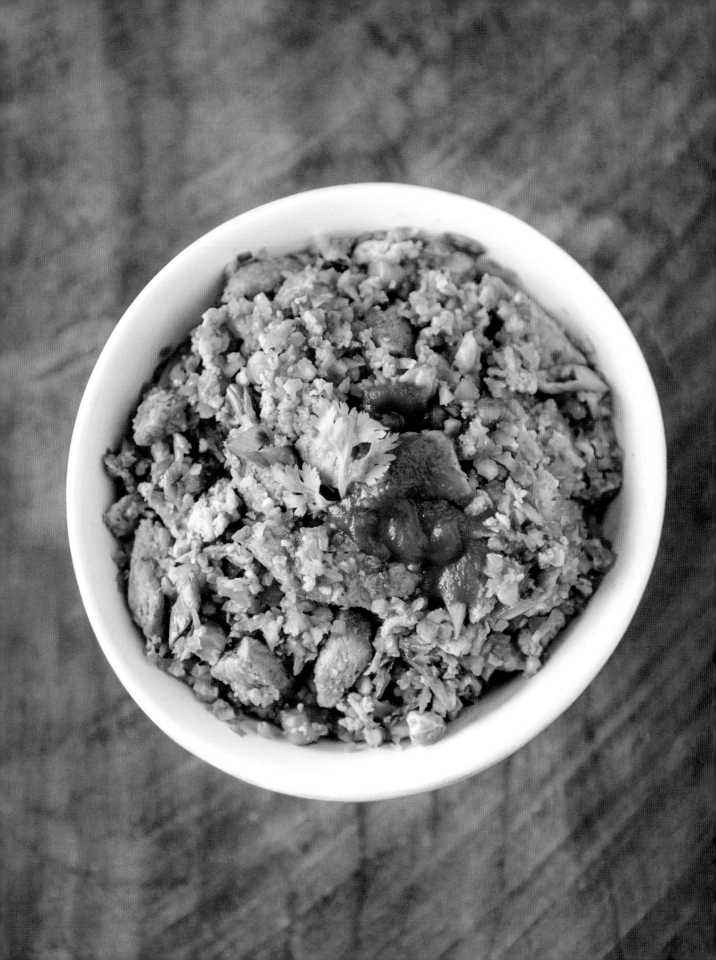

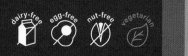

Mojo Pork Tenderloin

The citrus, garlic, and herbs in this classic Latin American–style marinade give pork tenderloin a bright, fresh flavor that will keep you coming back for more! Any leftovers make a fantastic addition to a salad the next day.

Yield: **10 servings** ◆ Serving Size: **4 ounces sliced tenderloin**

Prep Time: **10 minutes, plus at least 2 hours to marinate** ◆ Cook Time: **18 minutes**

For the marinade:

¼ cup extra-virgin olive oil

2 tablespoons apple cider vinegar

2 tablespoons lime juice

2 tablespoons orange juice

2 tablespoons chopped fresh cilantro

1 tablespoon grated lime zest

1 tablespoon grated orange zest

1 teaspoon dried oregano leaves

1 teaspoon granulated erythritol

1 teaspoon ground cumin

1 teaspoon kosher salt

½ teaspoon ground black pepper

3 cloves garlic, minced

3 pounds pork tenderloin, trimmed of silver skin membrane

1 tablespoon avocado oil or other light-tasting oil, for the pan

1 Whisk together the marinade ingredients in a medium-sized bowl. Remove ⅓ cup of the marinade for serving and refrigerate until needed. Add the pork to the remaining marinade and turn it to make sure it's well coated on all sides. Cover (it's fine for the pork to bend around the bottom of the bowl) and refrigerate for at least 2 hours or up to 24 hours. Remove the pork from the refrigerator 20 minutes before cooking and discard the marinade.

2 Heat the avocado oil in a large, heavy sauté pan with a lid over medium-high heat. Place the tenderloin in the pan and sear until golden brown, about 6 minutes per side. Cover and remove from the heat. Leave covered for another 6 minutes, or until a meat thermometer inserted in the thickest part of the meat reads 160°F. (As the tenderloin sits, the temperature will continue to rise due to carryover heat.)

3 Uncover and rest the tenderloin for another 10 minutes, then slice and serve with the reserved mojo marinade from the refrigerator.

4 Store leftovers in an airtight container in the refrigerator for up to 5 days. To reheat, microwave on high for only 1 minute (any longer and the meat will become tough) or in the oven at 375°F for 8 minutes, or until the desired temperature is reached.

Pro Tips:

Letting the meat come to room temperature before cooking ensures that the outside doesn't overcook while the inside stays raw.

If you slice into the meat while it's still piping hot, all of the juices will run out onto your cutting board, leaving you with dried-out meat. If you let the meat rest and cool for at least 10 minutes, the moisture (and flavor) will stay put and the meat will be tender and juicy.

Calories: 213 | Fat: 9g | Protein: 32g | Carbs: 0g | Fiber: 0g | Erythritol: 4g | **Net Carbs: 0g**

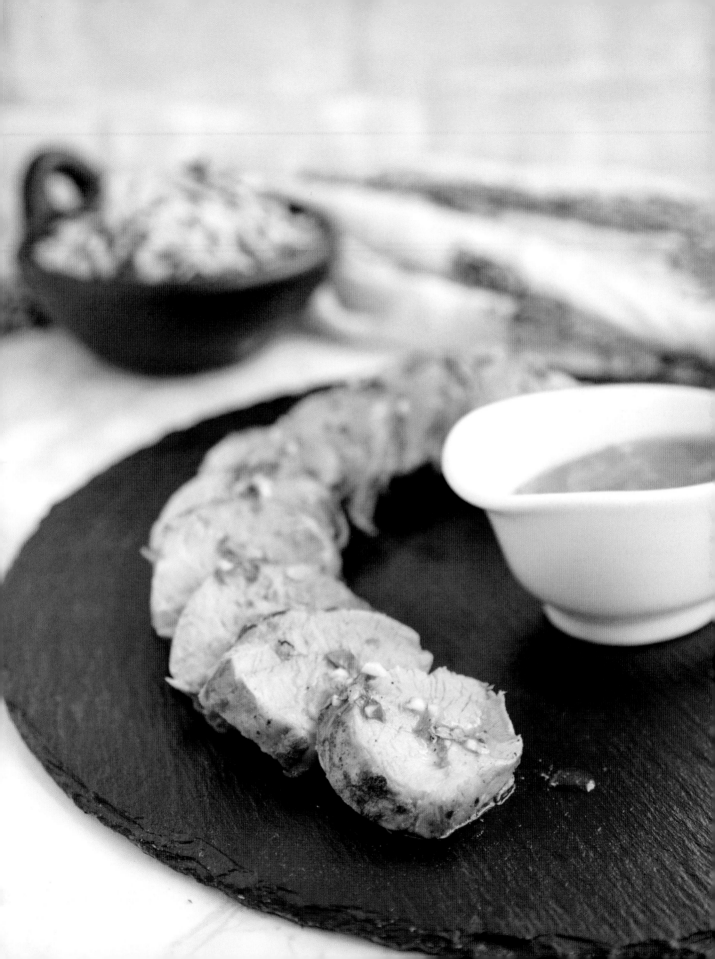

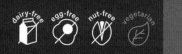

Pork Chili Verde

This pork chili has an entirely different personality and flavor profile than the Chili con Carne on page 182, but it's just as hearty and comforting. I love the bright zing from the tomatillos in the salsa verde!

Yield: **8 servings**   ◆   Serving Size: **1½ cups**   ◆   Prep Time: **10 minutes**   ◆   Cook Time: **1 hour 15 minutes**

2 pounds boneless pork shoulder (aka pork butt)

1 teaspoon kosher salt

¼ teaspoon ground black pepper

2 tablespoons avocado oil or other light-tasting oil

½ cup chopped onions

2 tablespoons chopped jalapeño peppers

1 tablespoon ground coriander

1 tablespoon ground cumin

1 tablespoon minced garlic

1 cup filtered water

1 cup salsa verde

1 Cut the pork into bite-sized pieces. Season with the salt and pepper.

2 Heat the oil in a small Dutch oven or heavy-bottomed pot over high heat for 2 minutes. Add the seasoned pork and cook, stirring occasionally, for about 8 minutes, until browned.

3 Reduce the heat to medium and add the onions, jalapeño peppers, coriander, cumin, and garlic to the pot. Cook for 5 minutes, or until the onions are translucent.

4 Add the water and salsa verde to the pot and stir well, scraping any bits off of the bottom of the pan. Cover and reduce the heat to low. Simmer for 1 hour, or until the pork is tender. Serve hot.

Serving Suggestion:
Serve with your choice of sour cream, cilantro, sliced avocado or guacamole, shredded cheddar cheese, finely diced red onions, and/or a side of Bacon & Cheddar Cornless Muffins (page 302).

Calories: 261 | Fat: 17g | Protein: 22g | Carbs: 3g | Fiber: 0.5g | **Net Carbs: 2.5g**

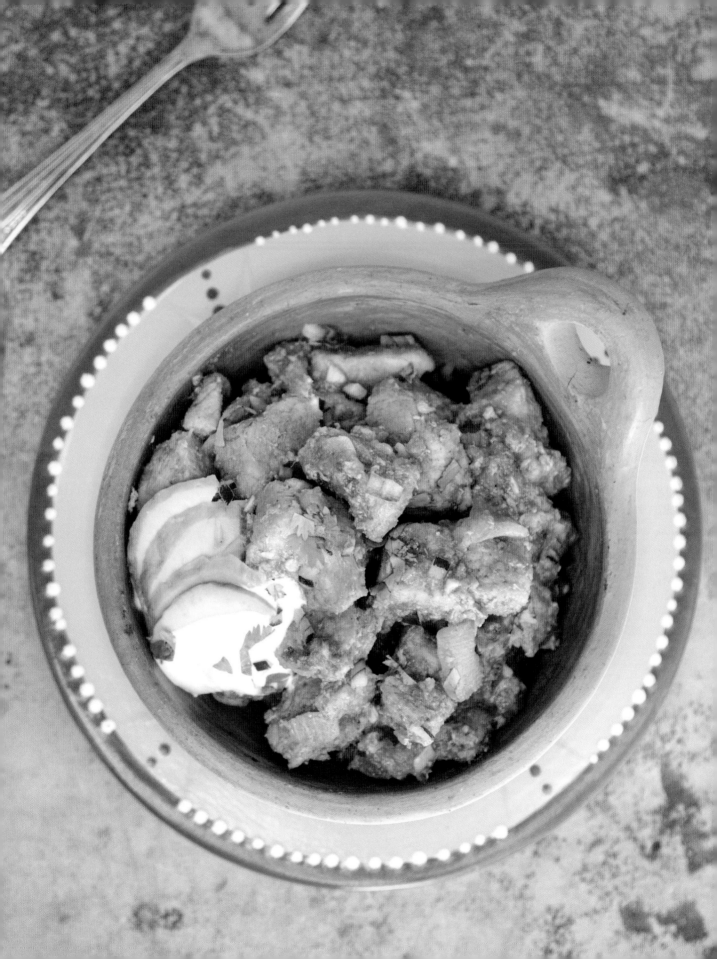

dairy-free egg-free nut-free vegetarian

Easy Sausage & Cauliflower Bake

This is one of those comforting casseroles that you can reheat all week and it just gets better and better! The flavors of the marinara and sausage soak into the nooks and crannies of the cauliflower, along with all that creamy cheese. If your family is on the fence about cauliflower, this recipe just might win them over!

Yield: **6 servings** • Serving Size: **1½ cups** • Prep Time: **10 minutes** • Cook Time: **20 minutes**

5 cups cauliflower florets (1 large head), cooked until fork-tender and well drained (see tip)

2 cups cooked and chopped Italian sausage (4 links)

1½ cups marinara sauce, store-bought or homemade (page 106)

¾ cup shredded whole-milk mozzarella cheese

¼ cup grated Parmesan cheese

¼ cup heavy whipping cream

1 tablespoon chopped fresh parsley

1 tablespoon chopped fresh basil, for garnish

1 Preheat the oven to 375°F.

2 Place all of the ingredients, except the basil, in a large bowl and mix well. Spoon into a 13 by 9-inch baking dish and spread evenly. Bake for 30 minutes, or until the cheese is melted and the sauce is bubbling.

3 Remove from the oven and let cool for 5 minutes. Garnish with the basil and serve hot.

Pro Tip:

It's important to drain the cooked cauliflower very well before you combine it with the other ingredients; otherwise, it will leach water into the sauce and dilute the flavors. This is especially important if you steam or boil the cauliflower to cook it. The best way I know to avoid waterlogged cauliflower is to microwave it in a dry bowl, uncovered, until fork-tender, which allows the extra moisture to evaporate. To cook the amount called for in this recipe, you'd need to microwave on high for 12 to 15 minutes.

Calories: 389 | Fat: 30g | Protein: 17g | Carbs: 14.5g | Fiber: 7.5g | **Net Carbs: 7g**

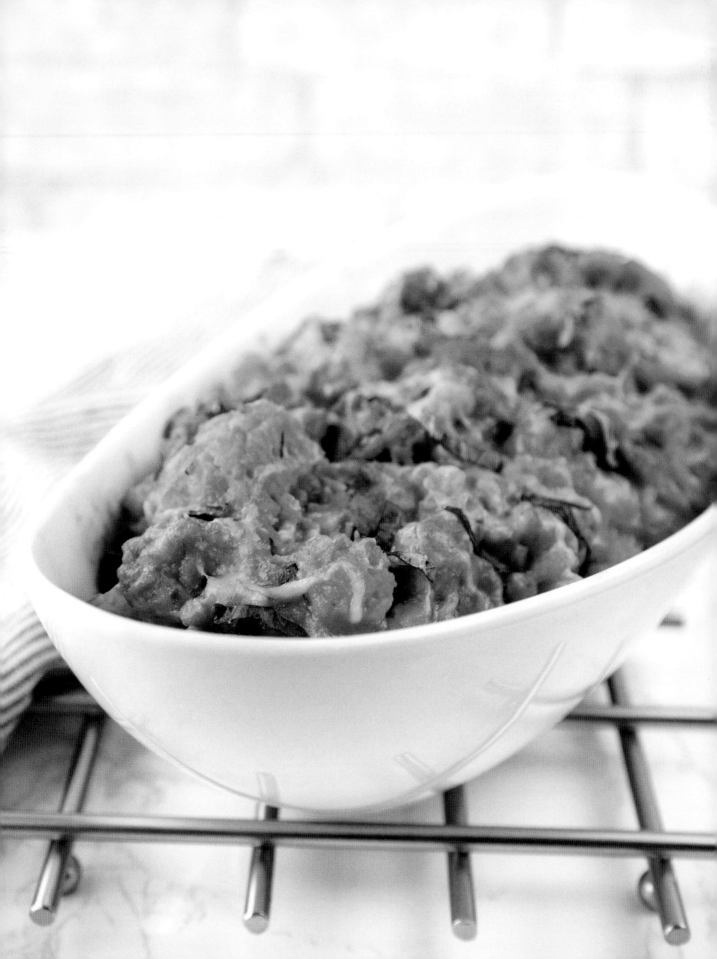

dairy-free egg-free nut-free vegetarian

Schnitzel with Sour Cream & Scallion Sauce

Don't let the name scare you off; *schnitzel* is just a fancy word for a meat cutlet that has been breaded and fried. This pork schnitzel is buttery and crunchy, but the real star is the tangy, creamy scallion sauce. Served with the Braised Red Cabbage on page 268, it makes for keto dinner bliss!

Yield: **4 servings** • Serving Size: **1 chop and 2 tablespoons sauce** • Prep Time: **12 minutes**

Cook Time: **8 minutes**

4 (6-ounce) boneless pork chops

2 tablespoons butter

1 large egg, beaten

⅓ cup Basic Breading (page 75)

⅓ cup dry sherry

2 ounces cream cheese (¼ cup)

¼ cup full-fat sour cream

¼ cup chopped scallions

1 small scallion, thinly sliced on the bias, for garnish (optional)

1 Place a 10-inch square sheet of plastic wrap on a large cutting board. Place a pork chop on the wrap, then cover with another 10-inch square sheet of plastic wrap. Pound the pork chop to ½-inch thickness with a mallet. Lift off the top wrap and remove the pork cutlet to a separate dish. Repeat with the remaining pork chops.

2 Melt the butter in a large nonstick skillet over medium heat. Dip the pork cutlets in the beaten egg and then in the breading, being sure to coat thoroughly. Fry the breaded cutlets in the hot butter for about 2 minutes per side, or until golden brown. Remove the pork from the skillet to individual plates or a serving platter.

3 Return the skillet to the stove over medium heat. Pour the sherry into the hot skillet and scrape up any bits. Simmer for 2 minutes, until reduced by half, then add the cream cheese and sour cream. Whisk until smooth and continue to simmer until thickened and slightly golden, about 2 minutes.

4 Remove from the heat and stir in the scallions. Serve the sauce over the warm pork schnitzel. Garnish with sliced scallions if desired.

Calories: 404 | Fat: 19g | Protein: 43g | Carbs: 5g | Fiber: 1g | **Net Carbs: 4g**

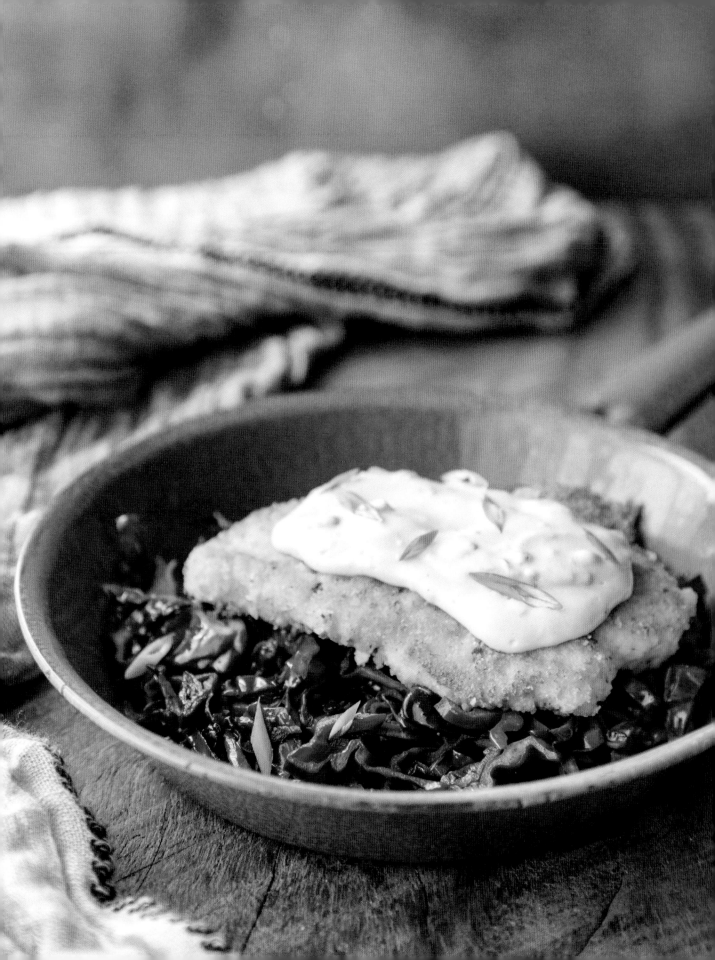

Bahn Mi Pork Burgers

dairy-free egg-free nut-free vegetarian

I know this looks like a lot of ingredients, but these burgers are not complicated to make, and the effort is well worth it, I promise! The blend of textures and the bright, fresh flavors are so unique, yet so harmonious, that you'll want to make these burgers over and over again. You won't miss the bun, but if your crew prefers it, you can easily serve the burgers on buns for everyone else.

Yield: **4 burgers** ◆ Serving Size: **1 burger** ◆ Prep Time: **15 minutes** ◆ Cook Time: **10 minutes**

For the burger patties:

1 pound ground pork

2 tablespoons chopped scallions

2 tablespoons fish sauce (no sugar added)

1 teaspoon granulated erythritol

1 teaspoon peeled and minced fresh ginger

1 teaspoon minced garlic

1 teaspoon toasted sesame oil

½ teaspoon cayenne pepper

For the pickled vegetables:

1 tablespoon granulated erythritol

1 tablespoon white vinegar

1 teaspoon fish sauce (no sugar added)

1 teaspoon lime juice

½ cup julienned radishes

½ cup sliced scallions

For the sauce:

⅓ cup sugar-free mayonnaise

1 tablespoon Sriracha sauce

1 teaspoon lime juice

8 red or green lettuce leaves

4 slices avocado

¼ cup fresh cilantro leaves, for garnish

¼ cup fresh mint leaves, for garnish

¼ cup fresh Thai or Italian basil leaves, for garnish

1   Place the burger ingredients in a medium-sized bowl and mix thoroughly with your hands. Form into 4 equal-sized patties about 1½ inches thick.

2   Heat a large nonstick skillet over medium-high heat for 2 minutes. Put the burger patties in the hot skillet and cook for 4 minutes per side, or until golden brown and cooked through. Remove the patties from the skillet and set aside.

3   Make the pickled vegetables: Whisk together the sweetener, vinegar, fish sauce, and lime juice in a medium-sized bowl. Add the radishes and scallions and toss to coat. Set aside.

4   Place all of the sauce ingredients in a small bowl and stir well. Set aside.

5   Assemble the burgers: Place 2 lettuce leaves on a plate. Top with a burger patty, then a generous dollop of the sauce. Next, add a slice of avocado and ¼ cup of the pickled veggies. Repeat with the remaining burgers and garnish each burger liberally with fresh cilantro, mint, and basil leaves before serving.

Calories: 495 | Fat: 44g | Protein: 21g | Carbs: 6g | Fiber: 2g | Erythritol: 4g | **Net Carbs: 4g**

Variation:

Bahn Mi Pork Salad. Rather than forming the meat into patties, you can cook the burger mixture in a skillet and crumble it over the rest of the ingredients salad style. This works well if you want to make it in advance and take it for lunch without having to reheat it.

Pork Chops with Dijon Tarragon Sauce

dairy-free · egg-free · nut-free · vegetarian

I think pork chops are really underrated, but I will say that this dish also lends itself well to being made with chicken breasts if you aren't a fan of pork. The pan sauce is super easy but very flavorful and really completes the dish.

Yield: **4 servings** • Serving Size: **1 pork chop and 2 tablespoons sauce**

Prep Time: **5 minutes** • Cook Time: **11 minutes**

4 (6-ounce) boneless pork chops

½ teaspoon kosher salt

⅛ teaspoon ground black pepper

2 tablespoons butter

⅓ cup heavy whipping cream

1 tablespoon chopped fresh tarragon

1 teaspoon Dijon mustard

½ teaspoon garlic powder

½ teaspoon onion powder

1 Season the pork chops on both sides with the salt and pepper. Melt the butter in a large sauté pan over medium-high heat. Cook the chops in the butter for 3 to 4 minutes per side for medium done chops. (When medium done, a meat thermometer will read 160°F when inserted in the middle of the chops.) Remove the pork chops from the skillet and set aside.

2 Add the cream, tarragon, mustard, garlic powder, and onion powder to the pan and whisk together until smooth. Reduce the sauce over medium heat for about 3 minutes, until thickened. Pour the sauce over the chops and serve warm.

Calories: 336 | Fat: 17g | Protein: 40g | Carbs: 0.5g | Fiber: 0g | **Net Carbs: 0.5g**

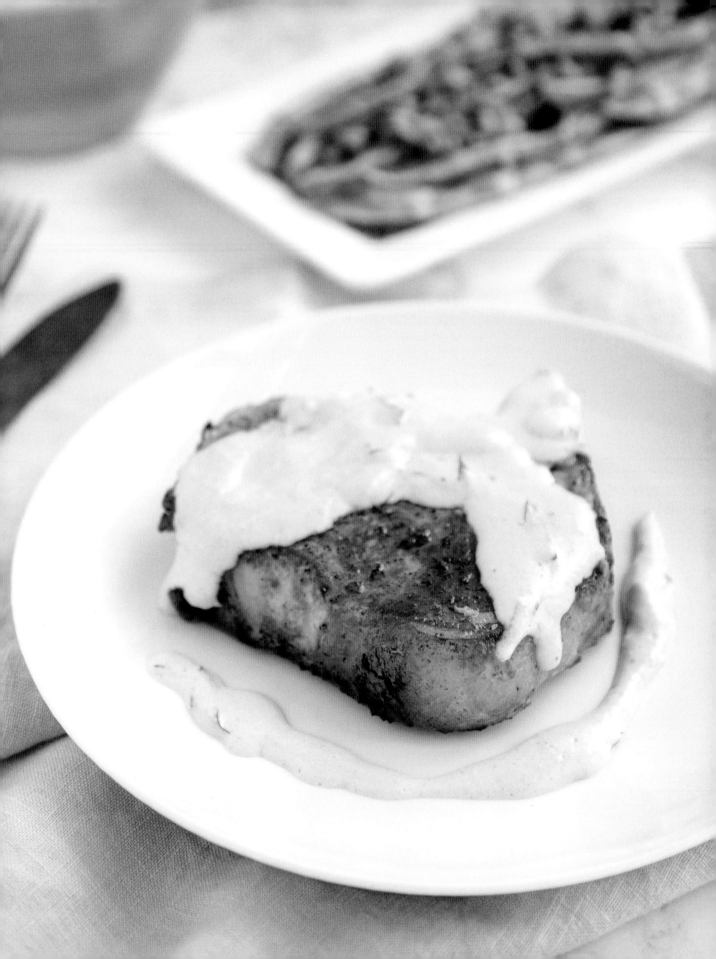

Easy Jerk Ribs

dairy-free · egg-free · nut-free · vegetarian

I have a love-hate relationship with ribs—I love to eat them and hate to make them because it seems to take *for-ev-er*! This relatively painless method produces melt-in-your-mouth, fall-off-the-bone ribs every time. I've provided you with a recipe so you can make them and invite me over. I'll bring the margaritas!

Yield: **4 servings** • Prep Time: **2 minutes** • Cook Time: **1 hour 45 minutes**

1 rack baby back ribs

¼ cup Jerk Seasoning (page 79)

2 teaspoons kosher salt

½ cup Easy Keto BBQ Sauce (page 104)

1. Preheat a grill to medium heat. Generously season the rack of ribs on both sides with the jerk seasoning and salt. Grill for 15 minutes per side over direct heat. The ribs should be browned and crispy looking on the outside.

2. Wrap the ribs loosely in foil and place on the grill over indirect heat. You may need to move coals to the side, or turn off one or two burners to create a flame-free space. With the lid closed, cook the ribs for 1 hour; the grill temperature should be about 350°F. After 1 hour, open the foil and baste the ribs on both sides with the BBQ sauce. Cook for 30 more minutes, or until the ribs are done to your desired tenderness. Cut into individual ribs to serve.

Alternative Method:

To bake the ribs, preheat the oven to 400°F. Line a sheet pan with foil. Generously season the rack of ribs on both sides with the jerk seasoning and salt. Place the ribs on the foil, meat side up, and bake for 30 minutes. Reduce the oven temperature to 325°F and cook for another hour. Brush the ribs on both sides with the BBQ sauce and cook for another 30 minutes, or until the ribs are done to your desired tenderness.

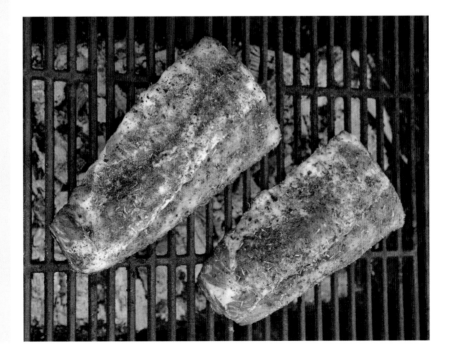

Calories: 390 | Fat: 27g | Protein: 26g | Carbs: 6g | Fiber: 2g | Erythritol: 7g | **Net Carbs: 4g**

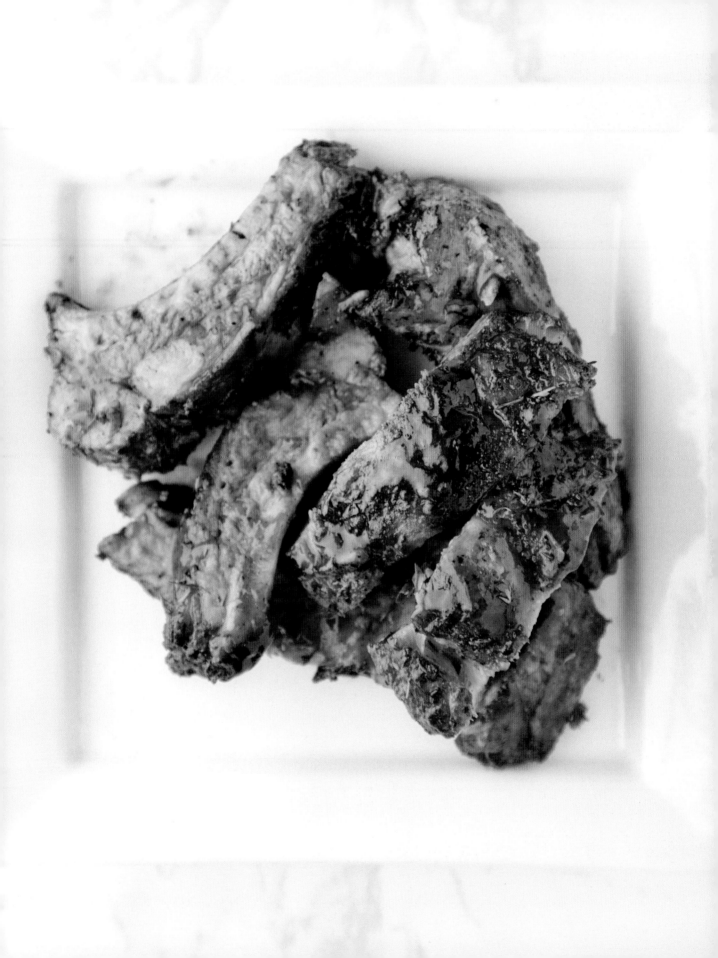

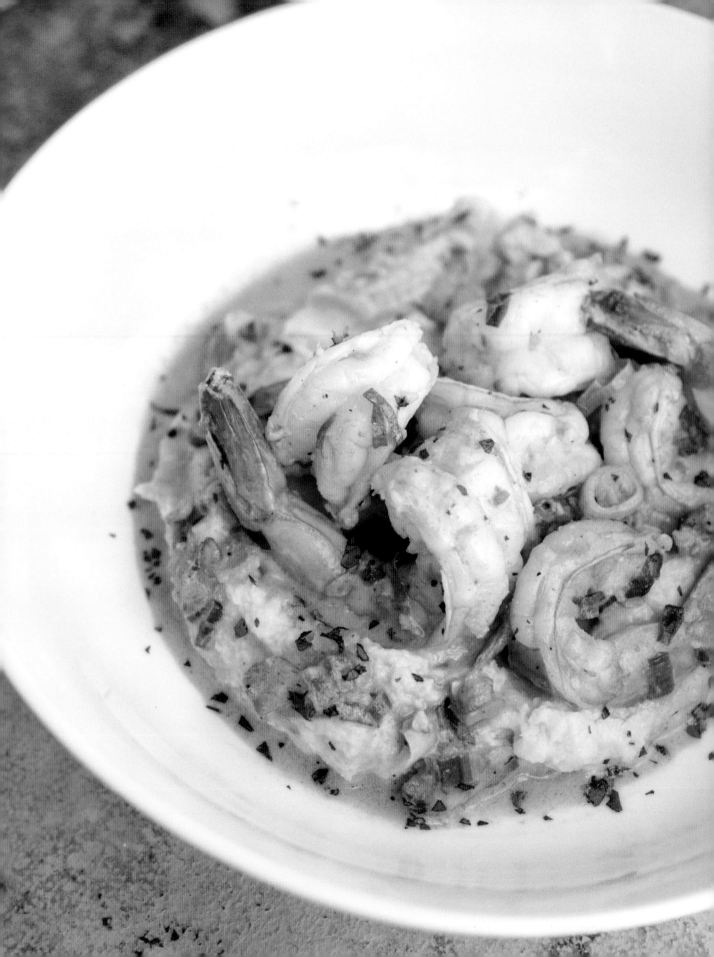

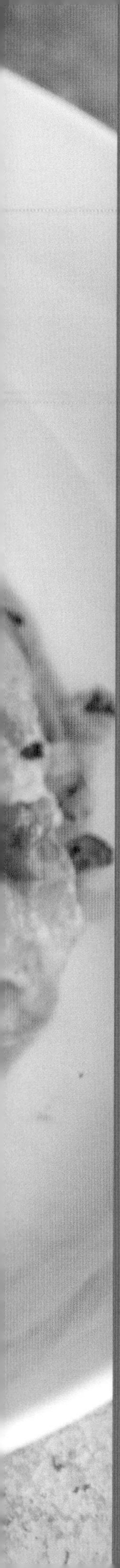

seafood

Cajun Fish Fingers / 222

Blackened Snapper / 224

Shrimp Caprese Salad / 225

Shrimp & Grits / 226

Spicy Tuna Cakes / 228

Niçoise Salad with Seared Tuna / 230

Shrimp Panang Curry / 232

Smoked Salmon Stacks / 234

Baked Mahi Mahi in Garlic Parsley Butter / 236

Fish Taco Bowl / 238

Shrimp Fajitas / 240

Creamy Lobster Risotto / 242

Spicy Shrimp-Stuffed Avocados / 244

dairy-free egg-free nut-free vegetarian

Cajun Fish Fingers

These aren't the sketchy freezer-burned fish sticks of your childhood. Crispy on the outside and boasting tender, flaky fish on the inside, these little gems will win over even the pickiest of eaters. Creamy remoulade makes a great dipping sauce for these fish fingers, but to change it up, I also love pairing them with Sweet Chili Sauce (page 105) for an extra kick!

Yield: **4 servings** ♦ Prep Time: **8 minutes** ♦ Cook Time: **10 minutes**

1½ pounds firm white fish fillets

¾ cup Basic Breading (page 75)

1 tablespoon Cajun Seasoning (page 76)

1 large egg, beaten

¼ cup avocado oil or other light-tasting oil, for the pan

½ cup Basic Remoulade (page 97), for serving (optional)

Lime wedges, for serving (optional)

1 Cut the fish fillets into strips about 4 inches long by 1 inch thick. Line a plate with paper towels.

2 Place the breading and Cajun seasoning in a medium-sized bowl and mix well. Dip the fish fingers into the beaten egg and then into the breading, rolling the fish to coat all sides.

3 Heat the oil in a large sauté pan over medium heat until shimmering, about 2 minutes. Fry the fish fingers in small batches until golden brown, about 2 minutes per side. Remove the fish to the lined plate and serve immediately. Serve with remoulade and lime wedges, if desired.

Calories: 467 | Fat: 35g | Protein: 35g | Carbs: 5g | Fiber: 2g | **Net Carbs: 3g**

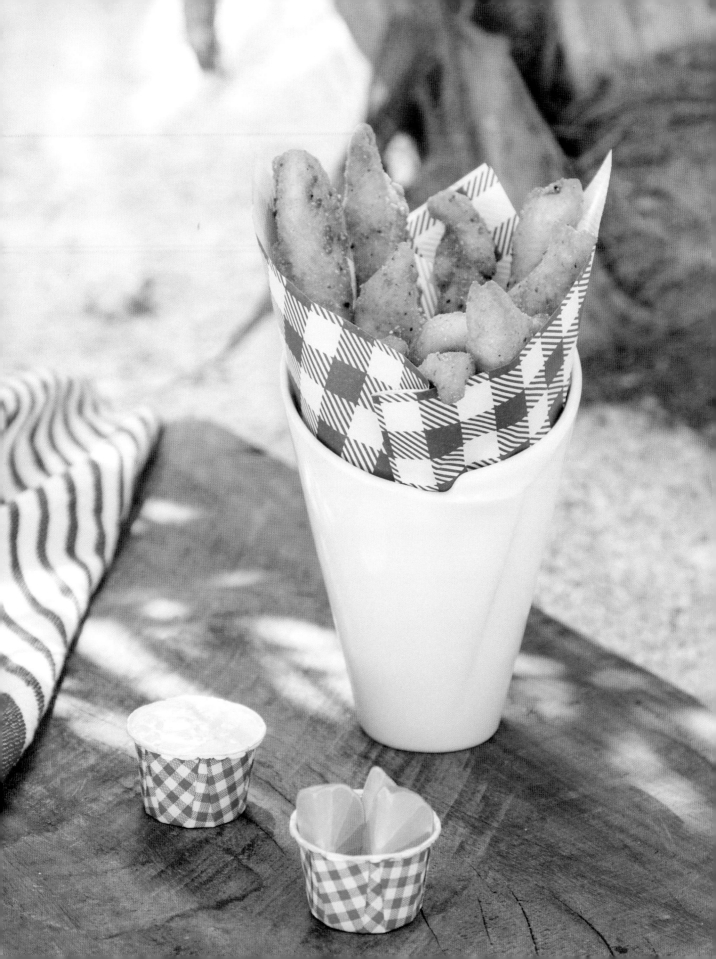

dairy-free · egg-free · nut-free · vegetarian

Blackened Snapper

This is one of those recipes that looks like it came out of a restaurant kitchen but takes only about ten minutes to make. Impress your guests—and have time to do your hair before they arrive, for a change—with this easy and delicious seafood masterpiece! Shown served with Quick Cucumber Pickles (page 114).

Yield: **4 servings** ◆ Prep Time: **5 minutes** ◆ Cook Time: **6 minutes**

4 (6-ounce) snapper or other white fish fillets

½ teaspoon kosher salt

¼ cup Blackening Seasoning (page 78)

2 tablespoons butter

1   Season the fish fillets with the salt, then coat them with the blackening seasoning on all sides.

2   Heat the butter in a medium-sized nonstick skillet over high heat until bubbling. Add the fish and cook for 2 to 3 minutes per side, until it becomes opaque and flakes easily. Remove from the pan and serve immediately.

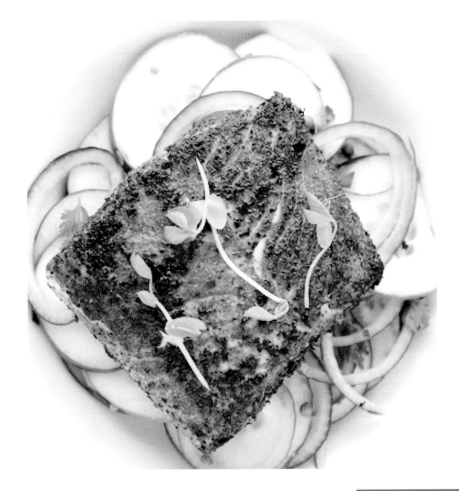

Calories: 241 | Fat: 9g | Protein: 36g | Carbs: 4g | Fiber: 2g | **Net Carbs: 2g**

Shrimp Caprese Salad

dairy-free · egg-free · nut-free · vegetarian

This recipe screams summertime and is perfect for picnics and barbecues. Just be sure to keep it chilled, as the dressing contains mayonnaise.

Yield: **4 servings** ◆ Serving Size: **1¼ cups** ◆ Prep Time: **12 minutes, plus 30 minutes to chill**

1 pound large shrimp, peeled, deveined, and cooked

1 cup halved cherry tomatoes

4 ounces fresh mozzarella, cut into 1-inch cubes

2 tablespoons chopped fresh basil, plus more for garnish if desired

1 batch Creamy Basil-Parmesan Vinaigrette (page 86)

1 Cut the shrimp in half lengthwise and place in a medium-sized salad bowl.

2 Add the tomatoes, mozzarella, and basil to the bowl. Pour the vinaigrette over the salad ingredients and toss to coat.

3 For best flavor, chill for 30 minutes before serving. Garnish the salad with additional chopped basil, if desired.

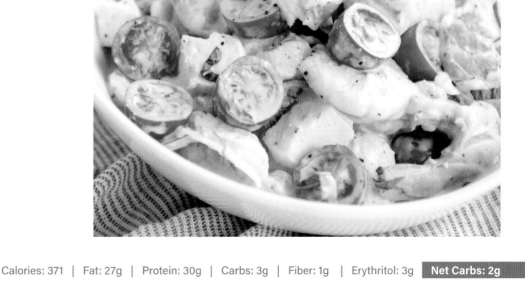

Calories: 371 | Fat: 27g | Protein: 30g | Carbs: 3g | Fiber: 1g | Erythritol: 3g | **Net Carbs: 2g**

Shrimp & Grits

When we lived in South Carolina, I had "real" Southern shrimp and grits for the first time, at a restaurant called Poogan's Porch in Charleston. It was a memorable experience, and I can still taste that incredible sauce in my mind. While this version isn't an exact replica, it hits all the same comfort food notes with the rich, silky sauce, succulent shrimp, and creamy, cheesy grits to soak it all up. Don't plan on having leftovers … I'm just saying.

Yield: **4 servings** • Serving Size: **1 cup shrimp served over ½ cup grits**

Prep Time: **8 minutes** • Cook Time: **15 minutes**

4 slices bacon, diced

1 tablespoon minced garlic

¾ cup chopped tomatoes

½ cup dry white wine

1 teaspoon Creole seasoning

¼ cup heavy whipping cream

1 pound large shrimp, peeled and deveined

¼ cup chopped scallions

Kosher salt and ground black pepper

1 tablespoon chopped fresh parsley, for garnish

2 cups Cheesy Cauliflower Grits (page 269), for serving

1 Cook the bacon in a large sauté pan over medium heat for 3 minutes, or until cooked but still soft. Add the garlic and cook for 1 minute, or until fragrant. Add the tomatoes, wine, and Creole seasoning and cook for 5 minutes, or until the liquid has reduced by half.

2 Pour in the cream and cook, stirring occasionally, for 3 minutes, or until slightly thickened. Stir in the shrimp and scallions and cook for 3 more minutes, or until the shrimp have just turned white and pink; don't overcook the shrimp or they will be tough and dry. Remove from the heat.

3 Taste and season with salt and pepper, if desired. Garnish with fresh parsley and serve over the cauliflower grits.

> **Pro Tip:**
> *For a fancier presentation, you can leave the tails on as I did, but if it's just the family, feel free to pinch the tails off before cooking for ease of eating.*

Calories: 448 | Fat: 25g | Protein: 35g | Carbs: 13g | Fiber: 6g | **Net Carbs: 7g**

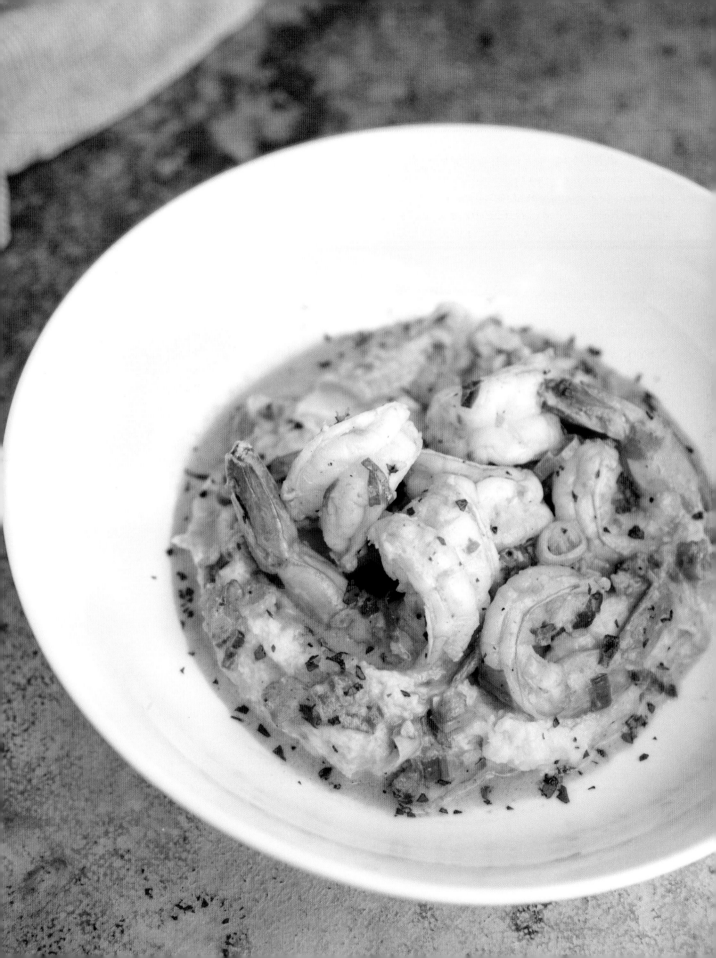

Spicy Tuna Cakes

dairy-free *egg-free* *nut-free* *vegetarian*

Recently, Mr. Hungry went fishing with some friends and brought back a bunch of small tuna. Because tuna lends itself so well to Asian flavors, I started experimenting with these fish cakes, and they were a hit! Our friends loved them, and even the pickier kids were big fans.

Yield: **12 cakes** ◆ Serving Size: **3 cakes** ◆ Prep Time: **10 minutes** ◆ Cook Time: **10 minutes**

3 tablespoons sugar-free mayonnaise

1 tablespoon Sriracha sauce

1 teaspoon wheat-free soy sauce

1 teaspoon coconut flour

1 pound fresh tuna, cut into ½-inch cubes

2 tablespoons white sesame seeds

1 tablespoon black sesame seeds

2 tablespoons avocado oil or other light-tasting oil, for the pan

1 In a mixing bowl, whisk together the mayonnaise, Sriracha, soy sauce, and flour until smooth. Add the tuna and stir to combine.

2 Combine the white and black sesame seeds and spread on a small plate.

3 Using your hands, form the tuna mixture into 12 small cakes about 2 inches in diameter. Gently dip both sides of the cakes in the sesame seeds to lightly coat them.

4 Heat the oil in a medium-sized nonstick sauté pan over medium heat. Cook the cakes in batches, 1 to 2 minutes per side, until golden brown. Serve warm.

Serving Suggestion:
Shown drizzled with Sweet Chili Sauce (page 105) and prepared wasabi on the side. You can purchase prepared wasabi in a tube or tin at most large grocery stores, or you can buy the powder and add water to make a thick paste.

Calories: 299 | Fat: 19g | Protein: 27g | Carbs: 2g | Fiber: 1g | **Net Carbs: 1g**

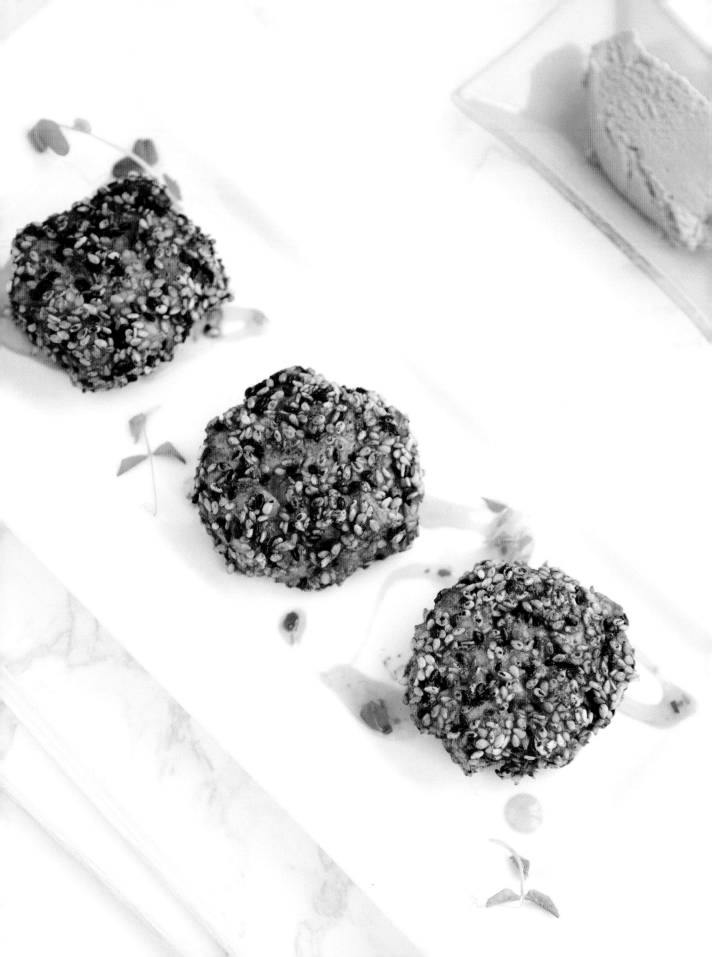

Niçoise Salad with Seared Tuna

dairy-free egg-free nut-free vegetarian

Niçoise is a classic French salad containing tuna, anchovies, haricots verts (basically fancy green beans), cooked potatoes, tomatoes, olives, and hard-boiled eggs and dressed with a Dijon vinaigrette. In this version, cauliflower stands in for the potatoes, and I used regular green beans because they are more readily available. If you can't get fresh tuna, skip the cooking part and just use canned tuna instead; it will still be delish. I skipped the anchovies and olives due to personal preference, but you can add them if you like.

Yield: **4 servings** ◆ Prep Time: **10 minutes** ◆ Cook Time: **8 minutes**

1 tablespoon sugar-free mayonnaise

1 teaspoon Dijon mustard

½ teaspoon kosher salt

¼ teaspoon ground black pepper

1 pound ahi tuna steaks

1 tablespoon avocado oil or other light-tasting oil, for the pan

2 medium heads red or green leaf lettuce, leaves washed and dried

8 hard-boiled eggs, peeled and quartered

2 cups cooked cauliflower florets

2 cups blanched green beans

2 large tomatoes, cut into wedges

For the Dijon vinaigrette:

¼ cup extra-virgin olive oil

¼ cup red wine vinegar

¼ cup sugar-free mayonnaise

1 tablespoon Dijon mustard

¼ teaspoon kosher salt

⅛ teaspoon ground black pepper

1 Combine the mayonnaise, mustard, salt, and pepper in a small bowl. Coat the tuna steaks on all sides with the mixture.

2 Heat the oil in a medium-sized nonstick pan over medium-high heat. Add the tuna steaks and sear for about 2 minutes per side for rare or 4 minutes per side to cook them through. Remove from the pan and set aside.

3 Place the lettuce leaves on a serving platter or divide them among 4 individual serving plates. Arrange the eggs, cauliflower, green beans, and tomato wedges around the outer edges on top of the lettuce.

4 Place the tuna steaks, whole or cut into pieces, in the center of the platter or plates.

5 In a medium-sized bowl, whisk together the vinaigrette ingredients. Drizzle over the salad just before serving.

Pro Tip:
Blanching usually involves submerging fruits or vegetables in boiling water for several minutes, then quickly transferring the food to ice water to halt the cooking process. It results in a slightly softened but still firm texture and an attractive bright-green color, and it's a common practice with green beans and asparagus intended for salads.

Calories: 546 | Fat: 37g | Protein: 16g | Carbs: 12g | Fiber: 6g | **Net Carbs: 6g**

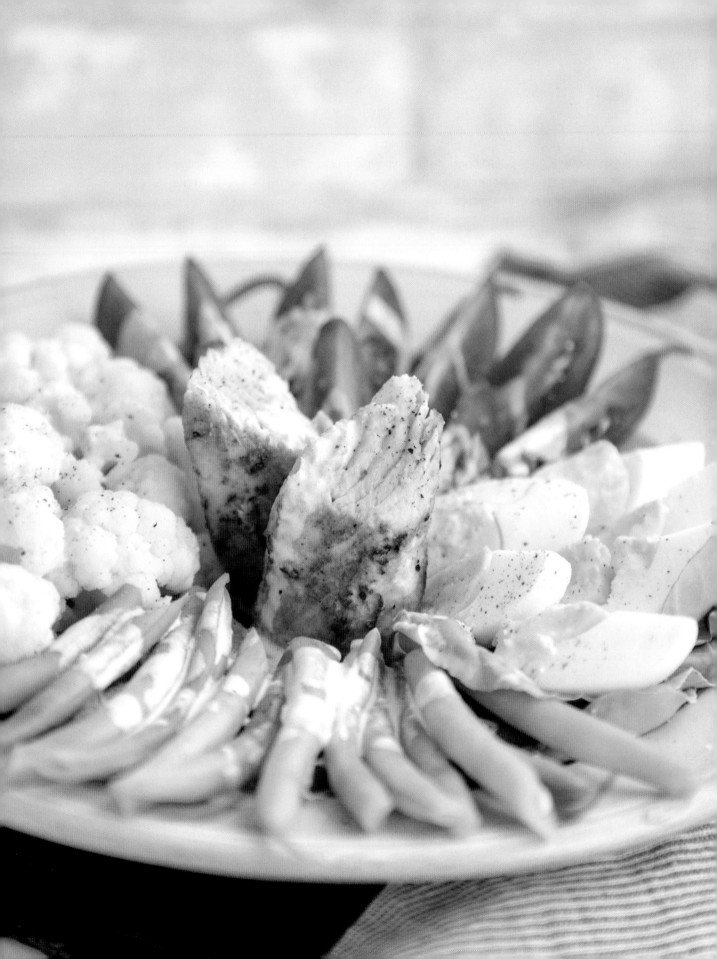

dairy-free egg-free nut-free vegetarian

Shrimp Panang Curry

Shrimp panang curry is my go-to order when we eat at Thai restaurants. It always tastes amazing in the moment, but then I regret it because all of that sugar and rice kicks me out of ketosis immediately. This version is just as spicy and sweet, with a creamy, luscious sauce and lots of shrimp, but instead of rice I serve it with daikon noodles made using a spiral slicer. Super fun and tasty, and it won't kick you out of ketosis!

Yield: **4 servings** ◆ Serving Size: **2 cups** ◆ Prep Time: **8 minutes** ◆ Cook Time: **15 minutes**

1 tablespoon coconut oil

3 tablespoons red curry paste

2 tablespoons natural peanut butter (no sugar added)

1 (14-ounce) can full-fat unsweetened coconut milk

2 tablespoons fish sauce (no sugar added)

2 tablespoons granulated erythritol

1 pound large shrimp, peeled and deveined

3 cups spiral-sliced daikon noodles (about 10 ounces)

½ cup sliced red bell peppers

1 teaspoon sliced Thai red chili peppers (optional)

1 tablespoon lime juice

¼ cup whole or chopped fresh cilantro leaves, for garnish (optional)

1 Heat the coconut oil in a large sauté pan over medium heat. Add the curry paste and peanut butter and cook for 2 minutes, stirring constantly. Add the coconut milk, fish sauce, and sweetener and cook for 10 more minutes, or until the sauce has thickened and coats the back of a spoon.

2 Add the shrimp, daikon noodles, bell peppers, and Thai chili peppers, if using, and cook for 3 minutes, or until the shrimp have just turned pink; don't overcook the shrimp or they will be tough and dry.

3 Remove from the heat and stir in the lime juice. Serve hot, garnished with cilantro, if desired.

Calories: 355 | Fat: 27g | Protein: 25g | Carbs: 9g | Fiber: 2g | Erythritol: 6g | **Net Carbs: 7g**

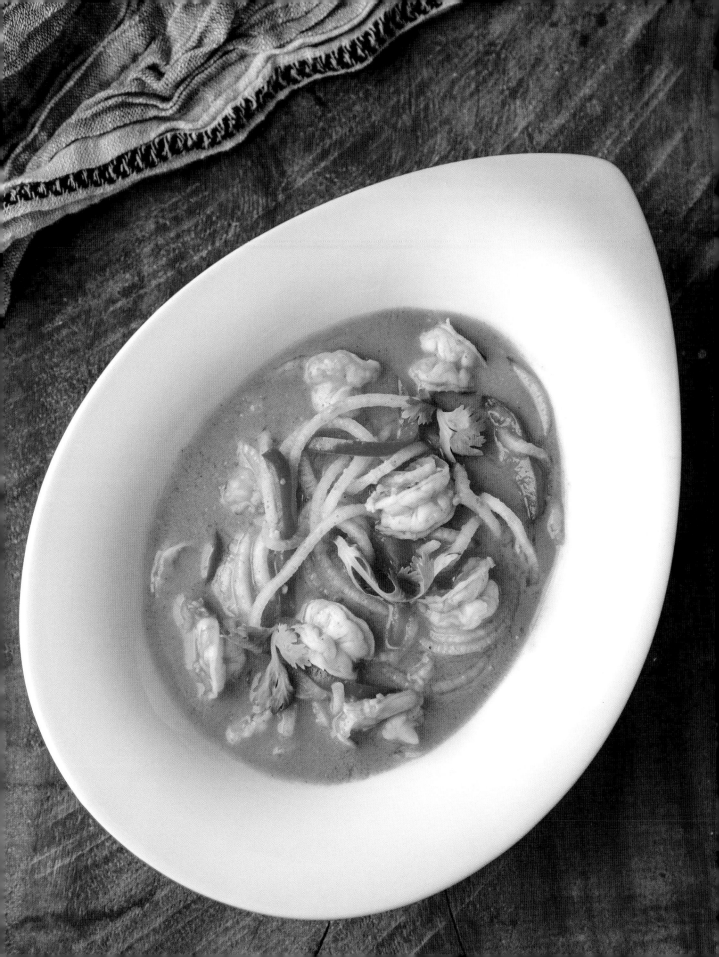

Smoked Salmon Stacks

Great for brunch, for a special lunch, or as a first course for dinner, this recipe doesn't involve any actual cooking. The salty, smoky lox pairs well with the sweet and tangy cucumber and onion and is nicely offset by the creamy avocado and lemon caper dressing. Bonus points for being pretty to look at, too!

Yield: **4 servings**   ◆   Serving Size: **1 stack**   ◆   Prep Time: **15 minutes**

8 ounces cold-smoked salmon (lox style)

1 cup diced cucumbers

1 tablespoon minced red onions

1 teaspoon granulated erythritol

1 teaspoon white vinegar

1 to 2 large ripe Hass avocados, halved and pitted

8 cups spring greens

8 tablespoons Creamy Lemon Caper Dressing (page 92)

1 Chop the salmon into ½-inch pieces.

2 Combine the cucumbers, onions, sweetener, and vinegar in a small bowl.

3 Remove the flesh from the avocados and chop into ½-inch pieces.

4 Assemble the stacks: Spread out 2 cups of spring greens on a salad plate. Pack one-quarter of the chopped salmon into a 4-inch ramekin or dish. Top the salmon with one-quarter of the cucumber-onion mixture, then one-quarter of the chopped avocados. Press the stack down gently to compact the layers but do not mash them out of shape. Carefully turn the ramekin over on the salad greens to unmold the stack.

5 Repeat Step 4 until you have four complete stacks. Drizzle 2 tablespoons of the dressing over each stack and serve.

Alternative Method:
If you don't have a ramekin or don't want to bother with stacking the ingredients, you can spread the greens on a large platter and then scatter the toppings over them and serve the dressing on the side.

Calories: 248 | Fat: 21g | Protein: 12g | Carbs: 5g | Fiber: 3g | Erythritol: 4g | **Net Carbs: 2g**

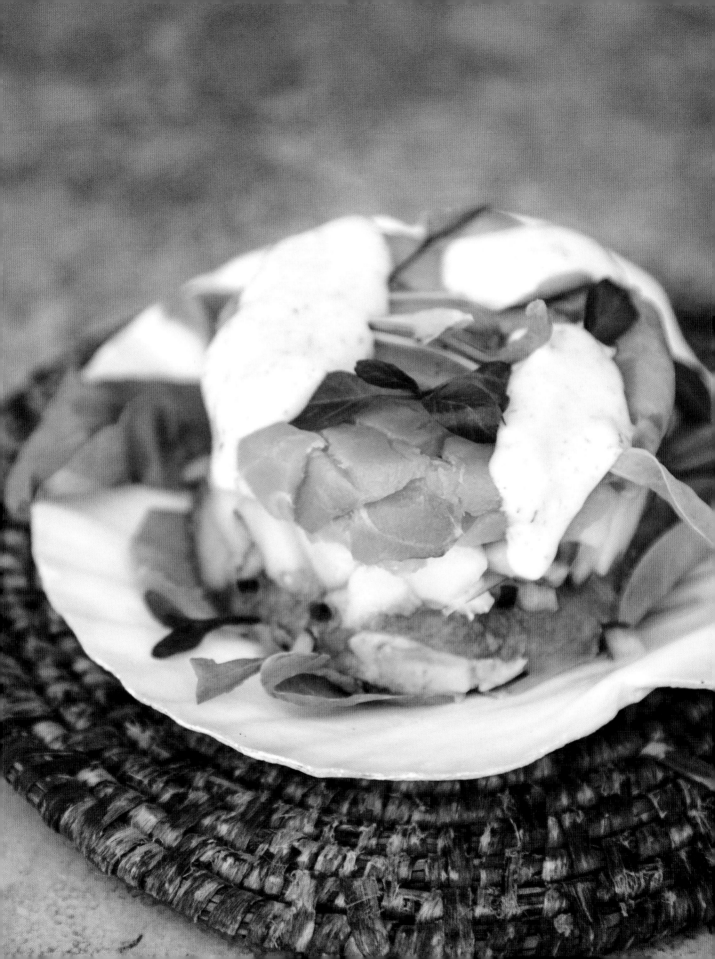

Baked Mahi Mahi in Garlic Parsley Butter

dairy-free · *egg-free* · *nut-free* · *vegetarian*

This is one of those healthy and super easy dinners that can be thrown together in minutes and tossed in the oven while you help your kids finish up their homework. If your brood isn't fond of fish, you can also make this recipe with chicken. Or turn it into a sheet pan dinner by adding some green beans and cherry tomatoes before baking.

Yield: **4 servings** ◆ Prep Time: **5 minutes** ◆ Cook Time: **15 minutes**

3 tablespoons butter, melted

2 tablespoons chopped fresh parsley

1 tablespoon grated lemon zest

1 tablespoon lemon juice

½ teaspoon kosher salt

½ teaspoon minced garlic

1 (1-pound) mahi mahi (or other firm white fish) fillet, cut into 4 pieces

¼ cup Keto Breadcrumbs (page 74)

1 Preheat the oven to 350°F.

2 Place the melted butter, parsley, lemon zest, lemon juice, salt, and garlic in a small bowl and mix well.

3 Place the fish fillets in a small casserole dish. Pour the butter mixture over the fillets. Top the fillets with the keto breadcrumbs. Bake for 15 minutes, or until the fish is flaky and opaque in the center and the tops are golden brown.

4 Remove the fillets from the oven and serve immediately.

Serving Suggestion:
Shown over Basic Cauliflower Rice (page 250).

Calories: 254 | Fat: 23g | Protein: 23g | Carbs: 2g | Fiber: 1g | **Net Carbs: 1g**

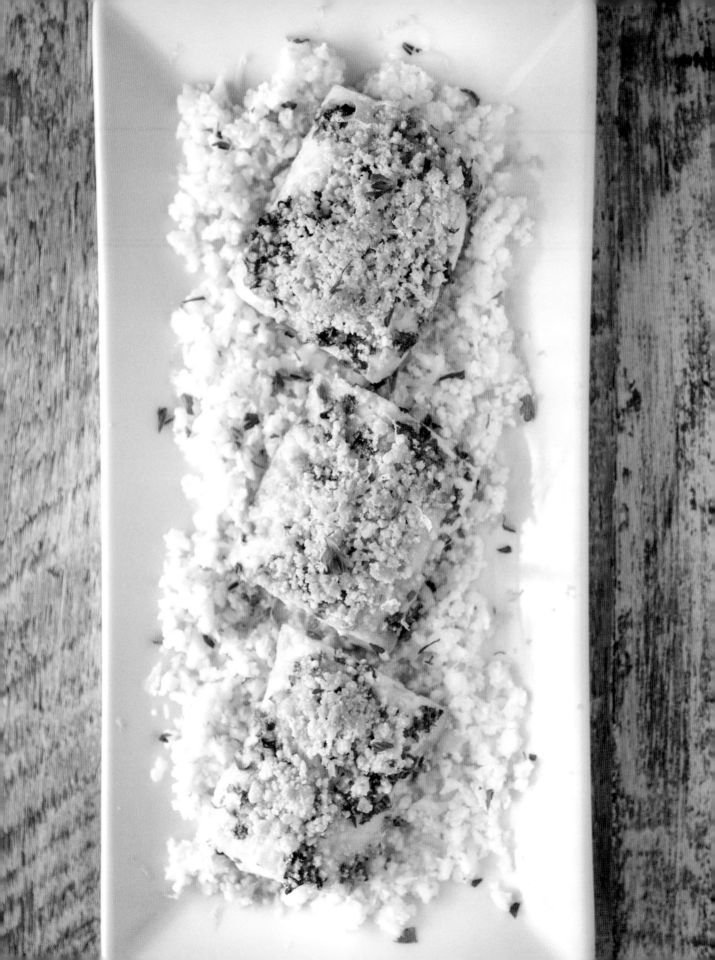

Fish Taco Bowl

Fish tacos are on almost every restaurant menu here in the Caribbean—which is great for me because I love them! If I'm being strict with my macros, I just scrape the toppings off the tortillas and sometimes ask for more cabbage on the side. This Fish Taco Bowl has all of my favorite fish taco flavors and textures, without the carbs.

Yield: **1 serving**   ◆   Prep Time: **8 minutes**   ◆   Cook Time: **8 minutes**

1 tablespoon avocado oil or other light-tasting oil, for the pan

1 (6-ounce) firm white fish fillet

½ teaspoon Cajun Seasoning (page 76)

½ cup shredded green cabbage

¼ cup shredded red cabbage

½ medium cucumber, sliced

½ Hass avocado, sliced

For garnish:

½ tablespoon chopped fresh cilantro

1½ teaspoons finely chopped red onions

2 lime wedges

1   Heat the oil in a medium-sized nonstick skillet for 2 minutes. Season the fish fillet on both sides with the Cajun seasoning.

2   Place the fish fillet in the hot oil and cook for 3 minutes per side, or until golden brown and cooked through. Remove the fish to a serving bowl.

3   Arrange the cabbage, cucumbers, and avocado slices around the fillet. Garnish with the cilantro, onions, and lime wedges before serving.

Calories: 367 | Fat: 21g | Protein: 37g | Carbs: 12g | Fiber: 7g | **Net Carbs: 5g**

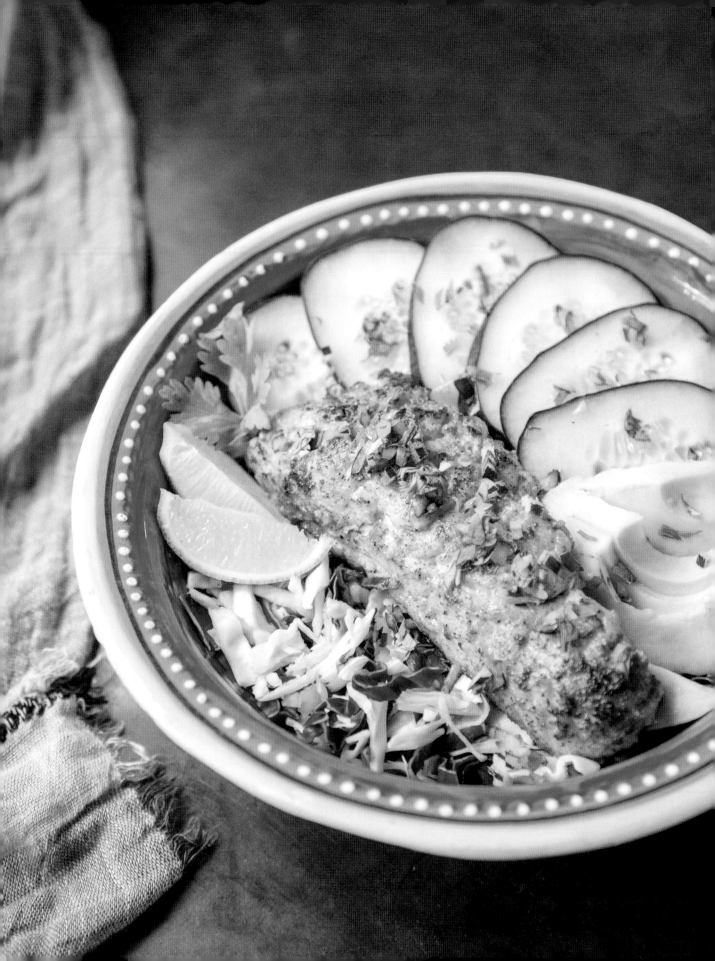

Shrimp Fajitas

I love the smell of fajitas being prepared in Mexican restaurants, and also how you can hear them sizzling on the little cast-iron skillet as the server hurries by to get them to a table. Fun fact about me: I never order fajitas for myself because I hate the taste of green bell peppers! This version is made with yellow and red bell peppers, which I love, and smells just as good as the restaurant version when it's cooking. The Cream Cheese Wraps are a perfect alternative to the typical flour tortillas—or you can skip them and serve the shrimp mixture over cauliflower rice (page 250). However you choose to serve them, adding a few spoonfuls of Restaurant-Style Salsa (page 292) is always a good idea!

Yield: **4 servings** ◆ Serving Size: **2 fajitas** ◆ Prep Time: **15 minutes** ◆ Cook Time: **6 minutes**

1 tablespoon avocado oil or other light-tasting oil, for the pan

1 cup sliced red bell peppers

1 cup sliced yellow bell peppers

½ cup sliced red onions

¼ cup seeded and julienned jalapeño peppers

1 tablespoon ground cumin

1 teaspoon chipotle powder

1 teaspoon ground coriander

1 teaspoon kosher salt

1 teaspoon minced garlic

½ teaspoon ground paprika

¼ teaspoon ground black pepper

1 pound extra-large shrimp, peeled and deveined

2 tablespoons chopped fresh cilantro, plus more for garnish

For the avocado crema:

¼ cup full-fat sour cream

2 tablespoons salsa verde

½ cup chopped avocado

2 batches Cream Cheese Wraps (page 70), for serving

1 Heat the oil in a large sauté pan over high heat. Add the bell peppers, onions, and jalapeño slices and sauté for 2 minutes, or until starting to brown.

2 Lower the heat to medium and add the cumin, chipotle powder, coriander, salt, garlic, paprika, and pepper and cook for 1 minute, or until fragrant and sizzling.

3 Add the shrimp and cook for 3 minutes, or until they have just turned white and pink; don't overcook the shrimp or they will be tough and dry. Remove from the heat and stir in the cilantro.

4 Make the avocado crema: Place the sour cream, salsa verde, and avocado in a small blender and blend for 30 seconds, or until smooth.

5 Assemble the fajitas: Divide the shrimp mixture among the 8 wraps and top with a generous drizzle of avocado crema. Garnish with some chopped cilantro and serve immediately.

6 The shrimp mixture, avocado crema, and wraps can be stored separately in the refrigerator for up to 5 days. Reheat the wraps for 15 seconds in the microwave before using. Reheat the shrimp mixture for 1 minute before assembling and serving.

Calories: 376 | Fat: 17g | Protein: 29g | Carbs: 10g | Fiber: 3g | Net Carbs: 7g

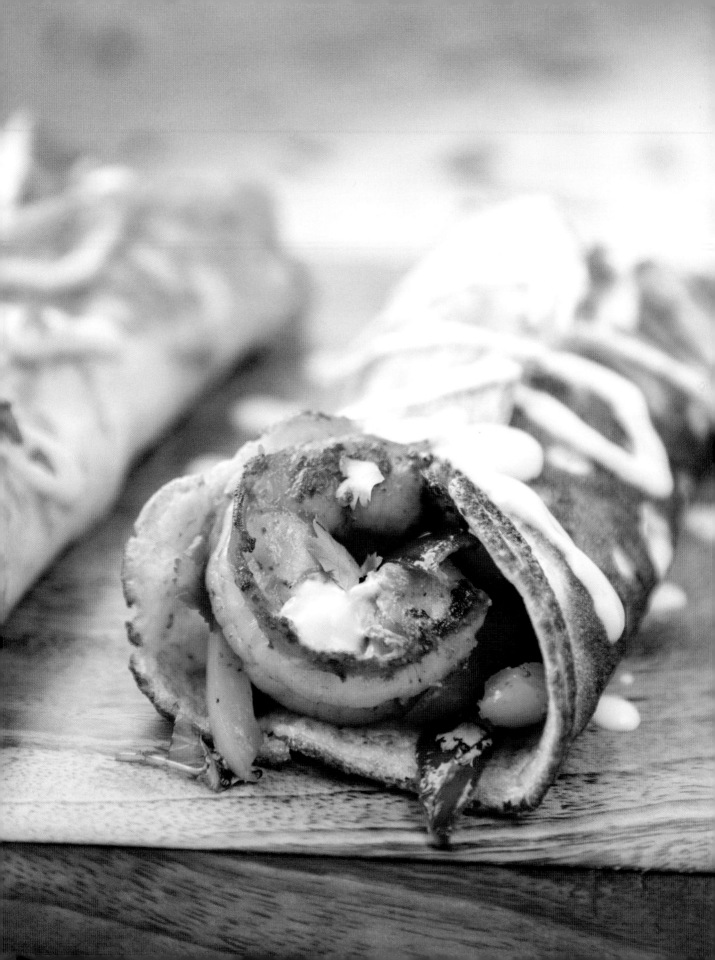

Creamy Lobster Risotto

dairy-free egg-free nut-free vegetarian

Our freezer is always well stocked with lobster tails thanks to Mr. Hungry's spearfishing hobby. But if you have a hard time obtaining lobster, shrimp works just as well in this creamy, decadent risotto made with riced cauliflower (see the variation below). It's perfect for date night, or you can double the recipe if you want to share it with friends.

Yield: **2 servings** ◆ Prep Time: **15 minutes** ◆ Cook Time: **18 minutes**

3 cups salted filtered water

3 (4-ounce) lobster tails

2 tablespoons butter

3 cups riced cauliflower (see page 250)

½ teaspoon kosher salt

¼ teaspoon ground black pepper

⅓ cup dry sherry

2 ounces mascarpone cheese (¼ cup)

¼ cup grated Parmesan cheese

2 tablespoons chopped scallions, plus more for garnish

1 Bring the water to a boil in a medium-sized saucepan. Add the lobster tails and boil for 5 minutes. Remove the lobster tails from the water and let cool. Reserve ¼ cup of the cooking water.

2 Remove the lobster meat from the tails and slice in half lengthwise (reserve two of the lobster tail shells for garnish, if desired). Keep two of the lobster tail halves intact for garnish and chop the other four halves into bite-sized pieces.

3 Melt the butter in a large sauté pan over medium heat. Add the riced cauliflower, salt, and pepper. Cook for 3 minutes, or until the cauliflower is starting to soften. Add the sherry and reserved lobster broth and cook for 3 minutes, or until the liquid is mostly absorbed. Stir in the mascarpone, Parmesan, scallions, and chopped lobster and cook for 2 more minutes.

4 Remove from the heat and divide between 2 serving bowls. Top each bowl with a lobster tail half, set inside the reserved shell, if desired. Garnish with additional chopped scallions and serve immediately.

Variation:

Creamy Shrimp Risotto. To make this recipe with peeled and deveined jumbo shrimp, replace the lobster broth with chicken or vegetable broth, then add the shrimp in Step 3, along with the cheese and scallions, and cook for about 3 minutes, until just done.

Calories: 449 | Fat: 30g | Protein: 41g | Carbs: 8g | Fiber: 3g | **Net Carbs: 5g**

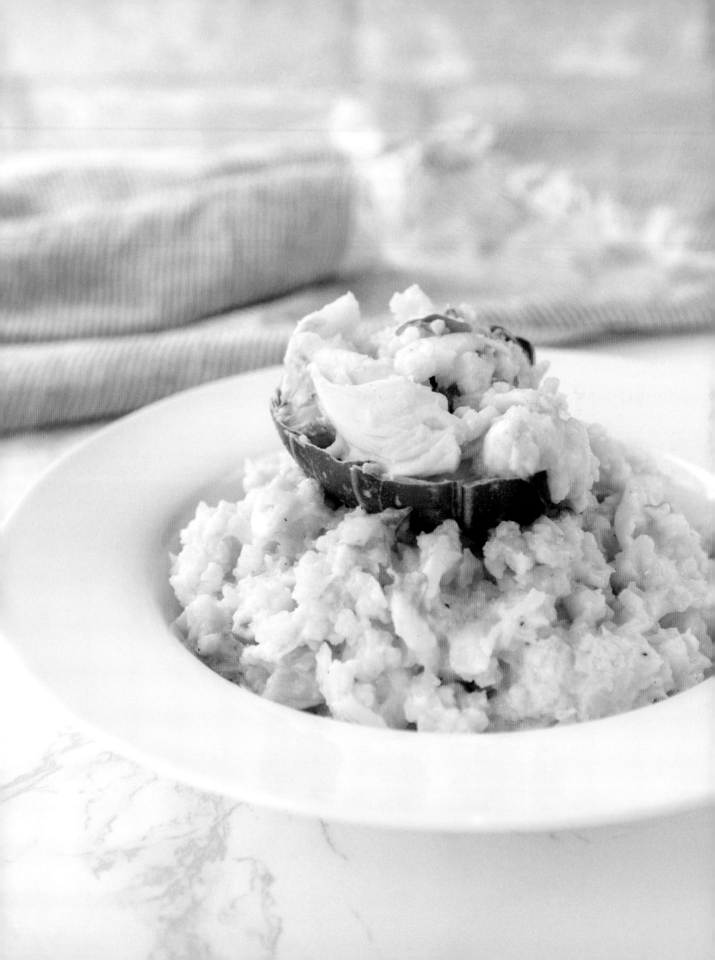

dairy-free egg-free nut-free vegetarian

Spicy Shrimp–Stuffed Avocados

Super easy to make, these stuffed avocados have all of your favorite sushi flavors without the carbs or the raw fish—perfect for brunch or a quick lunch at the office!

Yield: **4 servings**   •   Serving Size: **½ avocado and ½ cup spicy shrimp**

Prep Time: **5 minutes, plus 10 minutes to chill**

---

1 pound large shrimp, peeled, deveined, and cooked (tails removed)

⅓ cup sugar-free mayonnaise

2 tablespoons Sriracha sauce

1 teaspoon chopped fresh cilantro, plus more for garnish if desired

1 teaspoon lime juice

2 large ripe Hass avocados

1 Chop the shrimp into bite-sized pieces and place in a medium-sized bowl.

2 Add the mayonnaise, Sriracha, cilantro, and lime juice. Mix until well combined. Place in the refrigerator to chill for 10 minutes.

3 Just before serving, cut the avocados in half and remove the pits. Spoon ½ cup of the spicy shrimp mixture into each avocado half. Serve immediately, garnished with extra cilantro, if desired. If not consuming it right away, store the spicy shrimp mixture in the refrigerator for up to 5 days.

Calories: 334 | Fat: 29g | Protein: 15g | Carbs: 8g | Fiber: 5g | **Net Carbs: 3g**

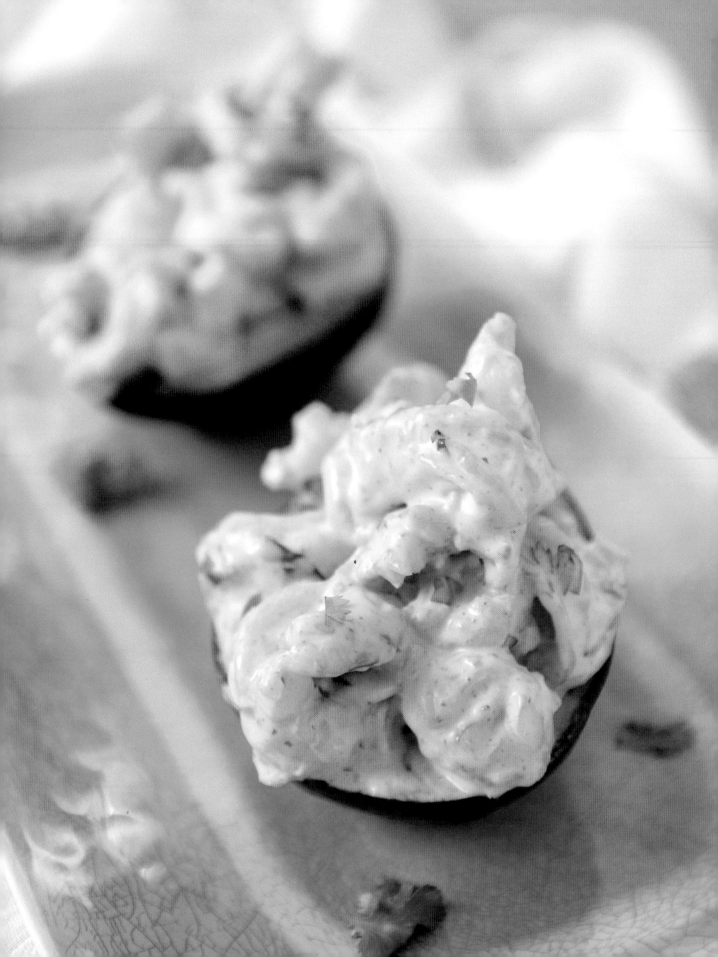

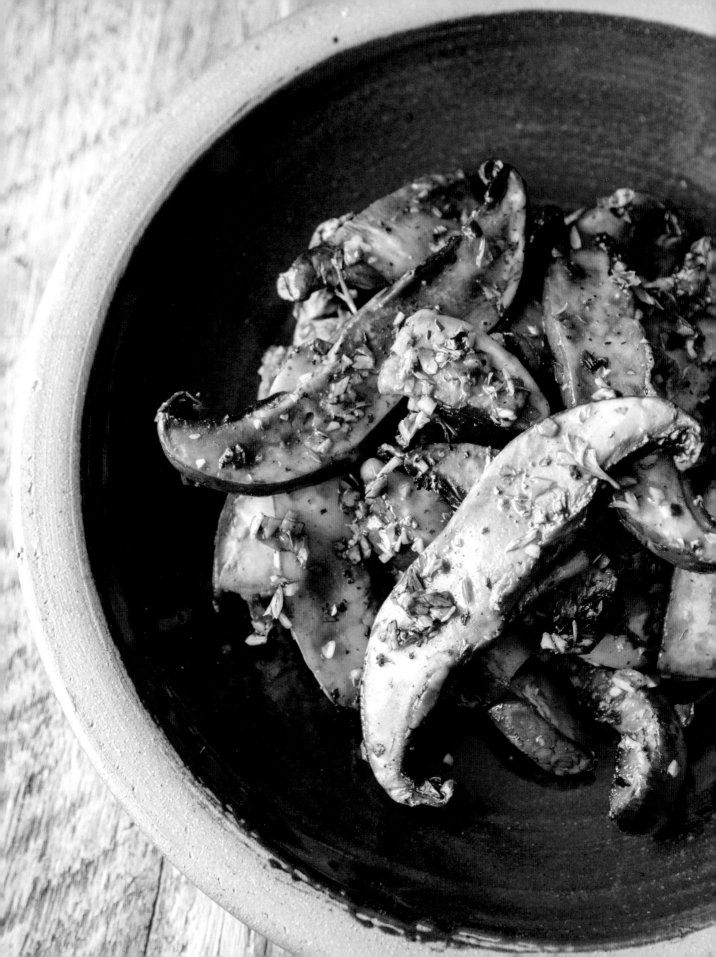

veggie mains & sides

How to Build the Perfect Keto Salad / 248

Basic Cauliflower Rice / 250

Basic Zucchini Noodles (Zoodles) / 252

Eggplant Parmigiana / 254

Cauliflower Risotto with Sherry & Hazelnuts / 256

Vegetarian Pad Thai / 258

Vegetable Lasagna / 260

Faux-tuccini Alfredo with Broccoli / 262

Zoodles with Creamy Roasted Red Pepper Sauce / 264

Faux-lafel / 266

Braised Red Cabbage / 268

Cheesy Cauliflower Grits / 269

Marinated Portobello Mushrooms / 270

Cheesy Cauliflower Puree / 272

Sweet Sesame Glazed Bok Choy / 274

Orange & Tarragon Coleslaw / 276

Creamed Spinach / 278

Sautéed Green Beans with Walnuts / 279

Spicy Jicama Shoestring Fries / 280

Sautéed Mushrooms / 281

How to Build the Perfect Keto Salad

You may notice that I don't have any typical salad recipes in this cookbook. It's not because I don't eat salad but because there are so many variations that it's easier to give you the tools to unleash your inner salad chef than to restrict you with a few recipes that you probably could have figured out on your own anyway.

With the many versatile salad dressing recipes in this book (see pages 86 to 94), you can make a bed of lettuce and low-carb veggies, then throw some of your favorite protein on top to turn it into a healthy and delicious keto lunch or dinner.

Not all salads are created equal, though. The following examples show both the wrong way and, more importantly, the right way to build the perfect keto salad.

Keto Salad Fail

You might have had the best intentions when making this tasty and technically healthy salad, but not paying attention to the carb counts of the ingredients you choose can add a lot of carbs and derail your keto efforts. You think you're on the right track with this salad—after all, you skipped your favorite raisins, peas, tortilla strips, and sweet salad dressing. You even used kale instead of iceberg lettuce for the health benefits! Let's see how it shakes out:

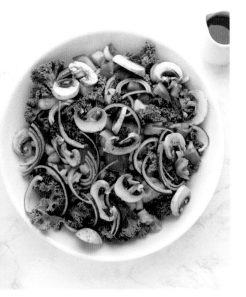

Ingredient	Net Carbs
2 cups chopped kale	10g
1 cup chopped tomatoes	5g
¼ cup diced red onions	3.5g
½ cup sliced cremini mushrooms	1.1g
2 tablespoons lemon juice	2.6g
1 tablespoon olive oil	0g

This pretty basic salad has 22.2 grams of net carbs. You just blew your budget for the entire day—on a salad!

Keto Salad Win

Let's see how being carb-savvy makes all the difference:

Ingredient	Net Carbs
2 cups spring greens	1.4g
½ cup sliced cucumbers	1.5g
½ cup sliced celery	0.9g
½ cup chopped avocado	1g
2 tablespoons chopped bacon	0g
2 tablespoons chopped hard-boiled egg	0.2g
2 tablespoons Bacon & Tomato Dressing (page 89)	0.5g

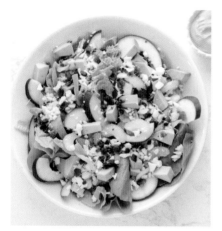

This huge salad, with lots of flavor and satiating fat, has 5.5 grams of net carbs. You just ate an entire healthy keto-friendly salad for around the same amount of carbs that's in a single cup of raw kale!

This dramatic example proves that paying attention to carbs on keto is very important and that seemingly small changes can make a huge difference. Veggies that are considered "free" or of no consequence on a low-fat or low-calorie diet can be high enough in carbs to kick you out of ketosis if you aren't measuring or are inadvertently making the wrong choices.

Salad Bar Tips

When eating out, the salad bar is often a great option for a keto-friendly meal. (See page 26 for more about eating out on keto.) Here are some helpful hints for making the best selections at salad bars:

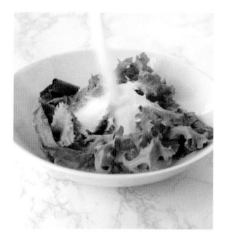

- Go with a creamy dressing like ranch, blue cheese, or Parmesan peppercorn. Avoid vinaigrettes, which can contain quite a bit of sugar.

- Avoid processed bacon bits, which usually contain fillers. If it looks like real cooked bacon, go for it!

- Skip the coleslaw; even in a creamy dressing, it's usually loaded with sugar.

- Never add peas, carrots, or beans.

- Avoid pickled vegetables because those are usually sugar-sweetened.

Basic Cauliflower Rice

Cauliflower rice is a blank canvas for so many delicious flavors, be they Asian, Mexican, or even Italian in some cases. There is no end to what you can do to it, so I've left it basic and unseasoned here. The recipes in this book that call for this rice all have a sauce or broth that will season the rice perfectly.

Yield: **6 servings** • Serving Size: **½ cup** • Prep Time: **5 minutes** • Cook Time: **6 minutes**

1 medium head cauliflower

1   Trim the cauliflower of any leaves and cut into florets, discarding the woody stems.

2   To rice the cauliflower, place the cauliflower florets in a blender and add enough water to cover. Pulse until the cauliflower resembles rice or large crumbles.

3   Pour the cauliflower and water through a large fine-mesh strainer. The water will pour out, leaving you with perfectly riced cauliflower.

4   To cook the riced cauliflower, transfer it to a medium-sized microwave-safe bowl. Microwave, uncovered, on high for 4 minutes. Stir and return the bowl to the microwave. Cook on high for 2 more minutes and stir again. Test for doneness and microwave for 1 more minute if you prefer it softer. Season as desired.

5   If not using the riced cauliflower immediately, store in an airtight container in the refrigerator for up to 5 days or in the freezer for up to 3 months. To reheat, thaw if frozen and microwave on high for 1 minute per cup of rice.

Calories: 10 | Fat: 0g | Protein: 1g | Carbs: 2g | Fiber: 1g | **Net Carbs: 1g**

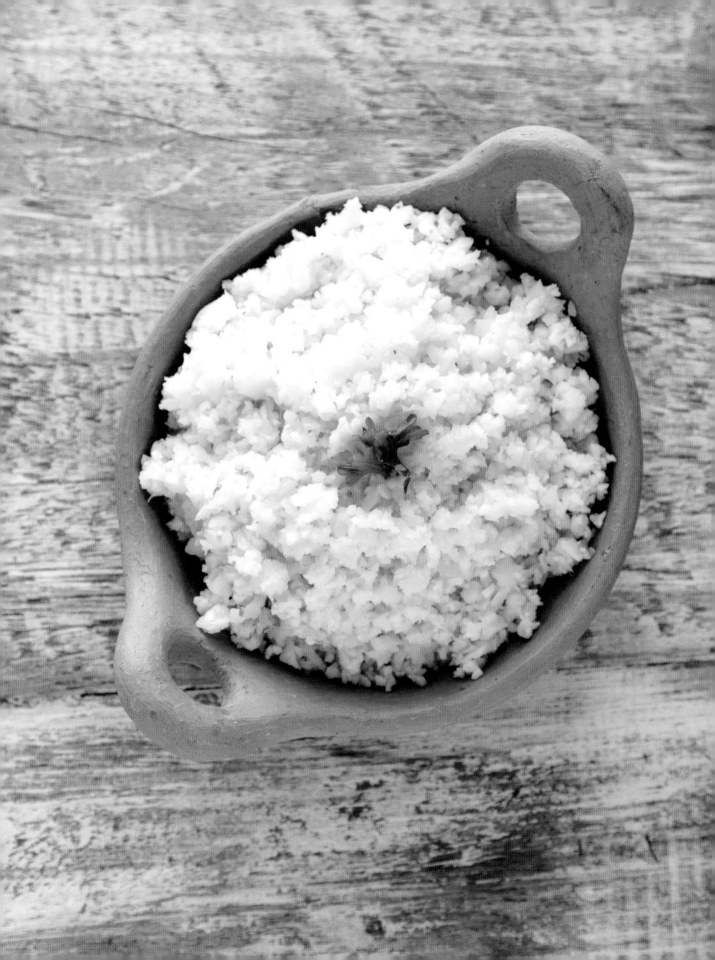

Basic Zucchini Noodles (Zoodles)

dairy-free egg-free nut-free vegetarian

I want to hug the person who first thought of turning zucchini into noodles. It's a truly genius idea that has kept me from giving in to regular pasta more times than I can count! Bonus points that zucchini is inexpensive and available year-round in most places. Making zoodles is also a fun job to get kids involved in the cooking process—just make sure they keep their hands away from the blades.

Yield: **4 servings** ◆ Serving Size: **1 cup** ◆ Prep Time: **5 minutes** ◆ Cook Time: **2 minutes**

2 medium zucchini

Special equipment:
Spiral slicer

1 Trim the ends from the zucchini. Following the manufacturer's instructions for your spiral slicer, cut the zucchini into noodles.

2 Place the zucchini noodles in a large microwave-safe bowl and microwave, uncovered, on high for 2 minutes. Meanwhile, line a colander with paper towels.

3 Remove the bowl from the microwave and place the zoodles in the lined strainer. Place another paper towel over the top of the zoodles and press down firmly for about 10 seconds to remove the excess moisture. Serve immediately, or store in an airtight container in the refrigerator for up to 3 days. To reheat, microwave on high for 1 minute per cup of zoodles.

Calories: 21 | Fat: 0g | Protein: 2g | Carbs: 4g | Fiber: 1g | Net Carbs: 3g

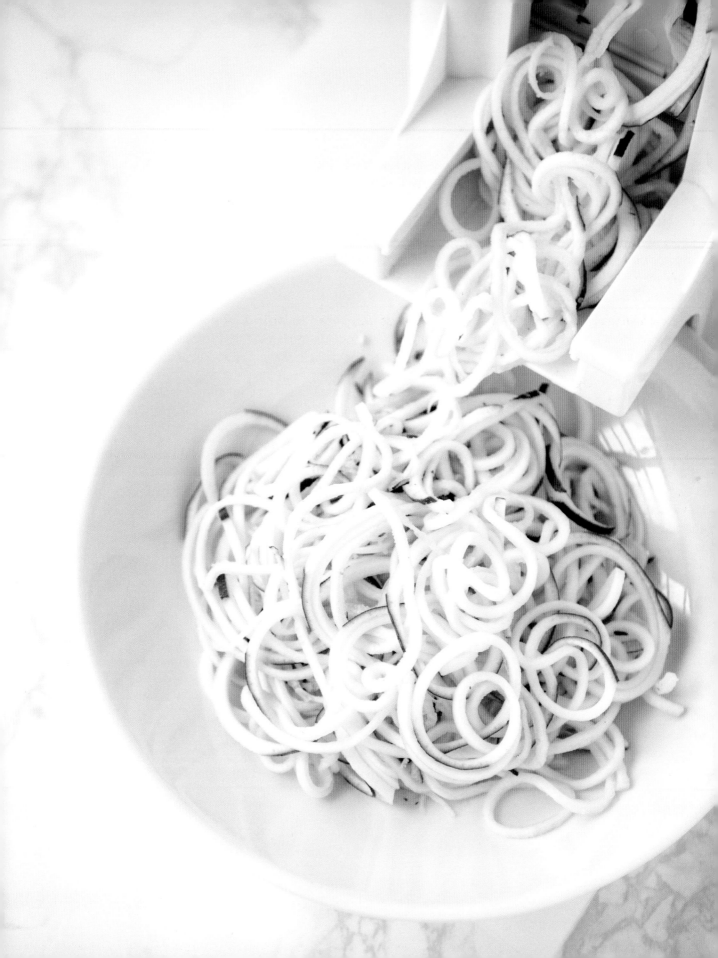

Eggplant Parmigiana

Eggplant parmigiana is one of my favorite meals. Crunchy on the outside, soft and creamy on the inside, it's comfort food in the extreme! This recipe calls for my basic breading, which uses seasoned almond flour and Parmesan cheese, in place of the traditional breadcrumb coating. You can assemble this as a casserole or, if you want to get fancy with it, in individual towers, as shown.

Yield: 4 servings • Prep Time: **10 minutes, plus 1 hour to sweat eggplant**

Cook Time: **45 minutes**

2 medium eggplants

Kosher salt

¼ cup extra-virgin olive oil, for frying

1 large egg, beaten

1 batch Basic Breading (page 75)

1½ cups marinara sauce, store-bought or homemade (page 106)

8 ounces fresh mozzarella cheese, cut into ¼-inch-thick slices

Fresh basil leaves, for garnish

1 Peel the eggplants and slice into ½-inch-thick rounds. Line a colander with paper towels and place a layer of eggplant slices in the colander. Generously sprinkle that layer with salt and place a paper towel on top of the salted eggplant to absorb the liquid. Repeat with the rest of the eggplant slices. Place the colander in the sink and let the eggplant sit for 1 hour.

2 Rinse the salt off of the eggplant and press the slices between more paper towels to remove as much moisture as possible.

3 Heat the olive oil in a large skillet over medium heat for 2 minutes. Line a plate with paper towels.

4 Preheat the oven to 375°F.

5 Dip the eggplant slices first in the beaten egg and then in the basic breading, being sure to coat both sides. Add the eggplant in batches to the hot oil and cook until golden brown, about 2 minutes per side. Remove the cooked slices to the lined plate and repeat until all of the eggplant slices are fried.

6 Spread a couple of tablespoons of marinara on the bottom of an 8-inch square baking pan. Cover with a layer of the fried eggplant slices.

7 Spread one-third of the remaining marinara onto the first eggplant layer, followed by one-third of the mozzarella cheese. Repeat 2 more times, until you have 3 layers.

8 Bake for 30 minutes, or until the cheese is browning and the sauce is bubbling. Cut into 4 equal-sized pieces, garnish with the basil, and serve hot.

Calories: 402 | Fat: 33g | Protein: 20g | Carbs: 16g | Fiber: 9g | **Net Carbs: 7g**

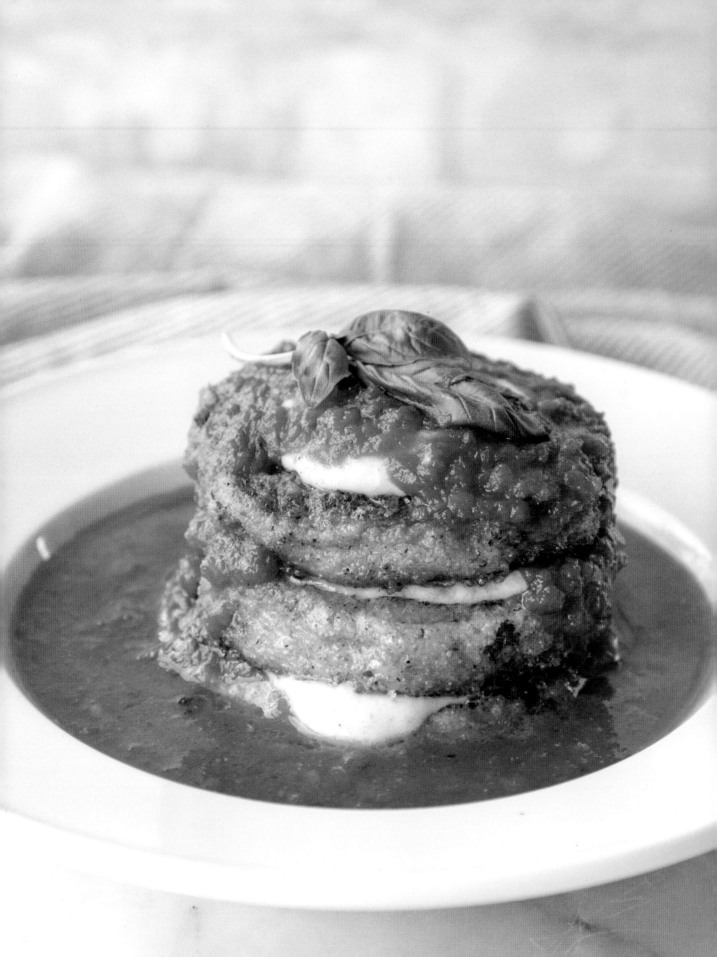

Cauliflower Risotto with Sherry & Hazelnuts

dairy-free · egg-free · nut-free · vegetarian

Creamy and rich, this cauliflower-based risotto is perfect for entertaining or special occasions but so easy and fast to make that you can indulge anytime. This is easily in the top ten of the most delicious keto recipes I've ever created, and I can't wait for you to try it!

Yield: **2 servings** ◆ Serving Size: **1⅓ cups** ◆ Prep Time: **5 minutes** ◆ Cook Time: **15 minutes**

2 tablespoons butter

½ teaspoon fresh thyme leaves, plus more for garnish if desired

½ teaspoon minced garlic

3 cups riced cauliflower (see page 250)

½ teaspoon kosher salt

¼ teaspoon ground black pepper

⅓ cup dry sherry

¼ cup grated Parmesan cheese, plus more for garnish if desired

¼ cup mascarpone cheese (2 ounces)

¼ cup chopped raw hazelnuts

1 Melt the butter in a large sauté pan over medium heat. Add the thyme and garlic and cook for 1 minute, or until fragrant.

2 Add the riced cauliflower, salt, and pepper and cook for 3 minutes, or until the cauliflower is beginning to soften. Add the sherry and cook for another 5 minutes, or until the cauliflower has absorbed almost all of the liquid.

3 Stir in the Parmesan and mascarpone cheeses and cook, stirring occasionally, until melted and creamy, about 3 minutes.

4 Stir in the hazelnuts, then remove from the heat. Garnish with thyme leaves and more Parmesan cheese, if desired. Serve hot.

Calories: 403 | Fat: 32g | Protein: 9g | Carbs: 11g | Fiber: 5g | **Net Carbs: 6g**

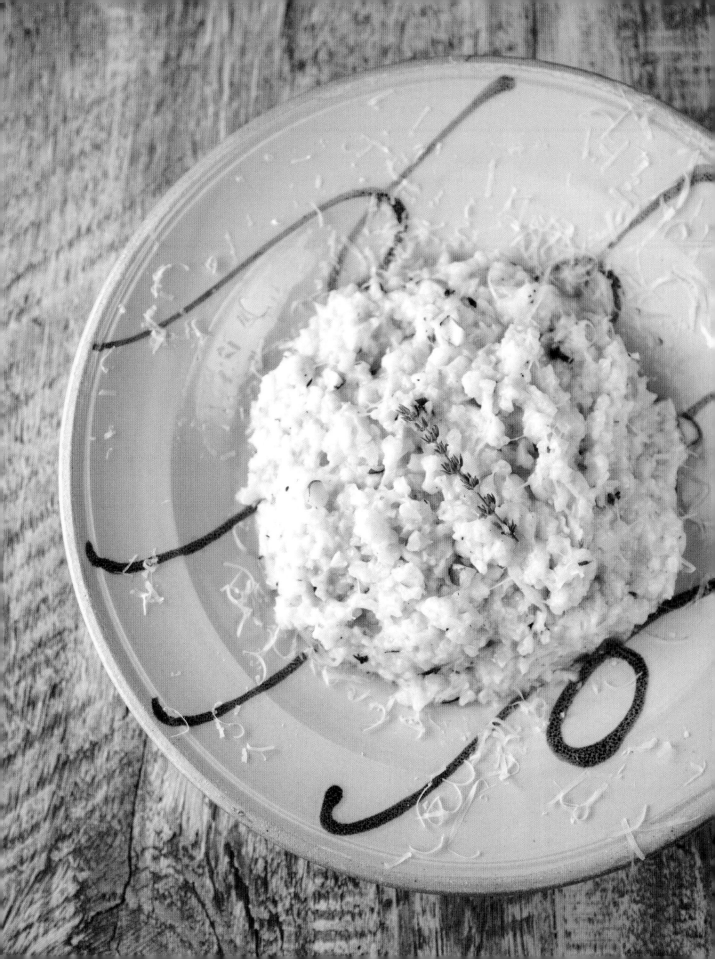

dairy-free egg-free nut-free vegetarian

Vegetarian Pad Thai

If you love Asian flavors like I do, then you'll be a huge fan of this keto pad Thai! It's loaded with crunchy vegetables and nuts, pungent fresh herbs, and a creamy almond butter sauce flavored with ginger and a hint of spice. Salty and sweet, this vegetarian pad Thai makes a great side, but it's also hearty enough to serve as a main dish. That being said, you can easily add some cooked chicken or shrimp if you like.

Yield: **3 servings as a main, 6 servings as a side** ◆ Serving Size: **2 cups as a main, 1 cup as a side**

Prep Time: **10 minutes**

2 cups spiral-cut daikon noodles

4 cups chopped napa cabbage

1 cup chopped red cabbage

¼ cup chopped fresh cilantro

¼ cup slivered almonds

For the dressing:

½ cup filtered water

¼ cup natural almond butter (no sugar added)

2 tablespoons peeled and minced fresh ginger

1 tablespoon fish sauce (no sugar added) or coconut aminos for strict vegetarian or vegan

1 tablespoon granulated erythritol

1 tablespoon lime juice

1 tablespoon toasted sesame oil

1 tablespoon wheat-free soy sauce

1 teaspoon minced garlic

½ teaspoon kosher salt

¼ teaspoon cayenne pepper

1 Combine the daikon noodles, cabbage, cilantro, and almonds in a large bowl.

2 Place the dressing ingredients in a small blender and blend until smooth. Pour the dressing over the vegetables and toss well to coat. Serve immediately.

3 Store any leftovers in an airtight container in the refrigerator for up to 5 days.

per 1-cup side dish serving: Calories: 145 | Fat: 10g | Protein: 5g | Carbs: 7g | Fiber: 3g | Erythritol: 2g **Net Carbs: 4g**

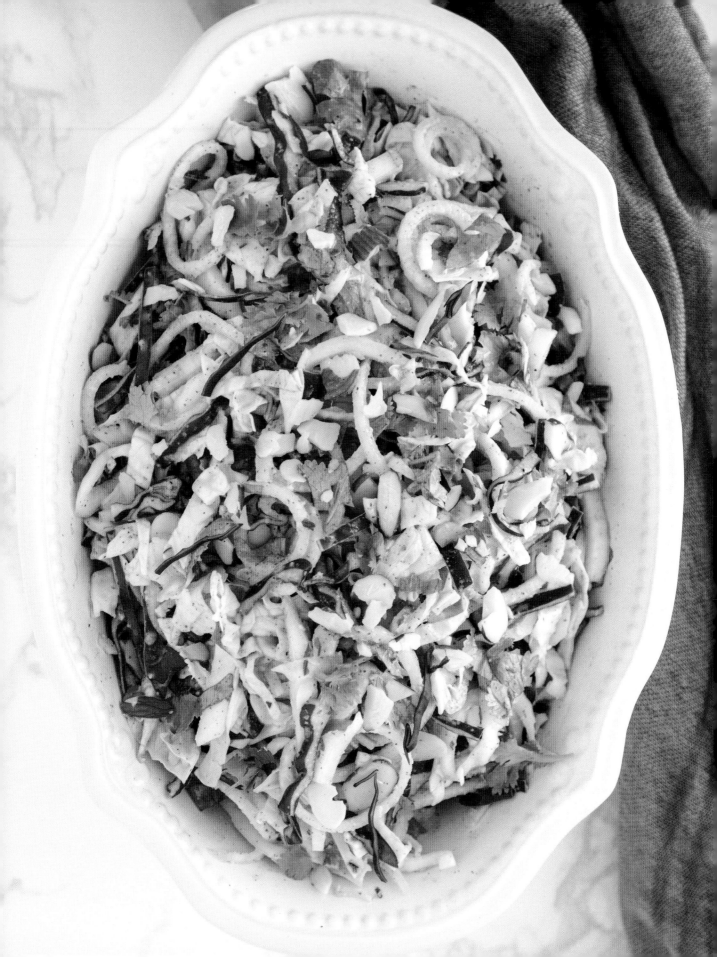

dairy-free egg-free nut-free vegetarian

Vegetable Lasagna

Who doesn't love a hearty, cheesy lasagna? In this version, my Cream Cheese Wraps stand in for the noodles, and it's virtually impossible to tell the difference. It's also loaded with healthy vegetables, but because they are chopped small and smothered in sauce and cheese, even my veggie-phobic guys always go for seconds!

Yield: **8 servings** ◆ Prep Time: **20 minutes** ◆ Cook Time: **1 hour 5 minutes**

For the vegetable filling:

2 tablespoons extra-virgin olive oil

1 tablespoon butter

1 cup chopped white mushrooms

2 cups chopped zucchini

1 cup frozen chopped spinach, thawed and drained

½ cup chopped yellow onions

1 tablespoon minced garlic

½ teaspoon kosher salt

¼ teaspoon ground black pepper

⅛ teaspoon ground nutmeg

For the cheese filling:

1½ cups whole-milk ricotta cheese

⅓ cup grated Parmesan cheese

1 large egg, beaten

½ teaspoon kosher salt

¼ teaspoon ground black pepper

1 tablespoon dried parsley leaves

3 batches Cream Cheese Wraps (page 70)

1½ cups marinara sauce, store-bought or homemade (page 106)

1½ cups shredded whole-milk mozzarella cheese

1 Make the vegetable filling: Heat the olive oil and butter in a large skillet over medium heat for 2 minutes. Add the mushrooms to the hot oil and cook, stirring occasionally, until golden brown and fragrant, about 5 minutes.

2 Add the zucchini, spinach, onions, garlic, salt, pepper, and nutmeg to the mushrooms and stir well. Cook 8 minutes, stirring occasionally, until the zucchini and onions have softened. Remove from the heat and set aside.

3 Make the cheese filling: Place the ricotta and Parmesan cheeses, egg, salt, pepper, and parsley in a medium-sized bowl and mix well.

4 Preheat the oven to 375°F. Grease the bottom and sides of an 8-inch springform pan.

5 Place 4 cream cheese wraps in the bottom of the greased pan. Make sure the bottom of the pan is completely covered; you may overlap them, if necessary, and cut off any extra.

6 Spread approximately one-half of the vegetable filling evenly over the wraps. Top with approximately one-half of the cheese filling, spread evenly, then top with ½ cup of the marinara and ½ cup of the mozzarella.

7 Start a new layer of 4 wraps, cutting off any excess. Spread the remaining vegetable filling evenly over the wrap layer. Top with the remaining cheese filling, spread evenly, then top with ½ cup of the marinara and ½ cup of the mozzarella.

Special equipment:

8-inch springform pan

Calories: 463 | Fat: 34g | Protein: 24g | Carbs: 10g | Fiber: 3g | **Net Carbs: 7g**

8 Add the final layer of wraps, cutting off any excess. Press down gently to remove any air space in the layers. Top with the remaining marinara and mozzarella.

9 Bake for 50 minutes, or until golden brown on top and bubbling at the edges. Remove the lasagna from the oven and let it rest for 30 minutes to firm up. When ready to serve, run a knife around the inside edge of the pan, then release the clamp and remove the side of the pan. Cut into wedges and serve warm.

Variation:

Classic Lasagna. To make this into a classic lasagna, simply omit the vegetable filling and replace it with a meat filling. Double the amount of marinara and add 1 pound of cooked ground beef and 4 links of cooked and chopped Italian sausage to the marinara. Assemble as follows: (1) 4 cream cheese wraps, (2) one-third of the cheese filling, (3) one-third of the meat sauce, (4) one-third of the mozzarella. Repeat twice and bake at 375°F as directed in Step 9.

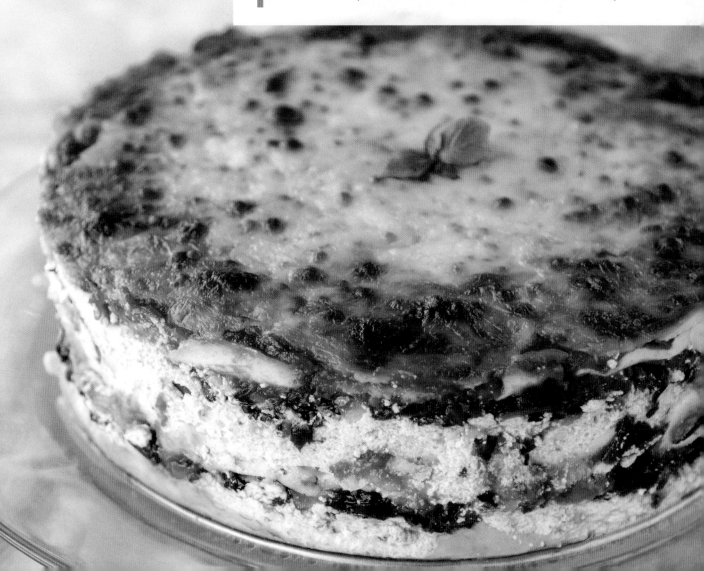

Faux-tuccini Alfredo with Broccoli

dairy-free *egg-free* *nut-free* *vegetarian*

This faux-tuccini Alfredo is always a crowd-pleaser and can be customized in a variety of ways, depending on your family's preferences. If your crew hates broccoli, then leave it out and serve the faux-tuccini with a salad or the vegetable of your choice on the side.

Yield: **4 servings** • Serving Size: **1½ cups** • Prep Time: **5 minutes**

1 batch Cream Cheese Noodles (page 72)

1 batch 5-Minute Alfredo Sauce (page 107)

2 cups broccoli florets

1 tablespoon water

Place the noodles and Alfredo sauce in a medium-sized bowl and gently fold to coat. Place the broccoli in a microwave-safe bowl with the water. Cover and microwave on high for 4 to 5 minutes, until fork-tender. Gently stir the cooked broccoli into the noodles and sauce and serve warm.

> **Note:**
> *This recipe is vegetarian, but you can easily add grilled chicken or shrimp if you prefer it with a protein.*

Calories: 400 | Fat: 36g | Protein: 12g | Carbs: 5.5g | Fiber: 1.5g | **Net Carbs: 4g**

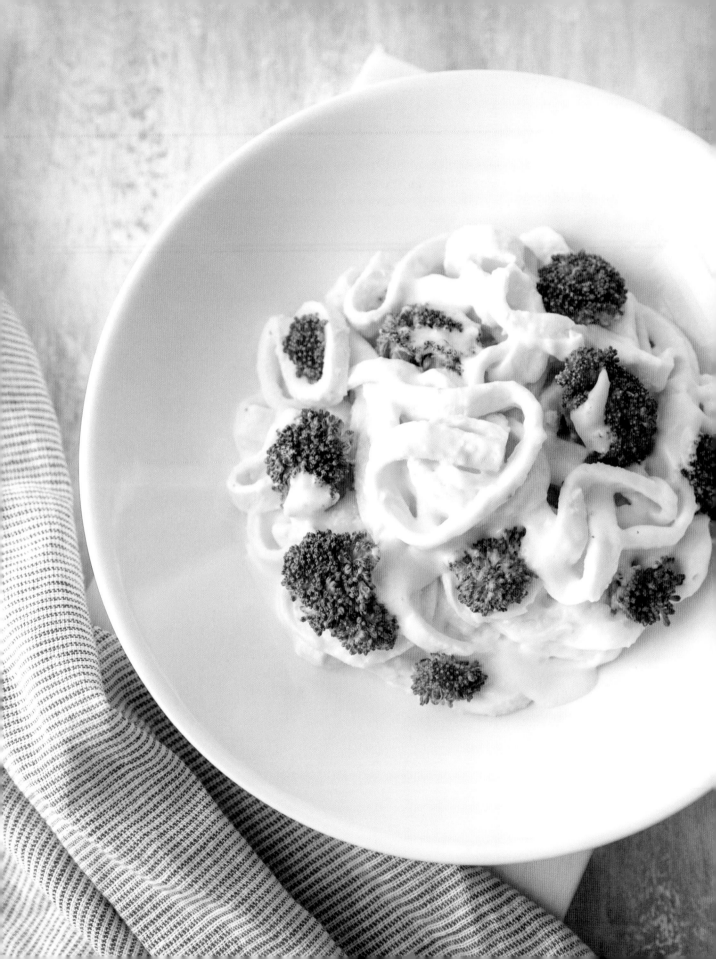

Zoodles with Creamy Roasted Red Pepper Sauce

This roasted red pepper sauce is so creamy and flavorful that I could eat it with a spoon. Paired with zoodles, it is my favorite weeknight meal—partly because it's so easy and fast to make, but mostly because it's straight-up delicious! A fantastic side dish or vegetarian main as is, it becomes over-the-top amazing with cooked Italian sausage mixed into it.

Yield: **2 servings as a main, 4 servings as a side** • Serving Size: **2 cups as a main, 1 cup as a side**

Prep Time: **5 minutes** • Cook Time: **1 minute**

¼ cup jarred roasted red peppers, drained

2 tablespoons grated Parmesan cheese

2 tablespoons heavy whipping cream

1 teaspoon minced garlic

⅓ cup mascarpone cheese (3 ounces)

Kosher salt and ground black pepper

4 cups Basic Zucchini Noodles (page 252)

1   In a small blender, blend the roasted red peppers, Parmesan, cream, and garlic until smooth, then transfer the mixture to a medium-sized microwave-safe bowl.

2   Add the mascarpone and microwave on high for 1 minute. Whisk until smooth. Season to taste with salt and pepper.

3   Add the zoodles to the sauce and toss to coat. Divide between 2 bowls and serve.

Note:
This recipe can easily be doubled or tripled for larger groups. To make it heartier, add cooked chicken or Italian sausage to the sauce before serving.

Family-Friendly Tip:
If serving this dish to nonketo family or friends, you can pour the sauce over cooked pasta for them and serve it over zoodles for yourself.

Variation:
Zoodles with Zesty Roasted Red Pepper Sauce. *To make this dish spicy, add ½ teaspoon of red pepper flakes to the sauce in Step 2.*

per 2-cup main dish serving: Calories: 283 | Fat: 24g | Protein: 6g | Carbs: 10g | Fiber: 3g | **Net Carbs: 7g**

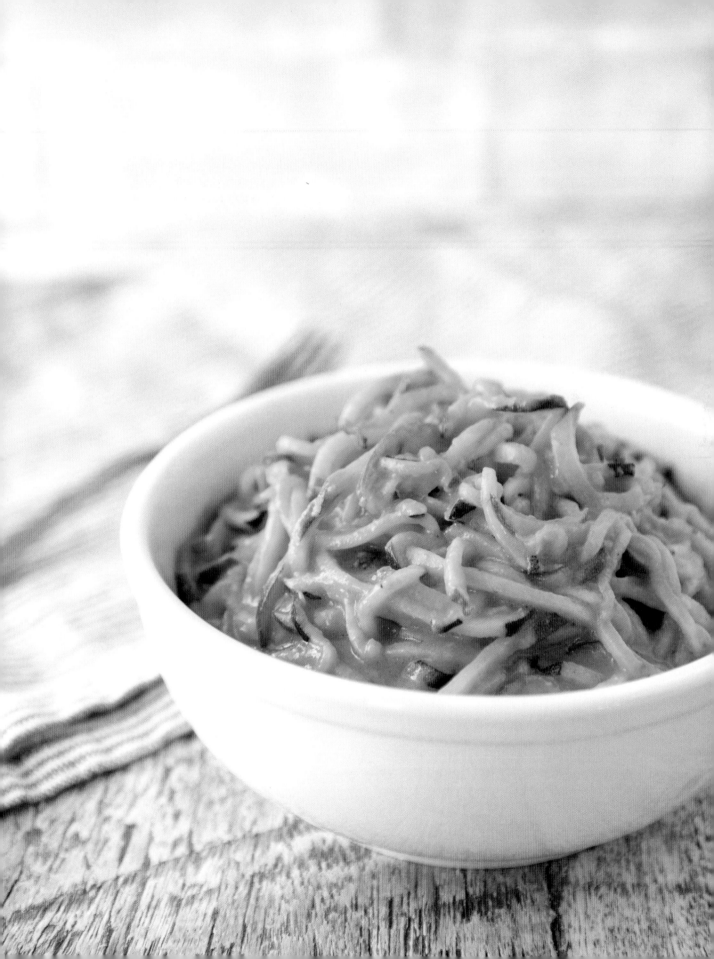

Faux-lafel

I created this recipe years ago when I was desperate for falafel one day. I thought the cauliflower and almonds might work, but even I was surprised at how authentic the "faux-lafel" were in both texture and flavor. Years and hundreds of blog comments later, this recipe is still insanely popular. Even sworn cauliflower-hater Mr. Hungry likes it and admits that he can't detect the cauliflower at all!

Yield: **4 servings** • Serving Size: **2 patties** • Prep Time: **8 minutes** • Cook Time: **16 minutes**

3 cups raw cauliflower florets

½ cup blanched slivered almonds

3 tablespoons coconut flour

2 tablespoons chopped fresh parsley

1 tablespoon ground cumin

1½ teaspoons ground coriander

1 teaspoon kosher salt

1 teaspoon minced garlic

½ teaspoon cayenne pepper

2 large eggs

¼ cup avocado oil or other light-tasting oil, for the pan

1   Place the cauliflower and almonds in a food processor and process until mostly smooth. Add the coconut flour, parsley, cumin, coriander, salt, garlic, cayenne, and eggs and pulse until well blended.

2   Form the mixture into 8 patties about 3 inches in diameter and 1 inch thick. Heat the avocado oil in a large nonstick skillet over medium heat.

3   Fry 4 patties at a time for about 4 minutes per side, until golden brown and crisp.

Serving Suggestion:

Serve the patties on shredded lettuce with sliced cherry tomatoes. Drizzle with the dressing of your choice and garnish with fresh parsley, if desired.

Calories: 247 | Fat: 19g | Protein: 10g | Carbs: 11g | Fiber: 5g | **Net Carbs: 6g**

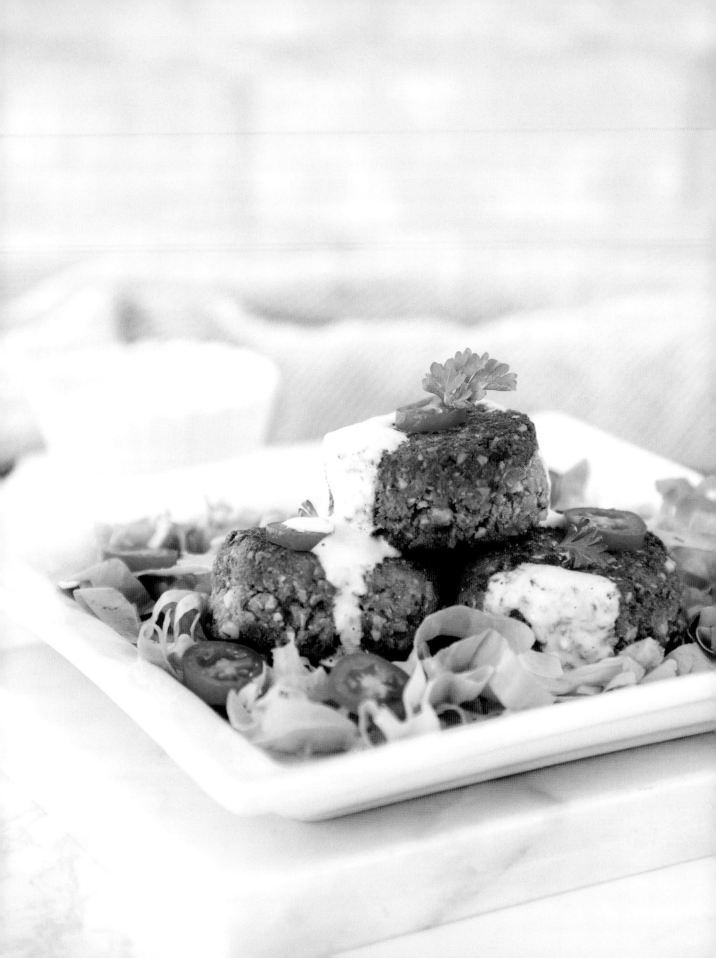

Braised Red Cabbage

Cabbage makes a great keto side dish because it contains a lot of nutrients, has a mild flavor, and is inexpensive. Cinnamon gives this braised red cabbage a homey and comforting vibe, but it isn't overly sweet or cloying. This dish reheats well for days, and the flavors get even better over time.

Yield: **4 servings** ◆ Serving Size: **¾ cup** ◆ Prep Time: **5 minutes** ◆ Cook Time: **10 minutes**

3 tablespoons butter

4 cups shredded red cabbage (1 medium head)

2 tablespoons granulated erythritol

2 tablespoons lemon juice

1 teaspoon ground cinnamon

½ teaspoon kosher salt

¼ teaspoon ground black pepper

Melt the butter in a large sauté pan. Add the cabbage, sweetener, lemon juice, cinnamon, salt, and pepper and cook over medium heat, stirring occasionally, until the cabbage is wilted and tender, about 8 minutes. Remove from the heat and serve.

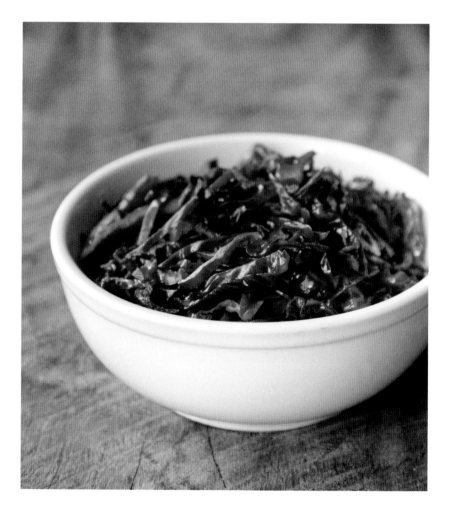

Calories: 102 | Fat: 9g | Protein: 1g | Carbs: 6g | Fiber: 2g | Erythritol: 2g | **Net Carbs: 4g**

Cheesy Cauliflower Grits

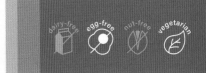

Stirring almond flour into cauliflower puree does a surprisingly good job of replicating the texture of real grits, and the extra cheese never hurts. These grits go great with a couple of runny eggs and a slice or two of bacon if you enjoy a Southern-style breakfast. My favorite way to eat this is in my Shrimp & Grits (page 226) because it soaks up that creamy sauce so well!

Yield: **4 servings** ◆ Serving Size: **½ cup** ◆ Prep Time: **5 minutes**

1 batch Cheesy Cauliflower Puree (page 272), hot

¼ cup shredded sharp cheddar cheese

2 tablespoons superfine blanched almond flour

1 teaspoon butter, melted, for serving (optional)

Place the cauliflower puree, cheese, and almond flour in a medium-sized bowl and stir until fully combined. Reheat in the microwave on high for 1 minute before serving if necessary. Drizzle melted butter on top before serving, if desired.

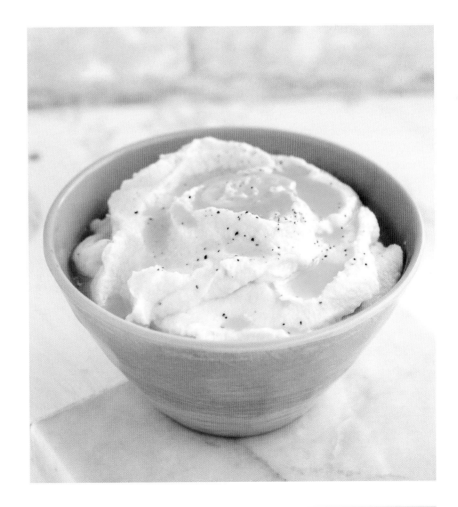

Calories: 172 | Fat: 15g | Protein: 8g | Carbs: 8g | Fiber: 4g | **Net Carbs: 4g**

dairy-free · egg-free · nut-free · vegetarian

Marinated Portobello Mushrooms

Don't be weirded out by the fact that these mushrooms aren't cooked. Once the marinade sinks in, they develop a meaty texture and an incredible flavor that makes them delicious on their own or as a topping for salads or a side to roasted meat. The red pepper flakes add a subtle amount of heat, but if you like your food really zesty, feel free to add more!

Yield: **2 servings** ◆ Serving Size: **1 cup** ◆ Prep Time: **5 minutes, plus 30 minutes to marinate**

2 large portobello mushroom caps

3 tablespoons extra-virgin olive oil

1 tablespoon balsamic vinegar (no sugar added)

1 tablespoon minced fresh parsley

½ teaspoon granulated erythritol

½ teaspoon kosher salt

½ teaspoon minced garlic

⅛ teaspoon ground black pepper

⅛ teaspoon red pepper flakes

1 Remove the stems from the mushroom caps and scrape off the inside ribs with a spoon. Slice the mushrooms into ¼-inch strips.

2 Place the oil, vinegar, parsley, sweetener, salt, garlic, black pepper, and red pepper flakes in a medium-sized bowl and whisk until fully combined. Add the mushrooms to the marinade and gently fold with a rubber spatula to coat the strips completely, being careful not to break the mushrooms into small pieces.

3 Marinate at room temperature for at least 30 minutes or up to 2 hours. Store in an airtight container in the refrigerator for up to 3 days.

Calories: 204 | Fat: 21g | Protein: 2g | Carbs: 3.5g | Fiber: 1g | Erythritol: 5g | **Net Carbs: 2.5g**

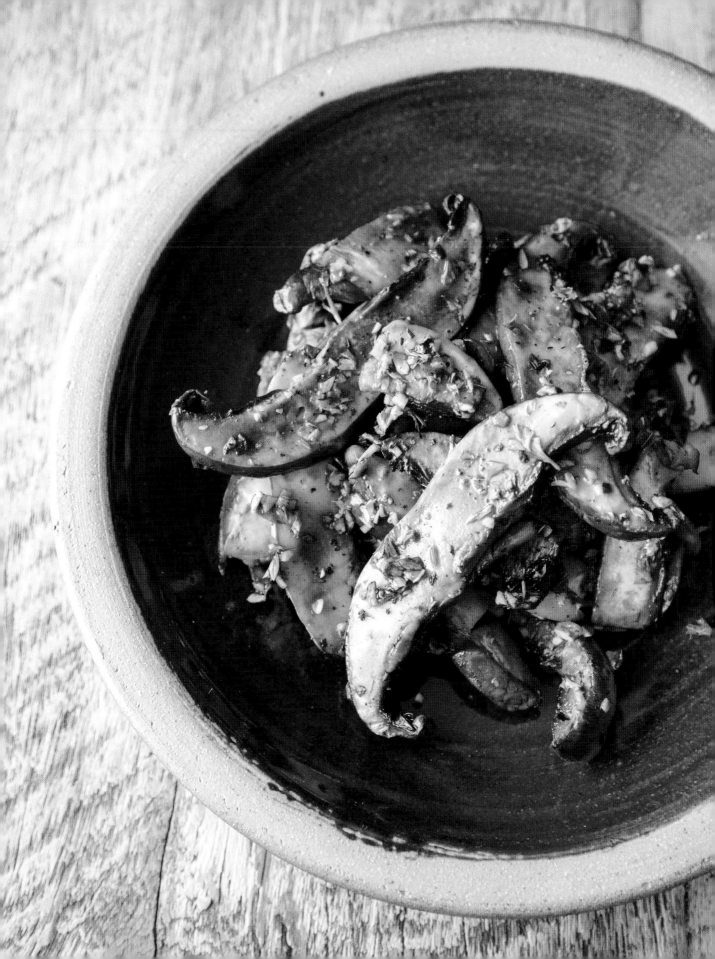

dairy-free egg-free nut-free vegetarian

Cheesy Cauliflower Puree

Still one of the most popular recipes on my blog, this cauliflower puree is different from others you may have tried. Microwaving the cauliflower uncovered steams a lot of moisture out of it before it gets blended, resulting in a thick and creamy texture rivaling that of traditional mashed potatoes. Using a strong cheese like Dubliner masks the cauliflower skunkiness and produces a sublime flavor that will win over even die-hard potato lovers!

Yield: **4 servings** • Serving Size: **½ cup** • Prep Time: **5 minutes** • Cook Time: **14 minutes**

5 cups raw cauliflower florets

2 tablespoons heavy whipping cream

1 tablespoon butter, plus more for serving if desired

½ teaspoon kosher salt

¼ teaspoon ground black pepper

⅛ teaspoon garlic powder

¼ cup shredded Dubliner or other sharp cheddar cheese

1 Place the cauliflower, cream, butter, salt, pepper, and garlic powder in a large microwave-safe bowl. Microwave, uncovered, on high for 6 minutes. Remove the bowl and stir well.

2 Return the bowl to the microwave and cook on high for another 8 minutes (again uncovered), or until the cauliflower is fork-tender. Remove the bowl from the microwave and transfer the cauliflower mixture to a blender or food processor.

3 Add the cheese and puree for 2 minutes, or until smooth, scraping the sides as necessary to puree all of the cauliflower. Taste and season with salt and pepper, if desired. Serve immediately, topped with more butter if you like.

4 Store in an airtight container in the refrigerator for up to 5 days. To reheat, microwave on high for 2 minutes per cup of puree. Stir and serve.

Calories: 145 | Fat: 11g | Protein: 6g | Carbs: 8g | Fiber: 4g | **Net Carbs: 4g**

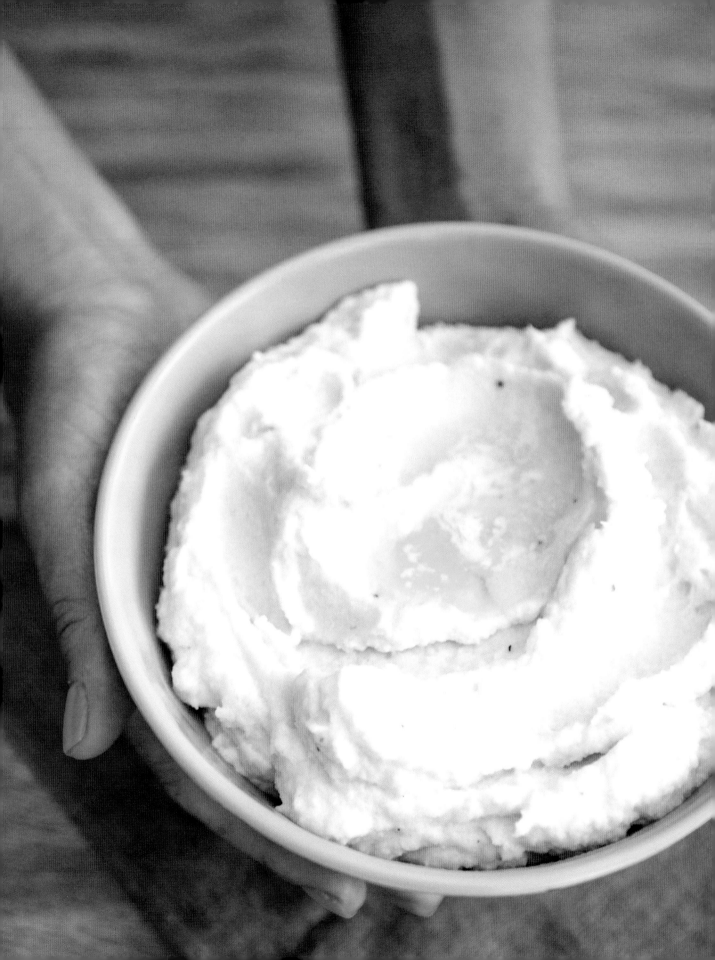

dairy-free egg-free nut-free vegetarian

Sweet Sesame Glazed Bok Choy

Bok choy has a mild flavor that to a lot of picky eaters isn't as offensive as spinach or kale. It gets by my guys easily when I prepare it with this sweet Asian-inspired sauce. We generally eat this dish hot, but I grabbed some of the leftovers out of the fridge on my way out the door one day, and it is surprisingly good cold as well. It would make a great addition to a salad to give it an Asian flair!

Yield: **4 servings** • Serving Size: **1 cup** • Prep Time: **5 minutes** • Cook Time: **17 minutes**

1 pound baby bok choy (see note)

¼ cup filtered water

3 tablespoons granulated erythritol

3 tablespoons unseasoned rice wine vinegar

3 tablespoons wheat-free soy sauce

½ teaspoon toasted sesame oil

1 tablespoon red pepper flakes

½ teaspoon xanthan gum

1 tablespoon sesame seeds, for garnish

1 Place the bok choy in a large microwave-safe bowl and add about ½ cup of water. Cover with plastic wrap and microwave on high for 5 minutes.

2 Remove the bowl from the microwave and uncover. Rinse the bok choy in cold water to stop the cooking process, then drain and set aside.

3 Place the water, sweetener, vinegar, soy sauce, and sesame oil in a large sauté pan and whisk until well blended. Cook over medium heat for 5 minutes, or until reduced by half.

4 Add the red pepper flakes and xanthan gum to the sauce and continue cooking, stirring occasionally, until the sauce has thickened enough to coat the back of a spoon, about 5 more minutes.

5 Add the bok choy to the sauce and stir gently to coat. Cook for 2 minutes, or until the bok choy is heated through. Garnish with sesame seeds and serve.

Note:
If you can't find bok choy or your family doesn't like it, this sauce works great with broccoli, cauliflower, or even zucchini. Throw in some chicken and serve it over cauliflower rice and it will feel like you're eating Chinese takeout!

Calories: 45 | Fat: 2g | Protein: 4g | Carbs: 4.5g | Fiber: 2.5g | Erythritol: 3g | **Net Carbs: 2g**

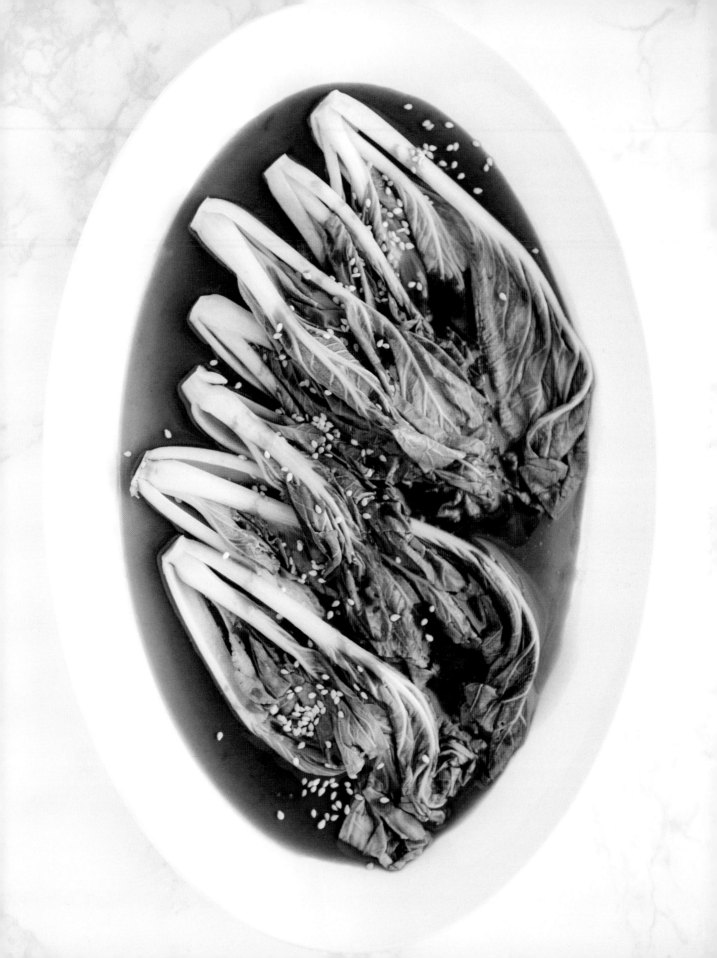

dairy-free egg-free nut-free vegetarian

Orange & Tarragon Coleslaw

This flavorful and refreshing coleslaw is easy to throw together and complements a wide variety of dishes. As an added bonus, dairy- and mayonnaise-free slaws like this one are perfect for picnics and BBQs because they won't spoil after sitting out for an hour or two on a hot day!

Yield: **8 servings** ◆ Serving Size: **½ cup** ◆ Prep Time: **10 minutes**

For the slaw:

3 cups thinly sliced or chopped white cabbage

1 cup thinly sliced or chopped red cabbage

½ cup thinly sliced scallions

1 tablespoon chopped fresh tarragon

For the dressing:

¼ cup extra-virgin olive oil

3 tablespoons apple cider vinegar

2 tablespoons granulated erythritol

2 tablespoons orange juice

1 tablespoon grated orange zest

1 teaspoon celery seeds

½ teaspoon kosher salt

¼ teaspoon ground black pepper

1 Combine the slaw ingredients in a large nonmetal bowl. Put the dressing ingredients in a separate small bowl and whisk together.

2 Pour the dressing over the slaw and mix well. Serve immediately or chill for a couple of hours before serving. Store in an airtight container in the refrigerator for up to 5 days.

Calories: 73 | Fat: 7g | Protein: 1g | Carbs: 3g | Fiber: 1g | Erythritol: 3g | **Net Carbs: 2g**

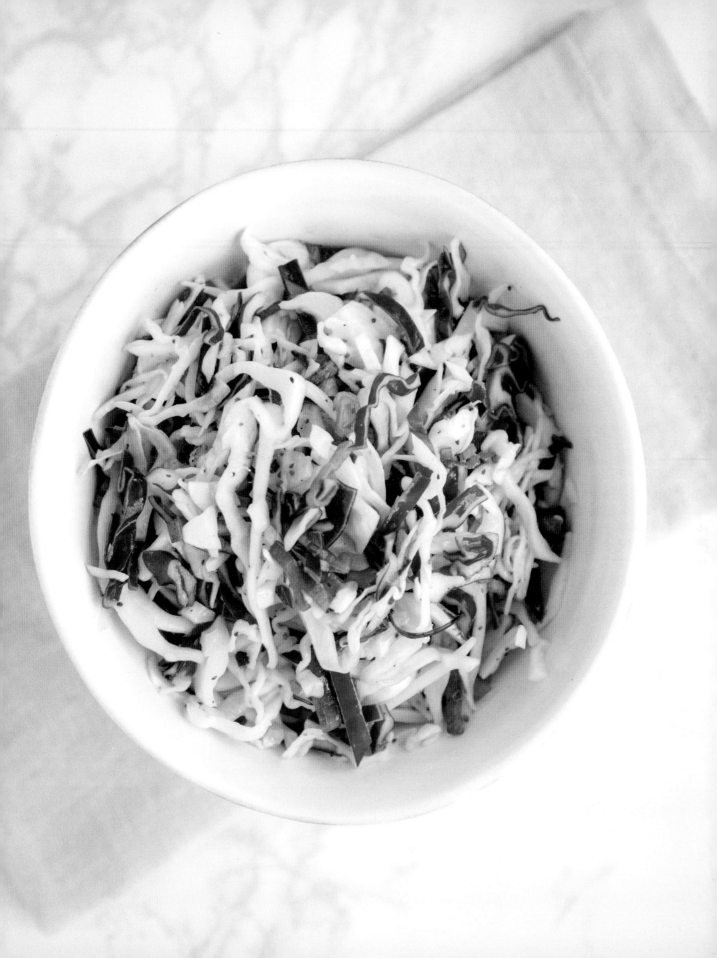

dairy-free egg-free nut-free vegetarian

Creamed Spinach

A steakhouse classic, creamed spinach is easy to make and easy to eat. This version is prepared entirely in the microwave and is ready in just a few minutes! Flavored with Parmesan cheese and a hint of nutmeg, it pairs perfectly with any steak or roasted meat.

Yield: **4 servings** ◆ Serving Size: **½ cup** ◆ Prep Time: **5 minutes** ◆ Cook Time: **6 minutes**

4 cups packed raw spinach leaves

4 ounces cream cheese (½ cup)

¼ cup grated Parmesan cheese

½ teaspoon garlic powder

½ teaspoon kosher salt

⅛ teaspoon ground black pepper

⅛ teaspoon ground nutmeg

1 Combine all of the ingredients in a medium-sized microwave-safe bowl. Microwave on high for 3 minutes, then stir.

2 Microwave on high for another 3 minutes. Stir until the spinach is creamy and all of the cheese has melted. Serve immediately.

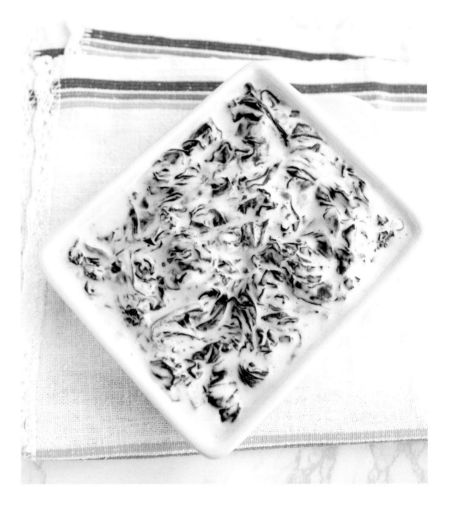

Calories: 135 | Fat: 11g | Protein: 5g | Carbs: 4g | Fiber: 1g | **Net Carbs: 3g**

Sautéed Green Beans with Walnuts

dairy-free   egg-free   nut-free   vegetarian

Green beans are inexpensive and widely available, so I make this recipe a lot. It's tasty and easy—two of my main criteria for side dishes these days! You can use any nuts you have on hand in place of the walnuts or omit them altogether if you aren't a fan or have an allergy.

Yield: **2 servings**   •   Serving Size: **1 cup**   •   Prep Time: **8 minutes**   •   Cook Time: **9 minutes**

1 tablespoon extra-virgin olive oil

8 ounces raw green beans, ends trimmed

1 tablespoon filtered water

3 tablespoons chopped raw walnuts

1 teaspoon minced garlic

½ teaspoon kosher salt

⅛ teaspoon ground black pepper

1. Heat the olive oil in a medium-sized sauté pan over medium heat. Add the green beans and water and sauté for 5 to 7 minutes, until the beans are bright green and tender.

2. Add the walnuts and garlic and sauté for 2 more minutes. Season with the salt and pepper. Serve immediately.

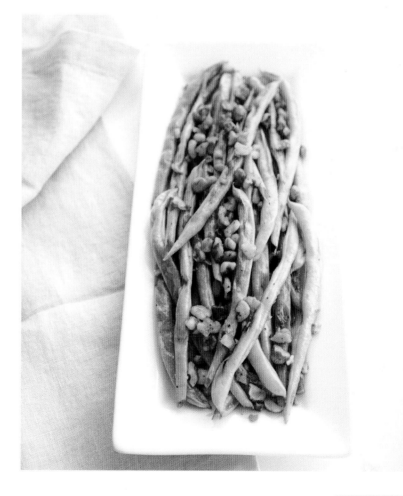

Calories: 169 | Fat: 14g | Protein: 4g | Carbs: 10g | Fiber: 5g | **Net Carbs: 5g**

dairy-free egg-free nut-free vegetarian

Spicy Jicama Shoestring Fries

I've experimented with jicama fries in different sizes and cuts, and this shoestring cut is the hands-down favorite. They stay crisper than thicker-cut fries, and there is a lot more seasoning-to-fry ratio, which my family likes. That being said, you can do your own experimenting; these fries are delicious in any size!

Yield: **4 servings** • Serving Size: **½ cup** • Prep Time: **5 minutes** • Cook Time: **15 minutes**

Avocado oil or other light-tasting oil, for frying

1 medium jicama, peeled and julienned

1 tablespoon Cajun Seasoning (page 76)

Kosher salt

1 Heat about 2 inches of the oil in a small Dutch oven or other heavy-bottomed pot over medium heat until it reaches 350°F, about 7 minutes. Meanwhile, line a plate with paper towels.

2 Fry the julienned jicama in 2 batches for 3 to 4 minutes per batch, or until golden and crisp. Remove the fries to the lined plate and toss immediately with the Cajun seasoning and salt to taste. Serve hot.

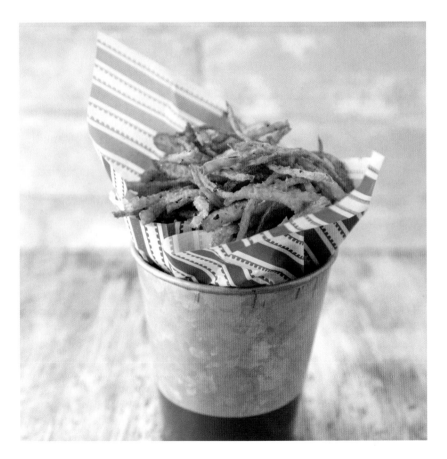

Calories: 148 | Fat: 14g | Protein: 1g | Carbs: 6g | Fiber: 3g | **Net Carbs: 3g**

Sautéed Mushrooms

dairy-free · egg-free · nut-free · vegetarian

This method brings out the unique toasty flavor that cooked mushrooms should have. Because mushrooms are high in moisture, it's important to cook them long enough for that moisture to evaporate—only then can they start browning and developing their best flavor. Of course, lots of butter doesn't hurt, either.

Yield: **4 cups** ◆ Serving Size: **¾ cup** ◆ Prep Time: **5 minutes**

Cook Time: **10 minutes**

¼ cup (½ stick) butter

8 ounces sliced white mushrooms (about 4 cups)

2 tablespoons extra-virgin olive oil

½ teaspoon kosher salt

¼ teaspoon ground black pepper

Melt the butter in a large sauté pan over medium-high heat. Add the mushrooms, olive oil, salt, and pepper and cook, stirring occasionally, for about 10 minutes, until the mushrooms are golden brown. Taste and season with more salt and pepper, if desired.

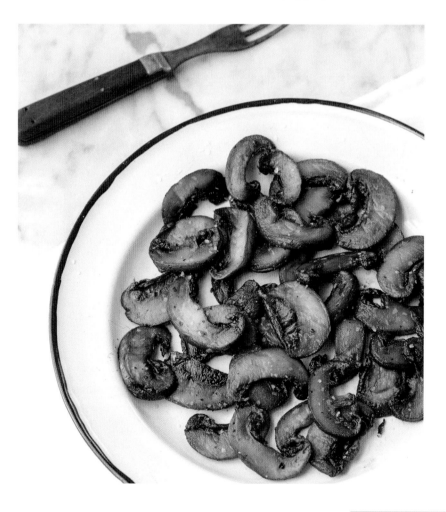

Calories: 174 | Fat: 19g | Protein: 2g | Carbs: 2g | Fiber: 1g | **Net Carbs: 1g**

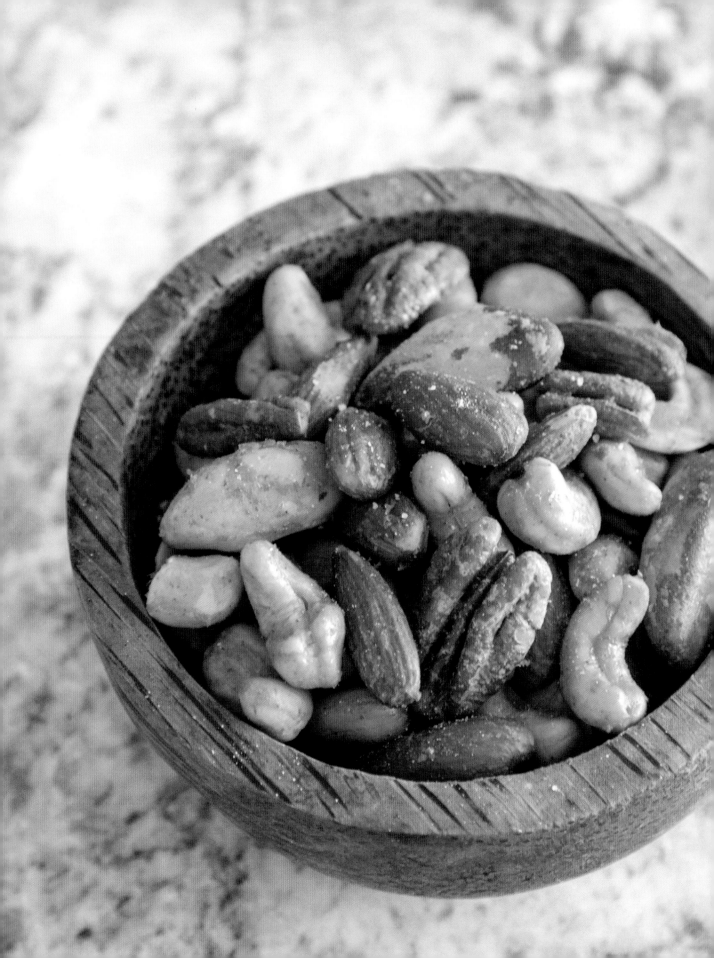

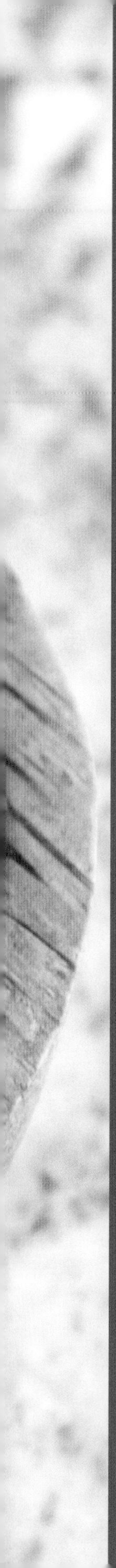

snacks & appetizers

Jalapeño & Cilantro Cauliflower Hummus / 284

Roasted Red Pepper Cauliflower Hummus / 286

Wasabi & Ginger Cauliflower Hummus / 288

Chipotle Deviled Eggs / 290

Restaurant-Style Salsa / 292

Easy Keto Guacamole / 293

Easy Nacho Dip / 294

Broccoli Cheddar Puffs / 296

Parmesan Crisps / 298

Keto Seed Crackers / 300

Buffalo Mixed Nuts / 301

Bacon & Cheddar Cornless Muffins / 302

dairy-free egg-free nut-free vegetarian

Jalapeño & Cilantro Cauliflower Hummus

When I created a classic cauliflower hummus for my blog a few years ago, I had no idea it would take off and become as popular as it did! I like this jalapeño and cilantro–flavored version even more than the original.

Yield: **2 cups** • Serving Size: **¼ cup** • Prep Time: **5 minutes, plus time to chill**

Cook Time: **15 minutes**

4 tablespoons avocado oil or other light-tasting oil, divided

3 cups raw cauliflower florets

2 tablespoons filtered water

1 teaspoon kosher salt, divided

3 tablespoons chopped fresh cilantro

3 tablespoons lime juice

2 tablespoons seeded and minced jalapeño peppers

1 tablespoon tahini

2 teaspoons minced garlic

For garnish (optional):

Extra-virgin olive oil

1 teaspoon seeded and minced jalapeño peppers

1   Cook the cauliflower: Place 2 tablespoons of the avocado oil, the cauliflower, water, and ¼ teaspoon of the salt in a large microwave-safe bowl and stir until the cauliflower is coated. Microwave on high for 12 to 15 minutes, until fork-tender.

2   Transfer the cauliflower to a food processor or blender and add the cilantro, lime juice, jalapeños, remaining 2 tablespoons of oil, tahini, garlic, and remaining ¾ teaspoon of salt. Blend until smooth. Taste and add more salt, if needed.

3   Spoon the hummus into a serving bowl and garnish with a drizzle of olive oil and minced jalapeños, if desired. Chill before serving. Store in an airtight container in the refrigerator for up to 1 week.

Serving Suggestion:
You can use fresh celery, cucumber, or bell peppers or low-carb crackers for dipping.

Calories: 84 | Fat: 8g | Protein: 2g | Carbs: 5g | Fiber: 2g | **Net Carbs: 3g**

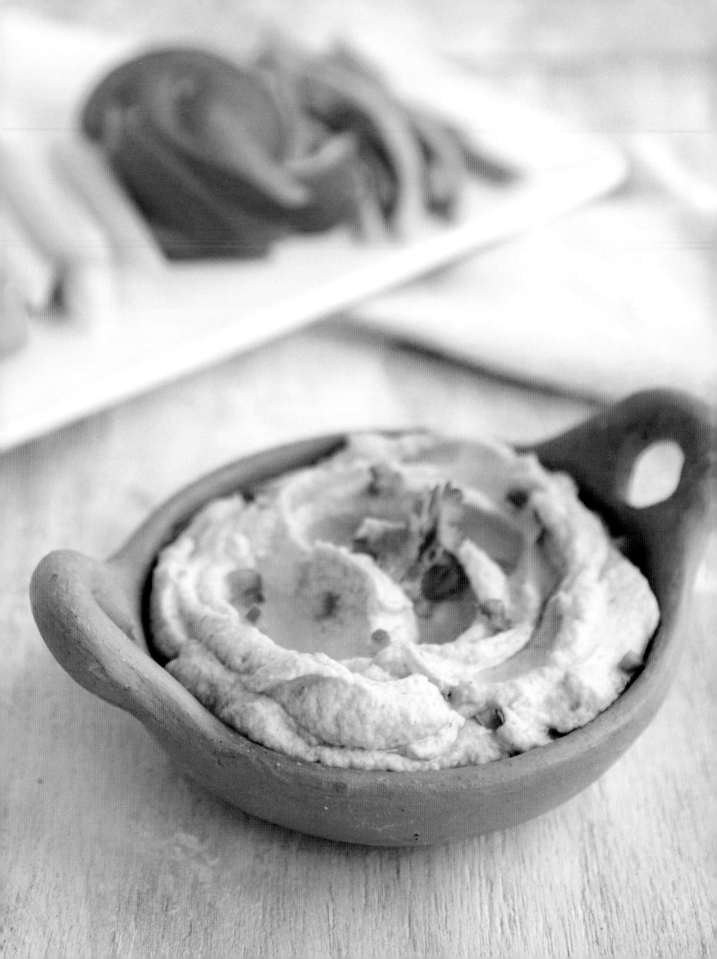

dairy-free • egg-free • nut-free • vegetarian

Roasted Red Pepper Cauliflower Hummus

Another version of my popular cauliflower hummus, but with a completely different flair. Roasted red peppers, basil, and lots of garlic give this one a punch of flavor that I really love!

Yield: **2 cups** • Serving Size: **¼ cup** • Prep Time: **5 minutes, plus time to chill**

Cook Time: **12 to 15 minutes**

3 cups cauliflower florets

3 tablespoons extra-virgin olive oil, divided

3 tablespoons filtered water, divided

1 teaspoon kosher salt, divided

⅓ cup jarred roasted red peppers, drained

1 tablespoon lime juice

1 tablespoon tahini

1½ teaspoons chopped garlic

1 tablespoon minced fresh basil

For garnish (optional):

Extra-virgin olive oil

1 tablespoon diced roasted red peppers

1 or 2 fresh basil leaves

1 Cook the cauliflower: Place the cauliflower, 2 tablespoons of the olive oil, 2 tablespoons of the water, and ¼ teaspoon of the salt in a large microwave-safe bowl and stir until the cauliflower is coated. Microwave on high for 12 to 15 minutes, until fork-tender.

2 Transfer the cauliflower to a food processor or blender and add the roasted red peppers, lime juice, tahini, remaining tablespoon of water, remaining tablespoon of olive oil, garlic, and remaining ¾ teaspoon of salt. Blend until smooth. Because the mixture is thick, you may need to stop the blender and stir it with a spoon a couple of times to get it to a smooth consistency.

3 Spoon the hummus into a serving bowl and stir in the basil. Taste and add more salt, if needed. If desired, garnish with a drizzle of olive oil, diced roasted red peppers, and fresh basil. Chill before serving. Store in an airtight container in the refrigerator for up to 1 week.

Serving Suggestion:
You can use celery, cucumber, bell peppers, Parmesan Crisps (page 298), or any low-carb crackers for dipping.

Calories: 91 | Fat: 7g | Protein: 3g | Carbs: 5g | Fiber: 2g | **Net Carbs: 3g**

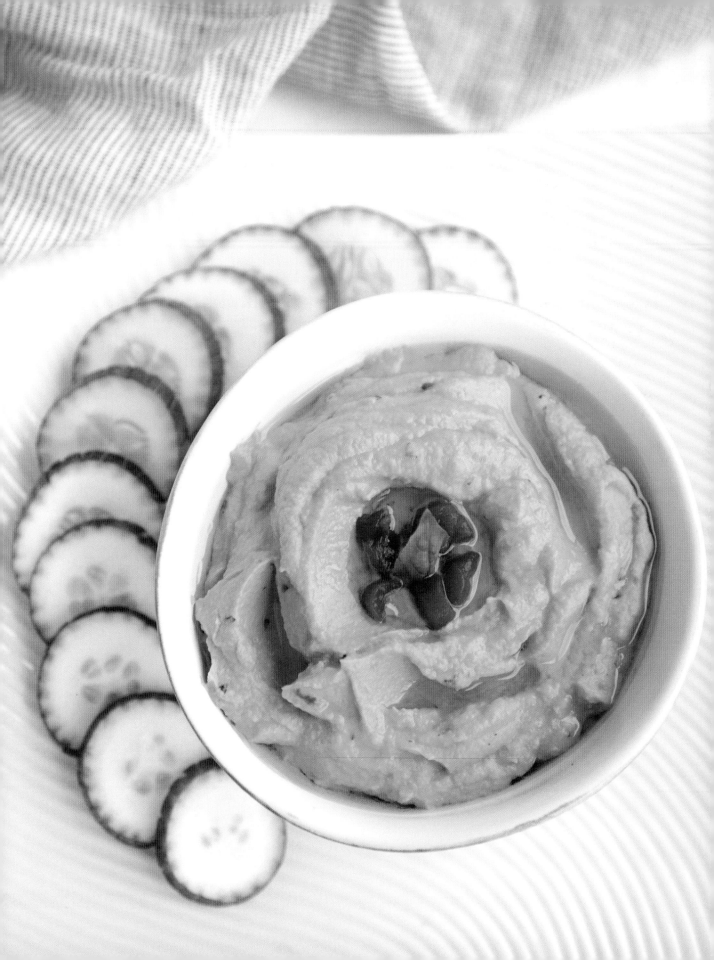

dairy-free egg-free nut-free vegetarian

Wasabi & Ginger Cauliflower Hummus

This Asian-inspired version is a little subtler than my classic cauliflower hummus, but the ginger and wasabi play well together with the sesame flavor of the tahini. I can't get enough of this hummus with radish chips for dipping!

Yield: **2 cups** • Serving Size: **¼ cup** • Prep Time: **5 minutes, plus time to chill**

Cook Time: **12 to 15 minutes**

3 cups cauliflower florets

4 tablespoons avocado oil or other light-tasting oil, divided

2 tablespoons filtered water

1¼ teaspoons kosher salt, divided

2 tablespoons tahini

1½ tablespoons wasabi powder

1½ tablespoons lime juice

1 tablespoon peeled and minced fresh ginger

1 teaspoon fish sauce (no sugar added) or coconut aminos for strict vegetarian or vegan

1 Cook the cauliflower: Place the cauliflower, 2 tablespoons of the oil, the water, and ¼ teaspoon of the salt in a large microwave-safe bowl and stir until the cauliflower is coated. Microwave on high for 12 to 15 minutes, until fork-tender.

2 Transfer the cauliflower to a food processor or blender and add the remaining 2 tablespoons of oil, the tahini, wasabi powder, lime juice, ginger, fish sauce, and remaining teaspoon of salt. Blend until smooth. Taste and add more salt, if needed.

3 Spoon the hummus into a serving bowl. Chill before serving. Store in an airtight container in the refrigerator for up to 1 week.

> **Serving Suggestion:**
> *You can use celery, radishes, cucumbers, or low-carb crackers for dipping.*

Calories: 70 | Fat: 2g | Protein: 2g | Carbs: 3g | Fiber: 1.5g | **Net Carbs: 1.5g**

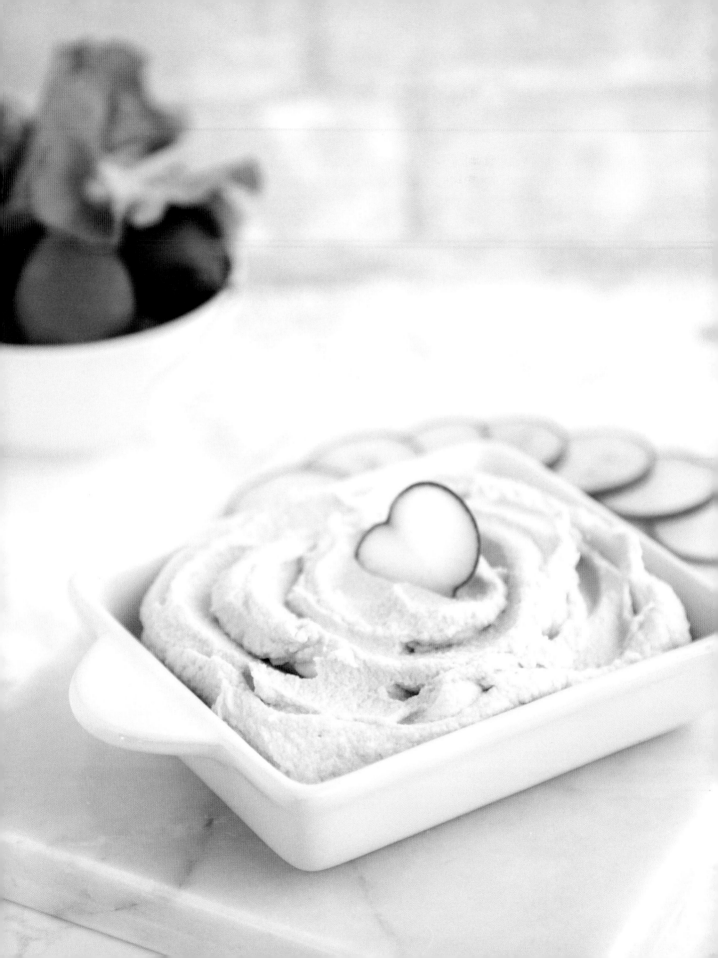

Chipotle Deviled Eggs

Deviled eggs are a classic appetizer, but they also make a fantastic keto lunch on the go! Mr. Hungry can't get enough of this smoky, spicy version flavored with canned chipotles.

Yield: **12 deviled eggs** ◆ Serving Size: **2 deviled eggs**

Prep Time: **10 minutes, plus time to chill** ◆ Cook Time: **12 to 15 minutes**

6 hard-boiled eggs, peeled

¼ cup sugar-free mayonnaise

2 tablespoons canned chipotles in adobo sauce

1 tablespoon lime juice

¼ teaspoon kosher salt

For garnish (optional):

Chipotle powder or paprika

Chopped fresh parsley

1   Cut the hard-boiled eggs in half lengthwise. Carefully remove the yolks with a spoon and place in a small blender; set the whites aside. Add the mayonnaise, chipotles, lime juice, and salt to the blender and blend for 30 seconds, or until creamy.

2   Transfer the yolk mixture to a resealable plastic bag and cut the tip off of one bottom corner to create a hole about ½ inch in diameter.

3   Squeezing the yolk mixture through the cut-off corner of the bag, pipe about 1 tablespoon of the filling into each egg white half. Sprinkle with chipotle powder or paprika and chopped parsley, if desired. Chill before serving. Store in an airtight container in the refrigerator for up to 5 days.

Calories: 134 | Fat: 12g | Protein: 6g | Carbs: 0.6g | Fiber: 0g | **Net Carbs: 0.6g**

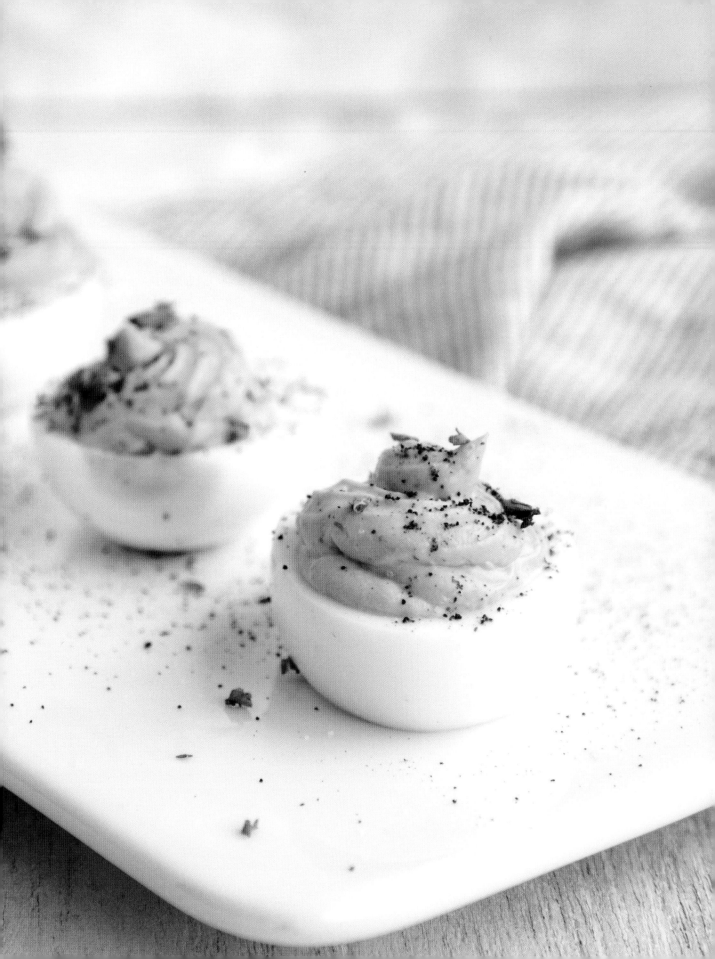

dairy-free egg-free nut-free vegetarian

Restaurant-Style Salsa

Do yourself a favor and stop purchasing store-bought salsa immediately! It takes just minutes to throw some ingredients in a blender and make a fresh, bright, restaurant-quality salsa at home.

Yield: **2 cups** ◆ Serving Size: **¼ cup** ◆ Prep Time: **5 minutes**

2 cups chopped fresh tomatoes

¼ cup chopped yellow onions

1 tablespoon chopped fresh cilantro

1 tablespoon lime juice

1 teaspoon kosher salt

1 teaspoon minced garlic

1 teaspoon seeded and chopped jalapeño peppers

¼ teaspoon ground black pepper

Place all of the ingredients in a blender and pulse for 30 seconds, or until the salsa reaches your preferred consistency. Taste and season with more salt and pepper if desired. Store in an airtight container in the refrigerator for up to 1 week.

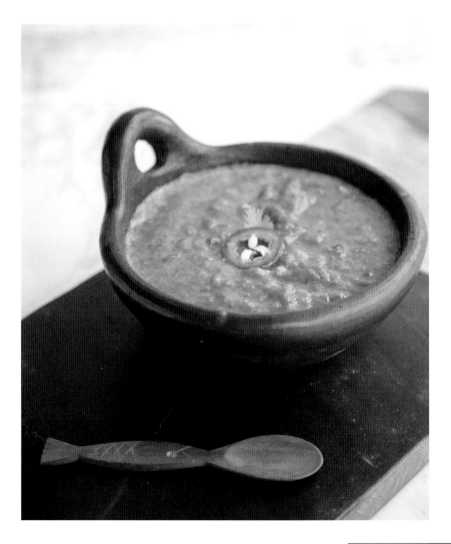

Calories: 12 | Fat: 0g | Protein: 0g | Carbs: 2.6g | Fiber: 0.6g | **Net Carbs: 2g**

Easy Keto Guacamole

dairy-free · egg-free · nut-free · vegetarian

Hungry Jr. has loved guacamole since he was a toddler, but he always called it "grockamolie," and that's how I still hear it in my head whenever he asks for it now. I make this for him (and me) often, and I feel good about all the healthy fats he's getting when he eats it. It's also delicious, so there's that.

Yield: **2 cups** • Serving Size: **¼ cup** • Prep Time: **5 minutes**

2 cups chopped avocados (about 4 medium avocados)

½ cup Restaurant-Style Salsa (page 292)

2 tablespoons chopped fresh cilantro

1 tablespoon lime juice

1 teaspoon minced garlic

1 tablespoon minced red onions

½ teaspoon kosher salt

¼ teaspoon chipotle powder

Place the avocados in a medium-sized bowl and mash with a fork until the desired texture is reached. Add the remaining ingredients and stir well. Store in an airtight container in the refrigerator for up to 3 days.

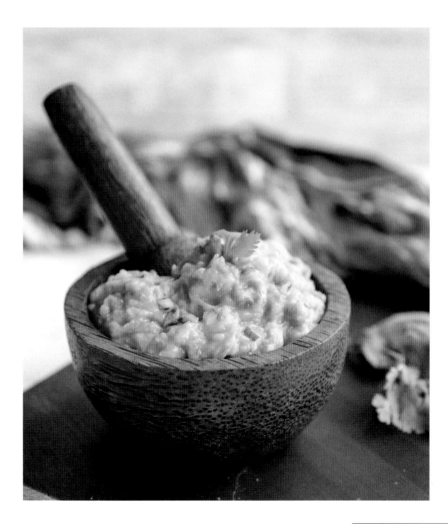

Calories: 51 | Fat: 4g | Protein: 1g | Carbs: 3g | Fiber: 2g | **Net Carbs: 1g**

Easy Nacho Dip

Nachos are one of my favorite foods, but they're problematic on keto because I haven't found a "chip" that stands up to the toppings and retains its crunch. This dip is what I go for when I want a nacho fix, and I eat it with pork rinds. That way I get the flavor and crunch of nachos and stay in ketosis.

Yield: **1½ cups** ◆ Serving Size: **¼ cup** ◆ Prep Time: **2 minutes** ◆ Cook Time: **3 minutes**

1 (8-ounce) package cream cheese

¾ cup shredded sharp cheddar cheese

⅓ cup Restaurant-Style Salsa (page 292)

Combine the cream cheese, cheddar cheese, and salsa in a medium-sized microwave-safe bowl. Microwave on high for 2 minutes, then stir. Microwave on high for 1 more minute. Stir until smooth and serve hot. Store in an airtight container in the refrigerator for up to 5 days. To reheat, microwave on high for 1 minute, or until melted and hot.

Note:
You can stir cooked chorizo or seasoned ground beef into this cheesy dip to make it even heartier.

Serving Suggestion:
This dip can be poured over a Beef Burrito Bowl (page 188) to make it even more saucy and decadent!

Calories: 188 | Fat: 17g | Protein: 6g | Carbs: 2.8g | Fiber: 0.3g | **Net Carbs: 2.5g**

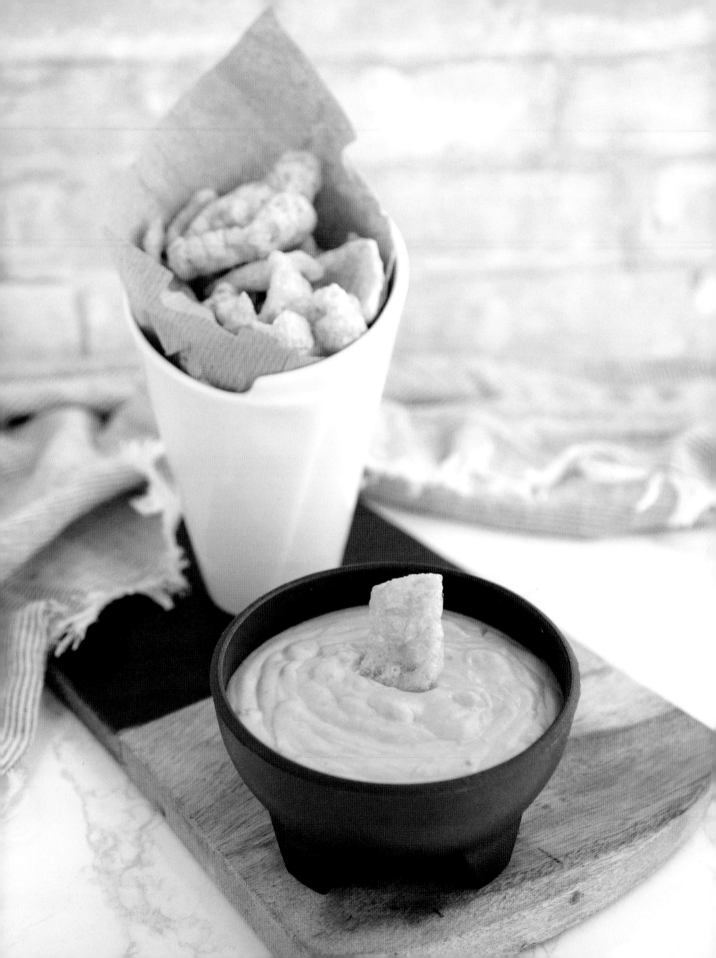

dairy-free egg-free nut-free vegetarian

Broccoli Cheddar Puffs

Similar in texture to a tot but lighter, these broccoli puffs have a delicious flavor that even children can appreciate. My son's issues with broccoli come mostly from the texture, so these puffs got by him with no problem! Shown with Tangy Feta & Dill Dressing (page 93).

Yield: **40 puffs** • Serving Size: **5 puffs**

Prep Time: **5 minutes, plus 30 minutes to chill** • Cook Time: **15 minutes**

2 cups cooked broccoli florets

1 cup shredded sharp cheddar cheese

1 cup superfine blanched almond flour

¼ cup (½ stick) butter, melted

2 large eggs

3 tablespoons heavy whipping cream

1 teaspoon ground paprika

1 teaspoon kosher salt

½ teaspoon garlic powder

½ teaspoon onion powder

¼ teaspoon ground black pepper

1 Place all of the ingredients in a blender or food processor and blend until mostly smooth. Chill for 30 minutes.

2 Preheat the oven to 350°F. The puffs can be baked in one batch using either two 24-well mini muffin tins or one 15 by 10-inch sheet pan. (You can also bake them in two batches if you have only one mini muffin tin.) If using two mini muffin tins, grease all of the wells in one of the pans, but only 16 wells in the second pan (to grease a total of 40 wells); if using a sheet pan, line it with parchment paper.

3 Fill each greased mini muffin cup with 2 tablespoons of the batter or use a medium-sized cookie scoop to drop the batter in rounds about ½ inch apart onto the lined sheet pan.

4 Bake for 15 minutes, or until slightly golden and firm. Remove from the oven and let cool slightly on the pan before removing from the pan and serving.

5 Store any leftovers in an airtight container in the refrigerator for up to 5 days or in the freezer for up to 3 months. To reheat, thaw the puffs, then microwave them on high, uncovered, for 30 seconds.

Calories: 237 | Fat: 20g | Protein: 9g | Carbs: 6g | Fiber: 3g | **Net Carbs: 3g**

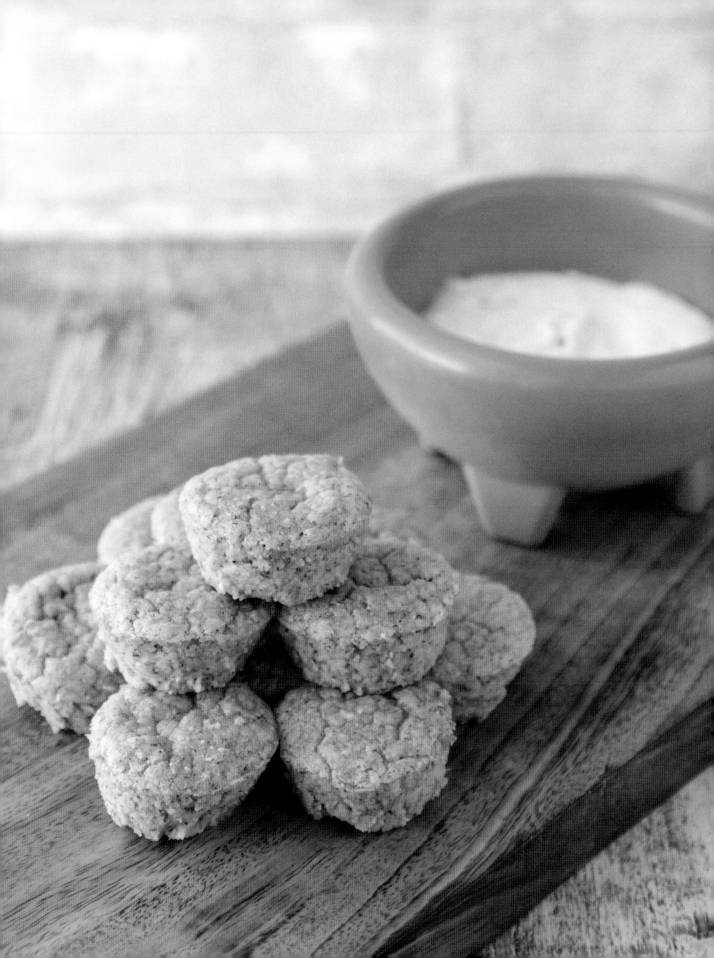

dairy-free egg-free nut-free vegetarian

Parmesan Crisps

You could pay seven dollars for a bag of around twenty Parmesan crisps at a store, or you can make these super-easy and economical Parmesan crisps by the hundreds at home for around the same price. They taste exactly like those little orange square cheese crackers you might remember eating as a kid.

Yield: **12 crisps** • Serving Size: **6 crisps** • Prep Time: **5 minutes** • Cook Time: **12 minutes**

⅓ **cup grated Parmesan cheese**

Special equipment:
Mini muffin tin

1 Preheat the oven to 375°F. Lightly grease 12 wells of a 24-well mini muffin tin.

2 Place 1½ teaspoons of the Parmesan in each mini muffin cup. Bake until golden brown, about 12 minutes.

3 Remove from the oven and let cool in the pan for 5 minutes to allow the chips to firm up. Once firm, they will easily pop out of the pan. Store in an airtight container for up to 1 week.

> **Family-Friendly Tip:**
> *This is a great recipe to have your kids help you make. It's a fun way to teach little ones how to use a measuring spoon and even how to count to twelve.*

Calories: 65 | Fat: 4g | Protein: 6g | Carbs: 1g | Fiber: 0g | **Net Carbs: 1g**

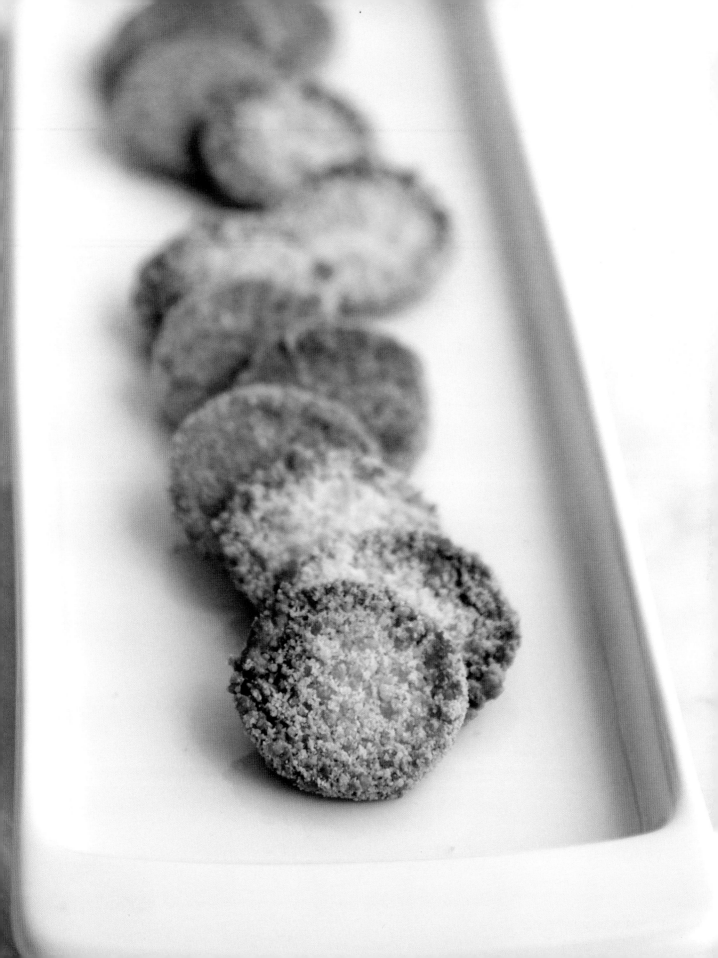

dairy-free *egg-free* *nut-free* *vegetarian*

Keto Seed Crackers

Low in carbs and super tasty, these little squares of goodness are great for dips or on a cheese tray. Because cheese without crackers is just so sad.

Yield: **15 servings** • Serving Size: **10 crackers** • Prep Time: **5 minutes, plus 20 minutes to soak**

Cook Time: **40 minutes**

1 cup shelled raw pumpkin seeds (pepitas)

1 cup shelled raw sunflower seeds

1 cup white sesame seeds

1 cup whole flax seeds

1 teaspoon kosher salt

1 teaspoon onion powder

1 teaspoon smoked paprika

½ cup filtered water

1 large egg white

1 Place all of the ingredients in a medium-sized bowl and stir well. Let sit at room temperature for 20 minutes.

2 Preheat the oven to 325°F. Line a 15 by 10-inch sheet pan with parchment paper.

3 Spread the mixture evenly on the parchment, pressing it flat with your hands or the back of a large metal spatula. Bake for 35 minutes, or until no longer wet in the center.

4 Remove from the oven and cut into 1-inch squares. Return the crackers to the oven and bake for 5 more minutes, until firm and crisp. Store in an airtight container for up to 1 week or freeze for up to 3 months.

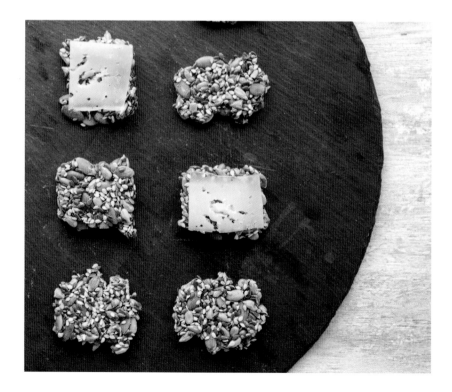

Calories: 198 | Fat: 15g | Protein: 9g | Carbs: 9g | Fiber: 6g | **Net Carbs: 3g**

Buffalo Mixed Nuts

dairy-free · egg-free · nut-free · vegetarian

When you want the flavor of Buffalo wings without all that tedious cooking, these Buffalo-flavored mixed nuts fit the bill. They are the perfect keto snack with cocktails or on game day!

Yield: **2 cups** • Serving Size: **¼ cup** • Prep Time: **5 minutes** • Cook Time: **20 minutes**

¼ cup hot sauce (such as Frank's RedHot)

3 tablespoons unsalted butter, melted

1 tablespoon Creamy Blue Cheese Dressing (page 90)

1 teaspoon granulated erythritol

2 cups fancy mixed nuts

1 Preheat the oven to 350°F. Line a 15 by 10-inch sheet pan with parchment paper.

2 Place the hot sauce, melted butter, dressing, and sweetener in a medium-sized bowl. Stir well until mostly smooth and uniformly orange in color. Add the nuts and stir to coat thoroughly in the sauce.

3 Spread the nuts on the lined sheet pan and bake for 20 minutes, or until the surface of the nuts is mostly dry. Remove from the oven and let cool slightly before transferring to a serving dish. Store in an airtight container in the refrigerator for up to 1 week.

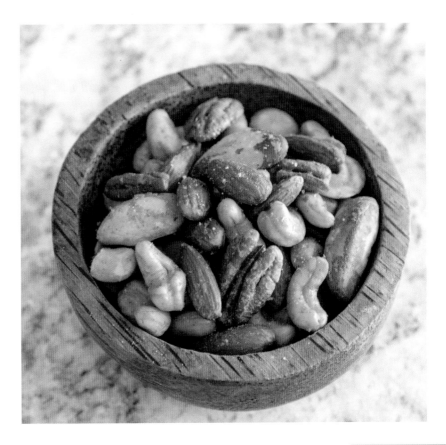

Calories: 216 | Fat: 20g | Protein: 5g | Carbs: 6g | Fiber: 2g | Erythritol: 1g | **Net Carbs: 4g**

Bacon & Cheddar Cornless Muffins

These muffins are fantastic with soup or chili, and also with bacon and eggs for breakfast when you want something that sticks to your ribs. Great flavor and a legit cornbread texture make these muffins a favorite in my house! While they taste great at any temperature, I like to eat them warm, with extra butter.

Yield: **6 muffins** ◆ Serving Size: **1 muffin** ◆ Prep Time: **8 minutes** ◆ Cook Time: **23 minutes**

5 tablespoons butter

1 tablespoon bacon grease

1 cup superfine blanched almond flour

⅓ cup shredded sharp cheddar cheese

⅓ cup unsweetened almond milk

2 tablespoons coconut flour

1 tablespoon granulated erythritol

2 teaspoons baking powder

½ teaspoon kosher salt

¼ teaspoon xanthan gum

2 large eggs

2 tablespoons chopped cooked bacon

1 Preheat the oven to 375°F. Grease or line 6 cups of a standard-size 12-well muffin tin.

2 Combine the butter and bacon grease in a medium-sized microwave-safe bowl. Microwave on high for 30 seconds, or until melted. Add the almond flour, cheddar cheese, almond milk, coconut flour, sweetener, baking powder, salt, xanthan gum, and eggs and mix well.

3 Spoon the batter into the muffin cups, filling them about two-thirds full. Sprinkle the bacon evenly over the tops of the batter. Bake for 22 minutes, or until a toothpick inserted in the center of a muffin comes out clean.

4 Remove the pan from the oven and let cool on a wire rack for about 10 minutes before removing the muffins. Store in an airtight container in the refrigerator for up to 5 days or in the freezer for up to 3 months.

5 To reheat, microwave on high for 30 seconds.

Calories: 300 | Fat: 27g | Protein: 10g | Carbs: 6g | Fiber: 3g | Erythritol: 2g | **Net Carbs: 3g**

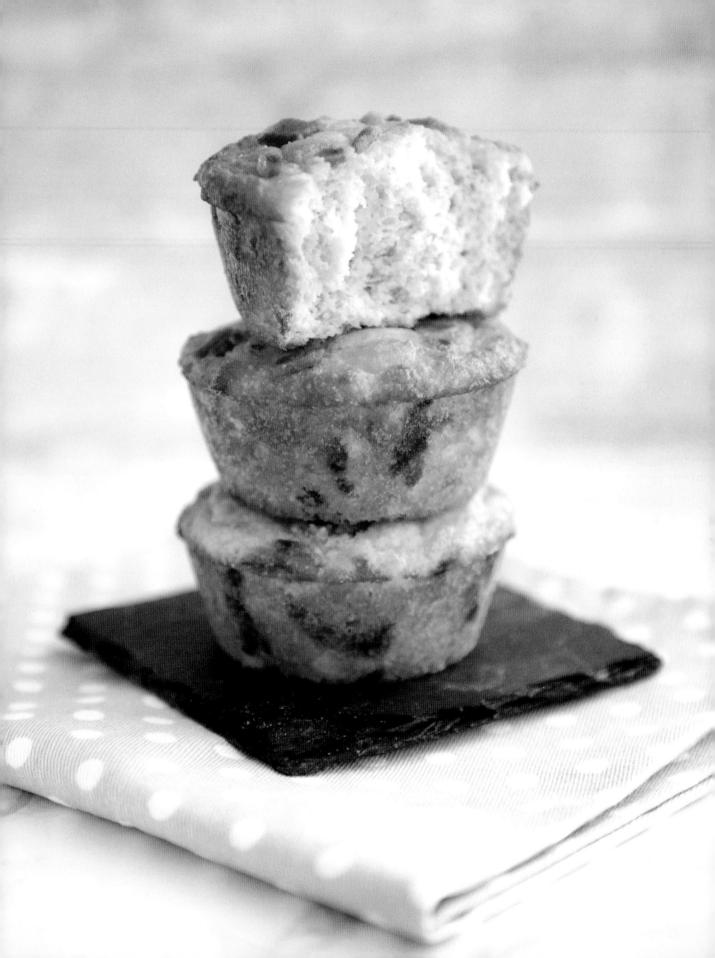

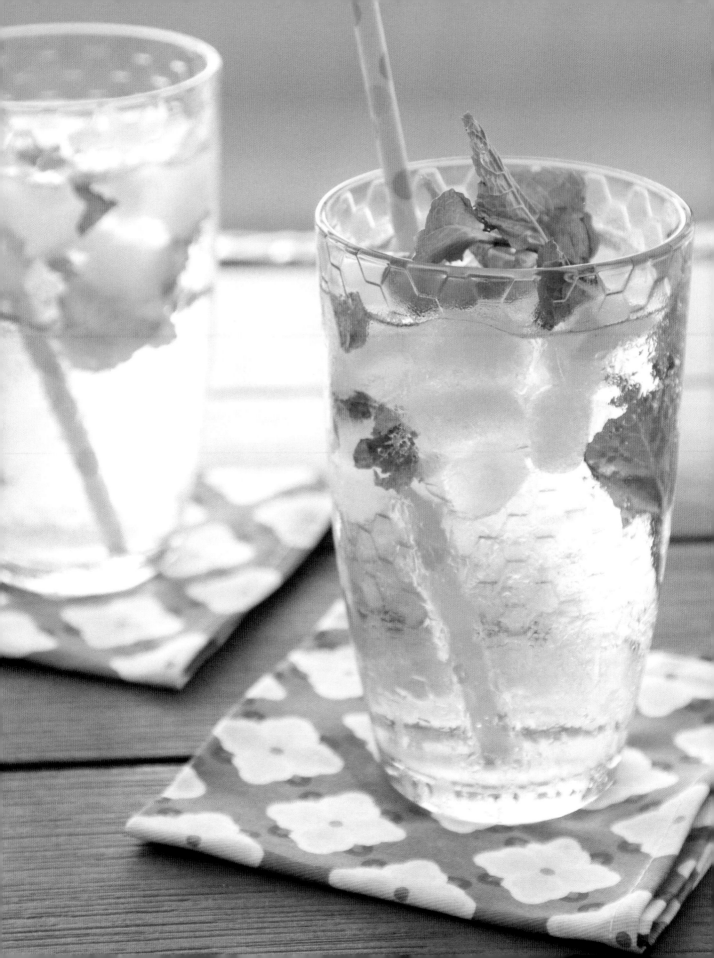

cocktails

Pink Grapefruit Martini / 306

Lemon Drop Martini / 308

Old-Fashioned / 309

Caipirinha / 310

Classic Mojito / 312

Blackberry Mojito / 314

Bourbon Sweetie / 316

Whiskey Sour / 317

Margarita / 318

Piña Colada / 320

Pink Grapefruit Martini

Refreshing and tart, this pretty pink cocktail is perfect for girl's night or a relaxing afternoon by the pool.

Yield: **1 serving** ◆ Prep Time: **2 minutes**

2 ounces premium vodka

1 ounce Grapefruit-Infused Simple Syrup (page 84)

1 ounce pink grapefruit juice

Grapefruit twist, for garnish (optional)

Place the vodka, simple syrup, and grapefruit juice in a cocktail shaker, along with 5 ice cubes. Cover and shake vigorously for 20 seconds. Strain the liquid into a chilled martini glass and garnish with grapefruit twist, if desired. Serve immediately.

> **Pro Tip:**
> *Because there is no ice in a martini when served, it's helpful to chill the martini glass in a bucket of ice water or in the freezer for at least 10 minutes before making the drink. The chilled glass will keep the drink cold for longer.*

Calories: 140 | Fat: 0g | Protein: 0g | Carbs: 3g | Fiber: 0g | Erythritol: 12g | **Net Carbs: 3g**

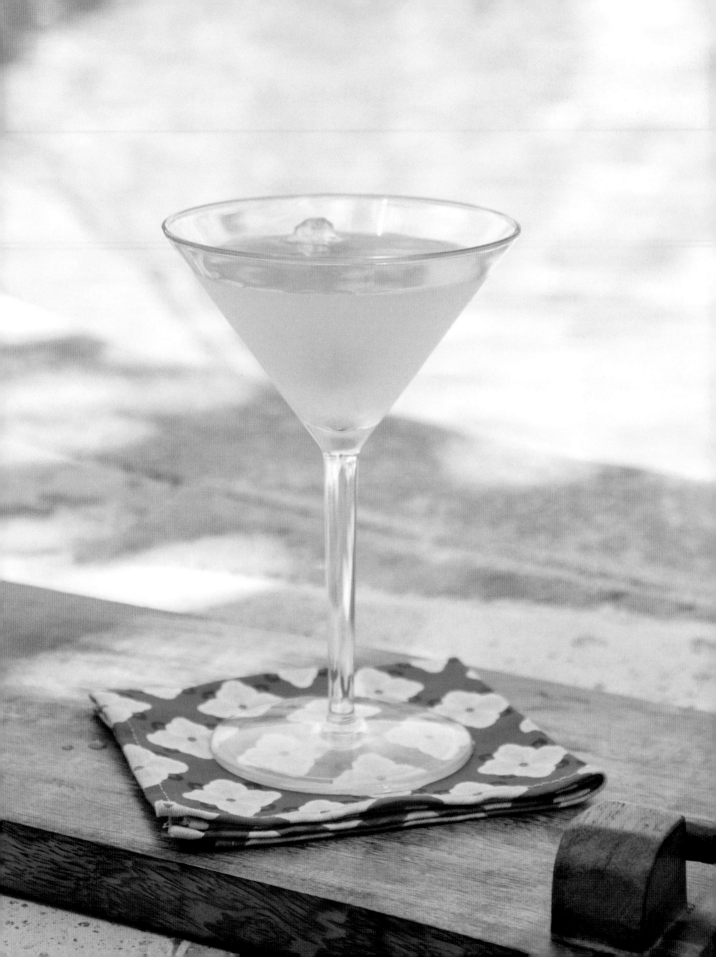

Lemon Drop Martini

dairy-free · egg-free · nut-free · vegetarian

When it comes to martinis, I'm usually a classic girl—very dry, straight up, extra olives. Every once in a while, though, I like to change it up. This Lemon Drop Martini is a fun alternative.

Yield: **1 serving** ◆ Prep Time: **2 minutes**

2 ounces premium vodka

1 ounce Lemon-Infused Simple Syrup (page 84)

1 tablespoon lemon juice

1 lemon slice, for garnish (optional)

Place the vodka, simple syrup, and lemon juice in a cocktail shaker, along with 5 ice cubes. Cover and shake vigorously for 20 seconds. Strain the liquid into a chilled martini glass and garnish with a lemon slice, if desired. Serve immediately.

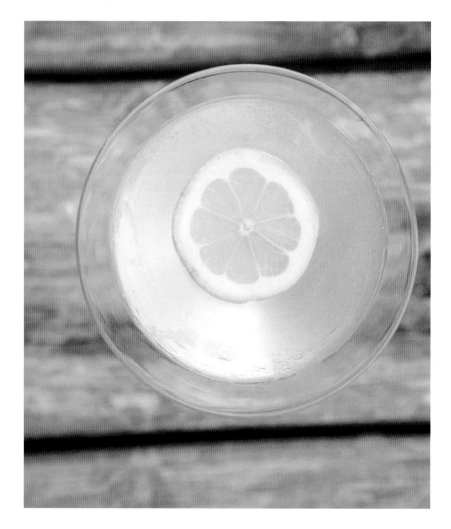

Calories: 132 | Fat: 0g | Protein: 0g | Carbs: 1g | Fiber: 0g | Erythritol: 12g | **Net Carbs: 1g**

Old-Fashioned

dairy-free · egg-free · nut-free · vegetarian

Drinking old-fashioneds makes me feel like a grown-up—all super sophisticated and stuff. However, I'm usually already in my flamingo pj's and watching Netflix, so it kind of ruins the effect…

Yield: **1 serving** • Prep Time: **2 minutes**

2 ounces bourbon

2 dashes bitters

1 tablespoon Orange-Infused Simple Syrup (page 84)

1 maraschino cherry, for garnish (optional)

1 orange slice, for garnish (optional)

Place the bourbon, bitters, and simple syrup in a cocktail shaker, along with 5 ice cubes. Cover and shake vigorously for 20 seconds. Pour into a 6-ounce glass tumbler and garnish with a maraschino cherry and an orange slice, if desired. Serve immediately.

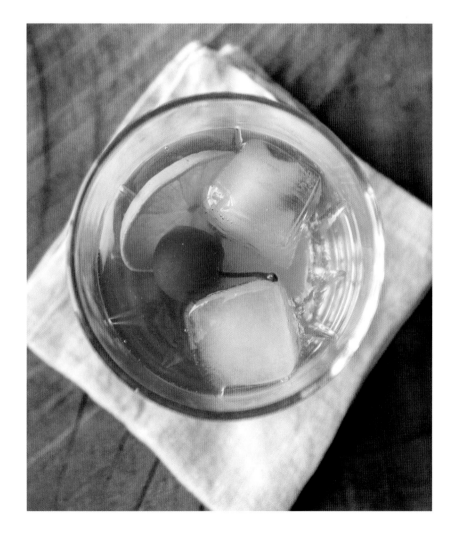

Calories: 143 | Fat: 0g | Protein: 0g | Carbs: 1g | Fiber: 0g | Erythritol: 6g | **Net Carbs: 1g**

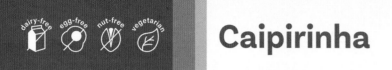
dairy-free egg-free nut-free vegetarian

Caipirinha

A classic Brazilian cocktail that a friend got me into years ago, the refreshing caipirinha gets its unique flavor from a sugarcane alcohol called cachaça. The traditional drink is loaded with sugar cubes, but I think this version, made with my keto Lime-Infused Simple Syrup, is just as good!

Yield: **1 serving** ◆ Prep Time: **2 minutes**

3 lime wedges, cut in half

1 tablespoon Lime-Infused Simple Syrup (page 84)

2 ounces cachaça

Place the lime pieces and simple syrup in a cocktail shaker and muddle with a wooden spoon or drink muddler. Add the cachaça and 5 ice cubes. Cover and shake vigorously for 20 seconds. Pour into a 6-ounce tumbler and serve immediately.

Pro Tip:
The word muddle *simply means "to crush"; this technique releases the flavor from whatever is being crushed. Citrus and other types of fruit, as well as herbs, are often muddled.*

Alternative Method:
If you don't have a wooden spoon or drink muddler, you can blend the limes, simple syrup, and cachaça together in a blender for 20 seconds, then pour the mixture through a strainer into a 6-ounce glass full of ice. This method works well for larger batches, too.

Calories: 134 | Fat: 0g | Protein: 0g | Carbs: 1g | Fiber: 0g | Erythritol: 6g | **Net Carbs: 1g**

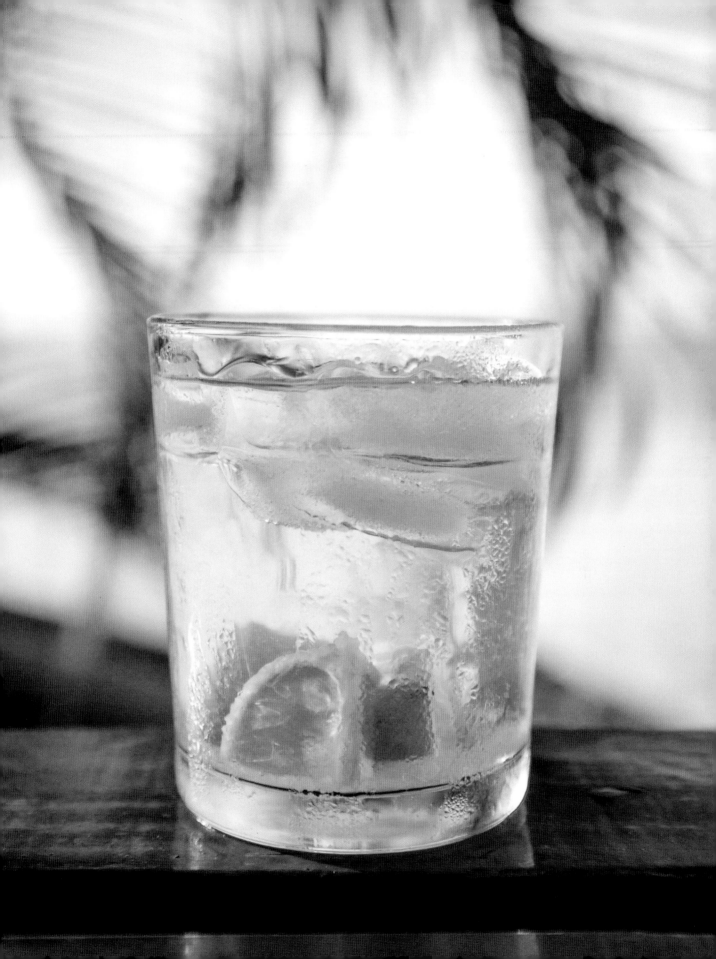

dairy-free · egg-free · nut-free · vegetarian

Classic Mojito

There's nothing better than a minty and lightly sweet guilt-free keto mojito by the pool on a hot day. Believe me, I speak from experience on this!

Yield: **1 serving** ◆ Prep Time: **2 minutes**

2 tablespoons fresh mint leaves

2 tablespoons Basic Simple Syrup (page 84)

2 ounces white rum

4 ounces unflavored seltzer water or club soda

Place the mint leaves in a tall 16-ounce glass and muddle with a wooden spoon or drink muddler. Pour in the simple syrup and white rum, then mix well. Add enough ice to fill the glass halfway. Pour in the seltzer and stir. Serve immediately.

Alternative Methods:

If you don't have a wooden spoon or drink muddler, you can briefly pulse the mint leaves, simple syrup, and rum together in a small blender; just be careful not to overblend it or the flavors and colors will be muddy. Then pour into a 16-ounce glass half full of ice and stir in the seltzer.

To make this drink for a group, you can prepare the mint, simple syrup, and rum in large quantities in a pitcher or jug and store in the refrigerator for up to 4 hours. Add the ice and seltzer to each drink individually right before serving.

Calories: 128 | Fat: 0g | Protein: 0g | Carbs: 0g | Fiber: 0g | Erythritol: 12g | **Net Carbs: 0g**

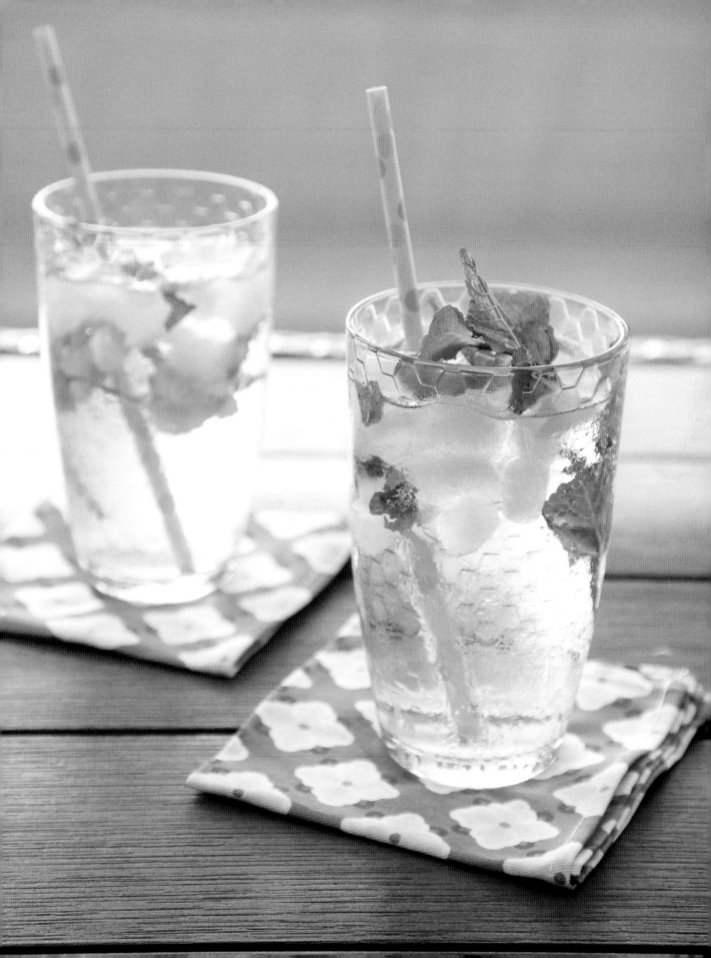

Blackberry Mojito

When you want to up your mojito game, this version with muddled blackberries has a pretty purple color and a lovely berry flavor.

Yield: **1 serving** ◆ Prep Time: **2 minutes**

5 fresh blackberries

2 tablespoons fresh mint leaves

2 tablespoons Basic Simple Syrup (page 84)

2 ounces white rum

4 ounces unflavored seltzer water or club soda

Place the blackberries and mint leaves in a tall 16-ounce glass and muddle them with a wooden spoon or drink muddler. Pour in the simple syrup and white rum, then mix well. Add enough ice to fill the glass halfway. Pour in the seltzer and stir. Serve immediately.

Alternative Methods:

If you don't have a wooden spoon or drink muddler, you can briefly pulse the blackberries, mint leaves, simple syrup, and rum together in a small blender; just be careful not to overblend it into a puree or the flavors and colors will be muddy.

To make this drink for a group, you can prepare the berries, mint, simple syrup, and rum in large quantities in a pitcher or jug and store in the refrigerator for up to 4 hours. Add the ice and seltzer to each drink individually right before serving.

Calories: 141 | Fat: 0g | Protein: 0g | Carbs: 5g | Fiber: 2g | Erythritol: 4g | **Net Carbs: 3g**

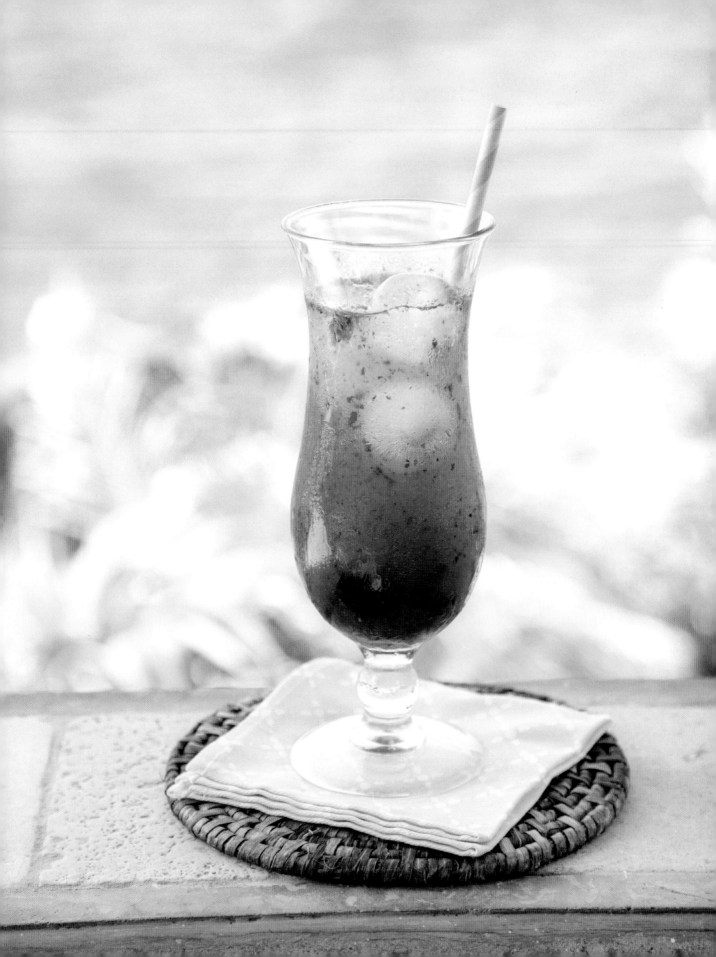

dairy-free egg-free nut-free vegetarian

Bourbon Sweetie

A combination of iced tea, lemon juice, and bourbon, this refreshing and delicious cocktail goes down super easy on a hot day. Maybe too easy, if you know what I'm saying!

Yield: **1 serving** ◆ Prep Time: **2 minutes**

2 ounces bourbon

4 ounces unsweetened iced tea

2 tablespoons Lemon-Infused Simple Syrup (page 84)

1 tablespoon lemon juice

1 lemon wedge, for garnish (optional)

1 maraschino cherry, for garnish (optional)

Place the bourbon, tea, simple syrup, and lemon juice in a cocktail shaker, along with 5 ice cubes. Cover and shake vigorously for 20 seconds. Pour into a 10-ounce tumbler and garnish with a lemon wedge and a cherry, if desired.

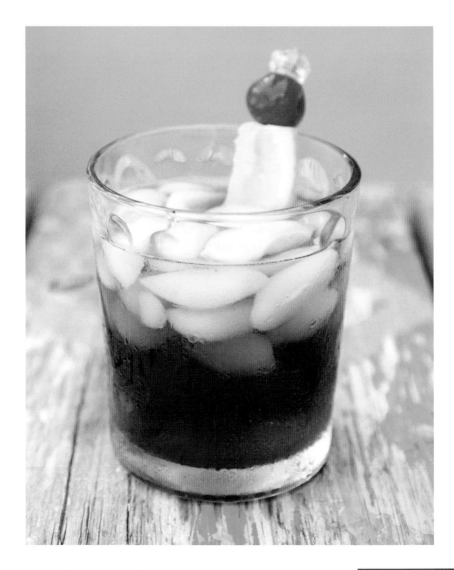

Calories: 130 | Fat: 0g | Protein: 0g | Carbs: 1g | Fiber: 0g | Erythritol: 12g | **Net Carbs: 1g**

Whiskey Sour

dairy-free egg-free nut-free vegetarian

When we were in our twenties, Mr. Hungry went through a whiskey sour phase, but he made them with that awful bottled sour mix that tastes mostly like chemicals. The real thing is so much better, and it's really easy to make!

Yield: **1 serving** ◆ Prep Time: **2 minutes**

2 ounces bourbon

1 tablespoon lemon juice

1 tablespoon Lemon-Infused Simple Syrup (page 84)

1 lemon wedge, for garnish (optional)

1 maraschino cherry, for garnish (optional)

Place the bourbon, lemon juice, and simple syrup in a cocktail shaker, along with 5 ice cubes. Cover and shake vigorously for 20 seconds. Pour into a chilled 6-ounce tumbler and garnish with a lemon wedge and a maraschino cherry, if desired. Serve immediately.

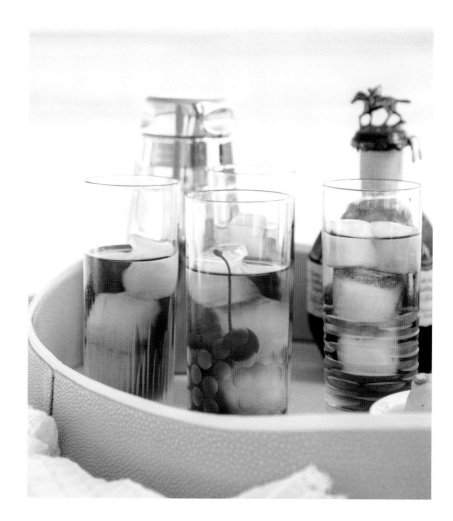

Calories: 135 | Fat: 0g | Protein: 0g | Carbs: 1g | Fiber: 0g | Erythritol: 6g | **Net Carbs: 1g**

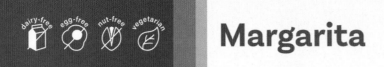

Margarita

Margaritas are typically made with triple sec, an orange-flavored liqueur that is high in sugar. This keto version uses sugar-free Orange-Infused Simple Syrup to achieve the same flavor without the carbs.

Yield: **1 serving** ◆ Prep Time: **2 minutes**

2 ounces premium white tequila

2 tablespoons lime juice

1 tablespoon Orange-Infused Simple Syrup (page 84)

1 lime slice, for garnish (optional)

Place the tequila, lime juice, and simple syrup in a cocktail shaker, along with 5 ice cubes. Cover and shake vigorously for 20 seconds. Pour into a margarita glass and garnish with a lime slice, if desired. Serve immediately.

> **Pro Tip:**
> *If you prefer a salted rim, before filling the glass, run a lime wedge around the rim of the glass and dip the rim of the glass into a shallow dish of coarse salt. The lime juice will be just enough glue to hold the salt on the rim. Pour your chilled drink into the glass and serve.*

Calories: 136 | Fat: 0g | Protein: 0g | Carbs: 2g | Fiber: 0g | Erythritol: 6g | **Net Carbs: 2g**

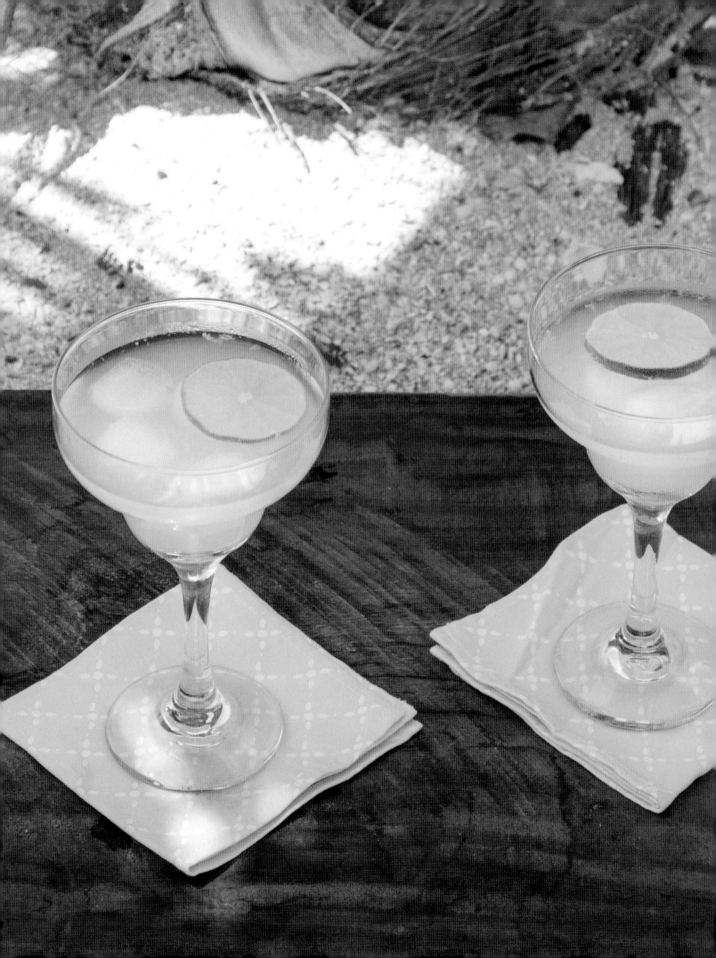

Piña Colada

The piña colada is the quintessential vacation drink, but there's no need to wait until your next Caribbean getaway to indulge. You can easily make this keto version at home and pretend you've got your toes jammed into the sand no matter what the time of year!

Yield: **1 serving** ◆ Prep Time: **2 minutes**

2 ounces dark rum

2 ounces full-fat unsweetened coconut milk

3 tablespoons Basic Simple Syrup (page 84), plus more to taste

1 tablespoon heavy whipping cream

1 teaspoon pineapple extract

1 pineapple wedge, for garnish (optional)

1 maraschino cherry, for garnish (optional)

Place all of the ingredients in a small blender, along with 10 ice cubes. Blend until smooth, about 1 minute. Taste and adjust the sweetness with more simple syrup, if desired. Pour into an 8-ounce tumbler and garnish with a pineapple wedge and a cherry, if desired. Serve immediately.

Calories: 230 | Fat: 11g | Protein: 0g | Carbs: 1g | Fiber: 0g | Erythritol: 18g | **Net Carbs: 1g**

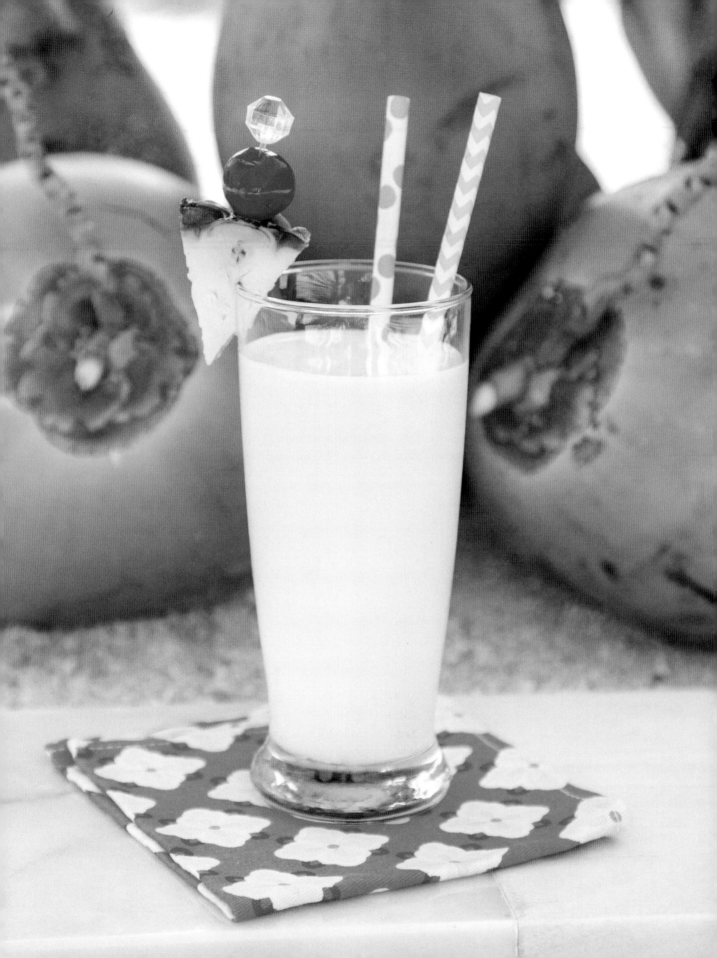

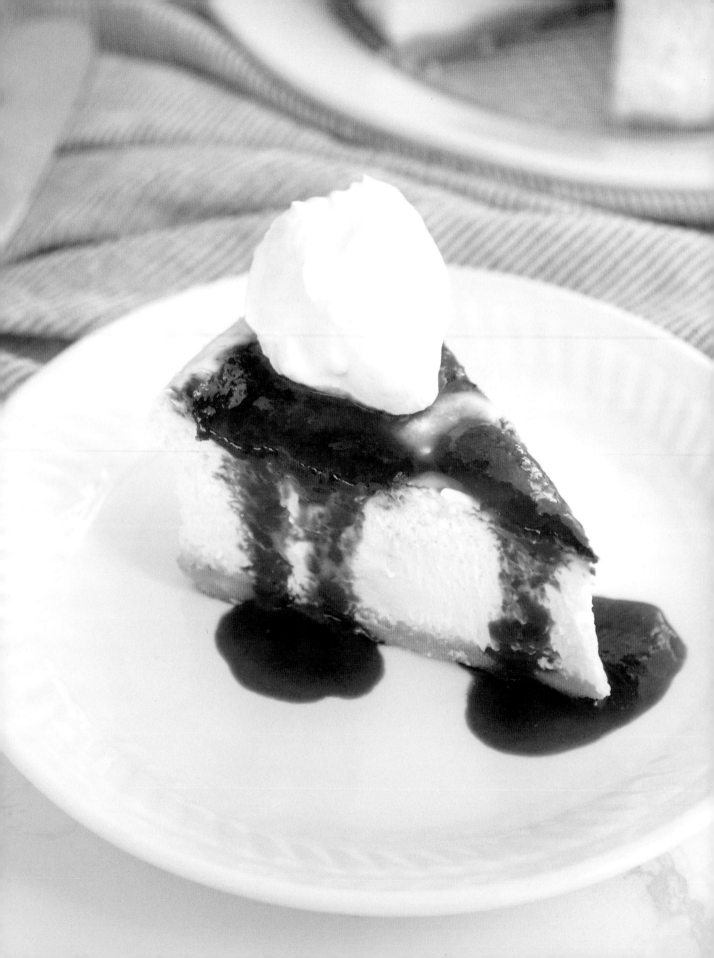

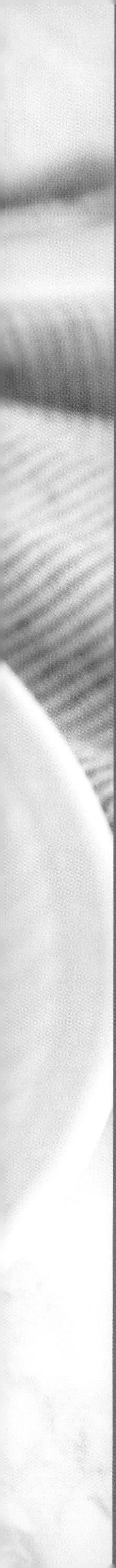

desserts

Chocolate Frosting / 324

Cream Cheese Frosting / 326

Basic Shortbread Dough / 328

Butter Rum Caramel Sauce / 330

Epic Chocolate Crunch Layer Cake / 332

Lemon Sour Cream Bundt Cake / 334

Pumpkin Spice Cupcakes / 336

No-Bake Sesame Cookies / 338

Pecan Shortbread Cookies / 340

Snickerdoodle Haystack Cookies / 342

Raspberry Swirl Cheesecake / 344

Triple Chocolate Cheesecake / 346

Coconut Tarts / 348

Coconut Paletas / 350

Chocolate Ice Cream / 352

Vanilla Ice Cream / 354

Affogato / 356

Chocolate Frosting

dairy-free egg-free nut-free vegetarian

Who doesn't love to steal a spoonful of rich and fluffy chocolate frosting out of the fridge with a spoon once in a while? Now you don't even have to feel guilty about it. If that isn't winning, I don't know what is! This chocolate frosting is also great on cakes, if you have any frosting to spare.

Yield: **4 cups** ◆ Serving Size: **2 tablespoons** ◆ Prep Time: **10 minutes, plus 1 hour to chill**

Cook Time: **2 minutes**

1½ cups heavy whipping cream

8 ounces unsweetened baking chocolate, chopped

¼ cup coconut oil

1¼ cups powdered erythritol

1 teaspoon pure vanilla extract

Pinch of kosher salt

1 Combine the cream, chocolate, and coconut oil in a medium-sized microwave-safe bowl. Microwave on high for 1 minute, then stir. Microwave on high for another minute and stir again. If the chocolate still isn't melted, microwave for 30 more seconds and stir until the chocolate is melted and the mixture is completely blended.

2 Stir in the sweetener, vanilla extract, and salt until the mixture is completely smooth. Place the bowl in the refrigerator to chill for 1 hour, or until firm.

3 Remove the bowl from the refrigerator and transfer the frosting to a mixing bowl. Using a handheld mixer, beat on low speed to break up the frosting, then gradually increase the speed to medium-high. Blend for 2 minutes, or until fluffy. Store in an airtight container in the refrigerator for up to 1 week or in the freezer for up to 3 months.

Alternative Method:
If you prefer a ganache-like frosting, chill the frosting until it is thickened but still pourable, about 15 minutes. Skip the beating in Step 3 and simply pour the cooled, but still liquid, mixture over your cake or dessert for a uniform glossy coating.

Calories: 88 | Fat: 9g | Protein: 1g | Carbs: 2g | Fiber: 1g | Erythritol: 8g | **Net Carbs: 1g**

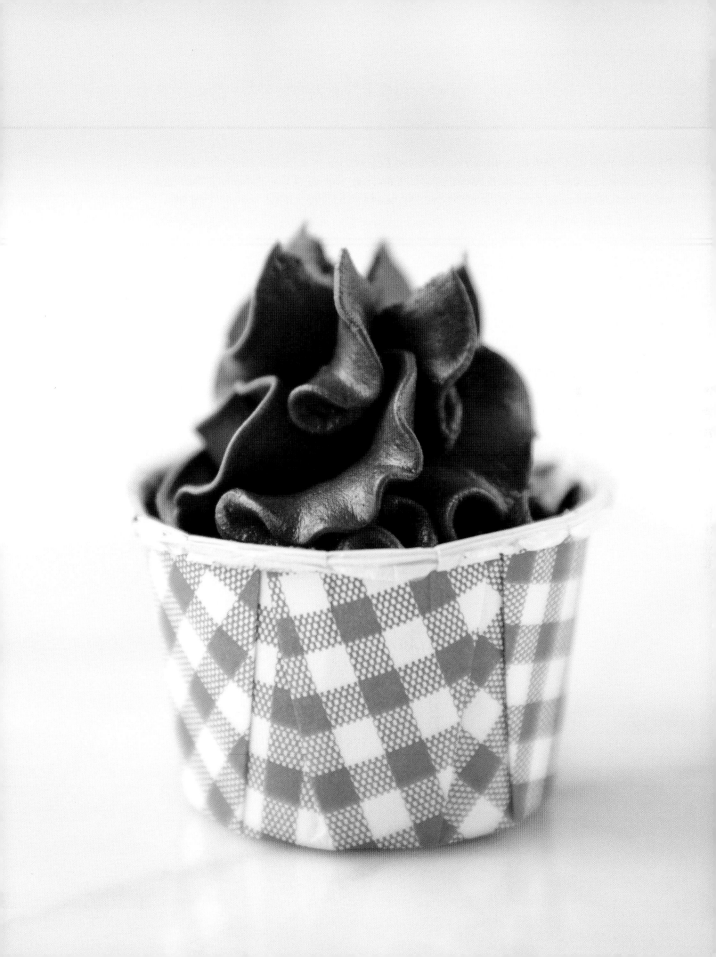

Cream Cheese Frosting

This cream cheese frosting is super versatile and can be used on a wide variety of cakes, cupcakes, and muffins and even as a crepe filling. Once chilled, it can be formed into balls and rolled in chopped nuts or toasted coconut to make a perfect fat bomb or a high-fat on-the-go snack!

Yield: **2 cups** ◆ Serving Size: **2 tablespoons** ◆ Prep Time: **10 minutes**

1 (8-ounce) package cream cheese, softened

½ cup (1 stick) butter, softened

⅔ cup powdered erythritol

½ teaspoon pure vanilla extract

1 In a medium-sized bowl, cream the cream cheese and butter with a handheld or stand mixer until light and fluffy.

2 Add the sweetener and vanilla extract and beat slowly until the sweetener is incorporated. Turn the speed up to high and beat for 2 minutes, or until fluffy. Use immediately or store in an airtight container in the refrigerator for up to 1 week or in the freezer for up to 3 months. Bring to room temperature before using.

Calories: 100 | Fat: 11g | Protein: 0g | Carbs: 1g | Fiber: 0g | Erythritol: 9g | **Net Carbs: 1g**

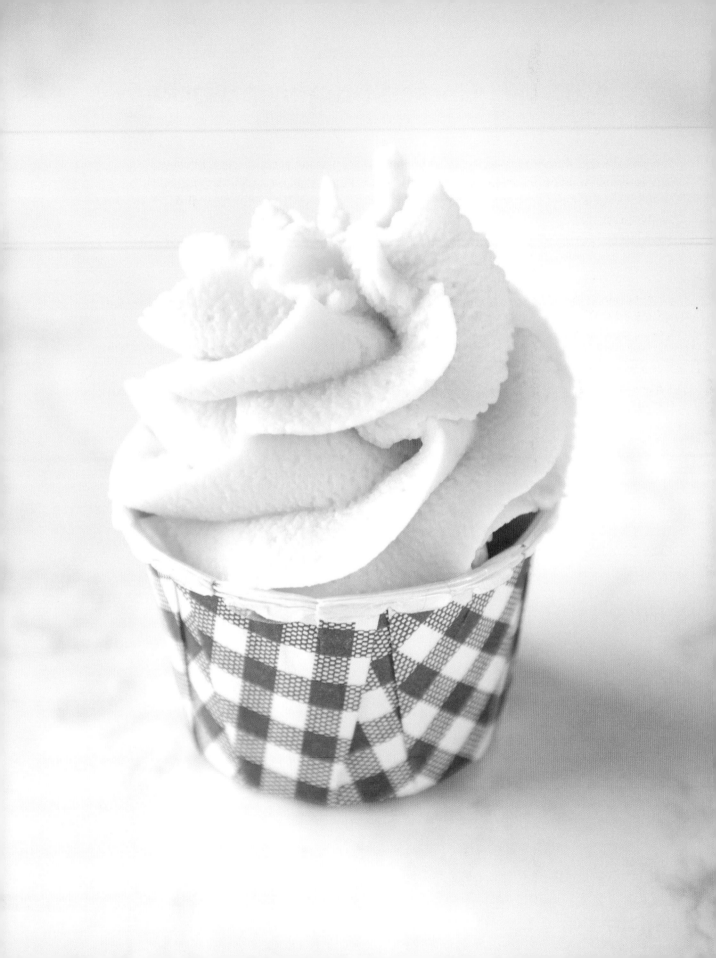

Basic Shortbread Dough

You can use this shortbread dough as is for a fantastic tart or pie crust or use it as a base for cheesecakes and bar cookie–style desserts. It also lends itself beautifully to any style of shortbread cookie (see page 340).

Yield: **two 10-inch or twelve 4-inch pie or tart crusts** • Prep Time: **2 minutes**

Cook Time: **8 minutes**

2 cups superfine blanched almond flour

6 tablespoons butter, melted

⅓ cup granulated erythritol

1 Place all of the ingredients in a medium-sized bowl. Mix well with a fork until a crumbly dough forms.

2 Form the dough into a ball and wrap tightly with plastic wrap. Chill until ready to use.

3 To form into pie or tart crusts, divide the dough into two balls for 10-inch pies, or twelve balls for 4-inch tarts.

4 Place the dough in tart or pie pans and use your fingers to press the dough evenly across the bottom and up the sides of the pans.

5 To par-bake the crust, place in a preheated 350°F oven for 8 minutes, or until lightly golden. Let cool, then fill and bake following the instructions in your recipe.

6 Store the wrapped dough in the refrigerator for up to 3 days or in the freezer for up to 3 months.

per crust: Calories: 1890 | Fat: 181g | Protein: 48g | Carbs: 48g | Fiber: 24g | Erythritol: 64g **Net Carbs: 24g**

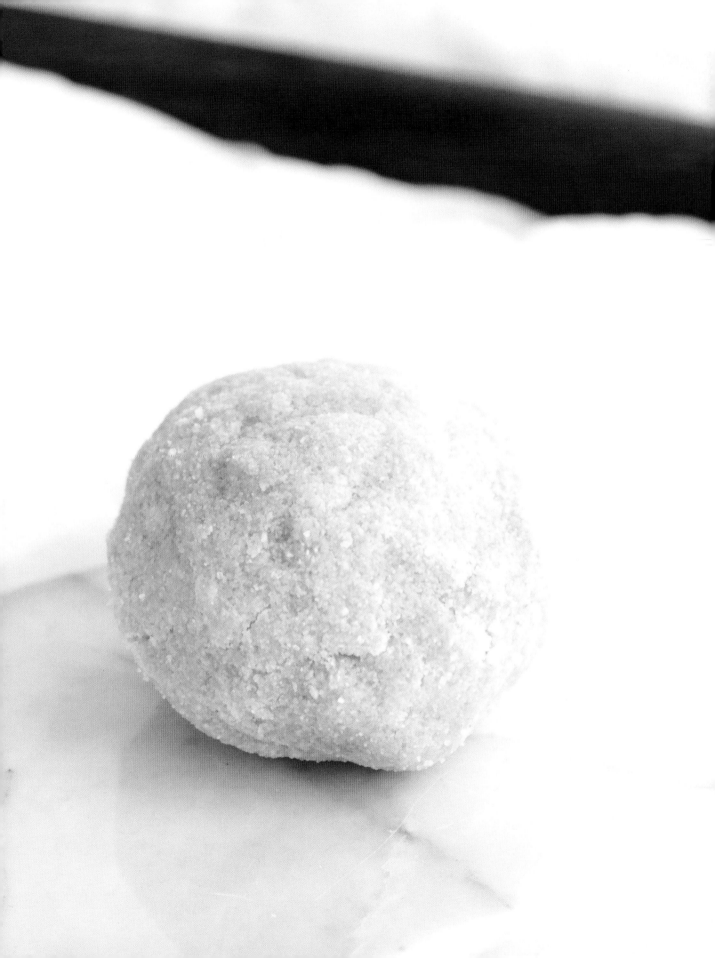

dairy-free egg-free nut-free vegetarian

Butter Rum Caramel Sauce

Is there anything caramel sauce isn't good on? I tested the theory—you know, for science. I can tell you with certainty that this sauce is good on low-carb cakes, ice cream, brownies, cream cheese pancakes, and even in coffee. Boom! I'll just leave that right there while you go try it. You're welcome.

Yield: ¾ cup • Serving Size: **2 tablespoons** • Prep Time: **3 minutes** • Cook Time: **12 minutes**

½ cup granulated erythritol

¼ cup (½ stick) butter

⅓ cup heavy whipping cream

¼ cup dark rum

¼ teaspoon xanthan gum

⅛ teaspoon kosher salt

1 Melt the sweetener and butter in a small saucepan over medium heat. Cook, stirring occasionally, for 8 minutes, or until liquid and bubbling.

2 Add the cream, rum, and xanthan gum. Cook, stirring constantly, for 4 minutes, or until the mixture reaches the desired color and thickness. Stir in the salt and let cool slightly before serving. Store in an airtight container in the refrigerator for up to 10 days.

Pro Tip:

If the caramel sauce solidifies or crystallizes while stored in the refrigerator, bring to room temperature and whisk before serving. If you don't want to wait (and I don't blame you), reheat in the microwave on high for 30 seconds to bring it back to a liquid state.

Calories: 139 | Fat: 13g | Protein: 0g | Carbs: 0g | Fiber: 0g | Erythritol: 16g | **Net Carbs: 0g**

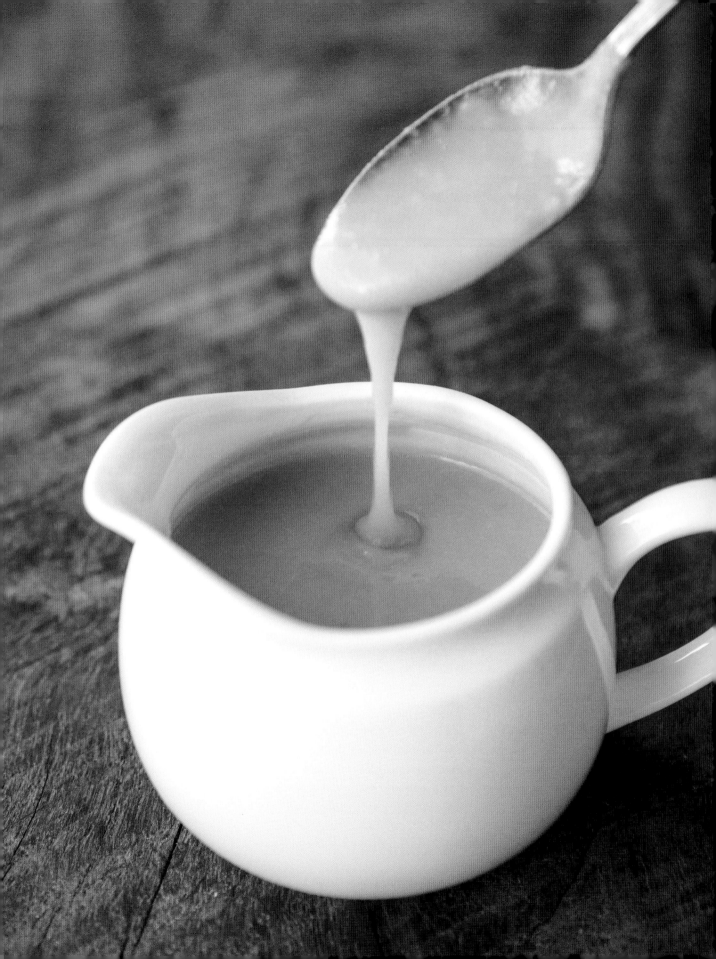

Epic Chocolate Crunch Layer Cake

dairy-free · egg-free · nut-free · vegetarian

I don't use the term *epic* lightly, but this is by far the best keto cake I've ever made. Not only is the cake unbelievably tender and fluffy and the frosting perfectly rich and chocolaty, but the cacao nib crunch is so on point that I want to put it on *everything*. Please go the extra mile to get some cacao nibs; the added texture and punch of chocolate that they give this cake is what transforms it from just awesome to truly epic. As always, use the highest-quality chocolate and cocoa powder that you can afford for best results.

Yield: one 9-inch double-layer cake (12 servings) ◆ Serving Size: **1 slice**

Prep Time: **15 minutes, plus 30 minutes to cool** ◆ Cook Time: **50 minutes**

2 cups granulated erythritol

1¾ cups unsweetened vanilla-flavored almond milk

1 cup (2 sticks) butter, melted but not hot

6 large eggs

2 ounces unsweetened baking chocolate, melted

2 teaspoons pure vanilla extract

3 cups superfine blanched almond flour

⅔ cup coconut flour

⅔ cup unsweetened cocoa powder

4 teaspoons baking powder

½ teaspoon xanthan gum

⅛ teaspoon kosher salt

For the cacao crunch:

⅔ cup cacao nibs

¼ cup granulated erythritol

1 batch Chocolate Frosting (page 324)

1 Preheat the oven to 350°F. Grease two 9-inch cake pans and line the bottoms with parchment paper rounds cut to fit.

2 Place the sweetener, almond milk, melted butter, eggs, melted chocolate, and vanilla extract in a blender and blend until smooth. Put the almond flour, coconut flour, cocoa powder, baking powder, xanthan gum, and salt in a large bowl and mix well.

3 Pour the wet ingredients from the blender into the bowl of dry ingredients, being sure to scrape the sides of the blender to get as much out as possible. Stir until the ingredients are well mixed.

4 Divide the batter evenly between the cake pans and smooth the tops with a rubber spatula. Bake for 50 minutes, or until a toothpick inserted in the center of a cake comes out clean. Let the cakes cool on a wire rack for 30 minutes.

5 Run a knife along the inside edge of one pan to free the cake from the sides. Carefully turn the pan over and release the cake into one hand, then place the cake upright on the rack. Repeat with the second cake. Let the cakes cool for 30 more minutes before frosting. If there is a noticeable bump on the top of your cake, you may slice it off with a knife to make it flat, if desired.

6 Make the cacao crunch: Place the cacao nibs and sweetener in a small blender and pulse for 30 seconds, or until the mixture resembles fine crumbs. Set aside.

7 Assemble and frost the cake: Place one cake right side up on a cake plate or pedestal. Spoon about 1 cup of frosting onto the middle of the cake. Spread with a metal spatula to the edges of the cake, but not down the sides.

Calories: 477 | Fat: 42g | Protein: 15g | Carbs: 20g | Fiber: 13g | Erythritol: 36g | **Net Carbs: 7g**

8   Sprinkle ½ cup of the cacao crunch evenly over the entire surface of the cake. Place the second cake upside down on top of the frosting and crunch layer. Frost the top and sides of the entire cake with about 2 cups of frosting, reserving about 1 cup for decorative piping, if desired.

9   Sprinkle the remaining cacao crunch around the outer edge of the cake. Decorate with the reserved frosting as desired. To serve, cut into 12 even slices. Store on a covered cake plate or pedestal in the refrigerator for up to 5 days or in the freezer for up to 3 months.

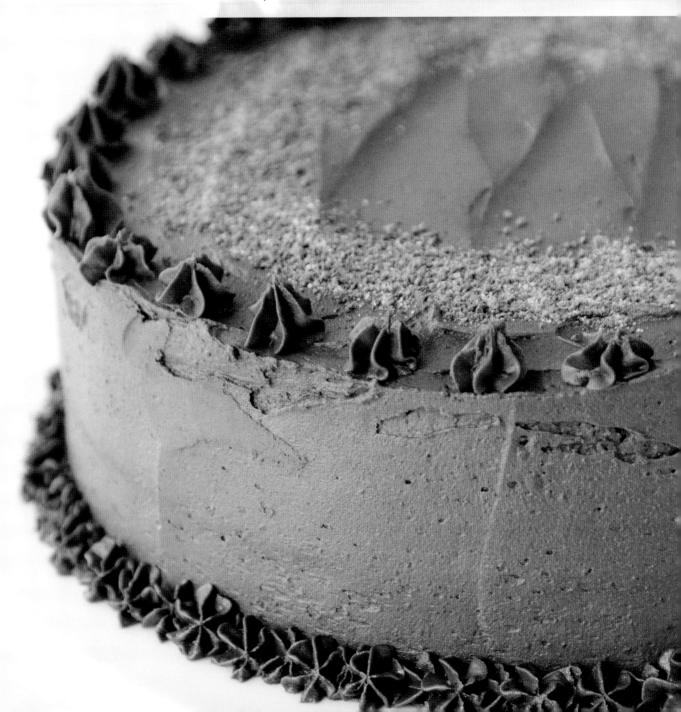

Lemon Sour Cream Bundt Cake

dairy-free · egg-free · nut-free · vegetarian

This tangy, melt-in-your-mouth cake is *life* when paired with a cup of coffee during those golden few alone minutes right before the after-school homework, what's for dinner, and "When was the last time you took a bath, child?" craziness. Maybe make that two cups of coffee...

Yield: **1 Bundt cake (12 servings)** ◆ Serving Size: **1 slice**

Prep Time: **8 minutes, plus 30 minutes to cool** ◆ Cook Time: **55 minutes**

For the cake:

1½ cups superfine blanched almond flour

1 cup full-fat sour cream

¾ cup granulated erythritol

½ cup coconut flour

½ cup (1 stick) unsalted butter, softened

3 large eggs

3 tablespoons lemon juice

1 tablespoon grated lemon zest

2 teaspoons baking powder

½ teaspoon pure vanilla extract

¼ teaspoon xanthan gum

Pinch of kosher salt

For the glaze:

½ cup powdered erythritol

3 tablespoons lemon juice

Special equipment:

Bundt pan

1. Preheat the oven to 350°F. Grease a 12-cup Bundt pan with butter or coconut oil.

2. Place the cake ingredients in a commercial-grade blender or a food processor and blend until smooth. The mixture will be thick, so you'll have to scrape down the sides with a rubber spatula a few times to get it to blend until smooth.

3. Spoon the batter into the greased Bundt pan and spread it evenly. Bake for 55 minutes, or until a toothpick inserted in the center of the cake comes out clean.

4. Remove from the oven and let cool on a rack for at least 30 minutes before unmolding onto a cake plate or pedestal.

5. Meanwhile, place the glaze ingredients in a small bowl and stir until well blended and pourable. If it's too thin, add more sweetener; if it's too thick, add more lemon juice. It should be just thin enough to pour in an even stream with no clumps.

6. Unmold the cake and pour the glaze evenly over the top. Cut into 12 even slices when ready to serve. Store on a covered cake plate or pedestal in the refrigerator for up to 1 week or in the freezer for up to 3 months.

> **Pro Tip:**
> *Because so much of the flavor in this cake comes from the lemon juice, be sure to use freshly squeezed instead of lemon juice from a bottle. I've made it both ways, and there is a huge difference in the quality of the flavor when you use fresh juice.*

Calories: 229 | Fat: 21g | Protein: 6g | Carbs: 7g | Fiber: 3g | Erythritol: 14g | **Net Carbs: 4g**

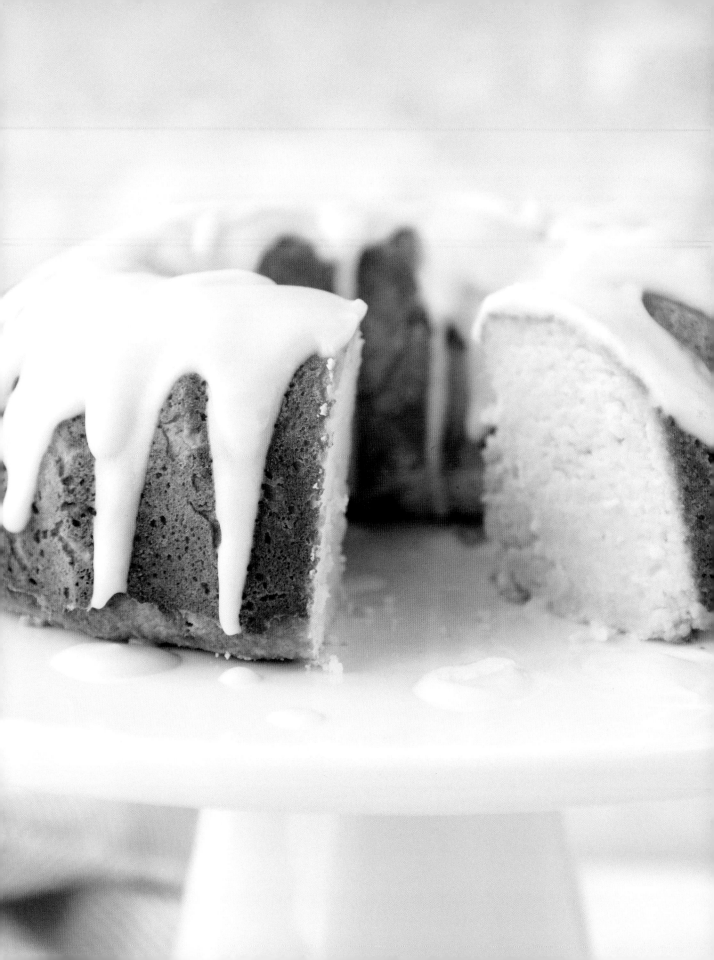

dairy-free egg-free nut-free vegetarian

Pumpkin Spice Cupcakes

I may currently live in perpetual summer weather in the Caribbean, but as a native New Englander, I still have a Pavlovian response when October hits, and I want to pumpkin all the things. Because pumpkin puree isn't a common ingredient here, I paid eleven dollars for a can of it to make you these truly delicious cupcakes. It was absolutely worth it!

Yield: **8 cupcakes** • Serving Size: **1 cupcake**

Prep Time: **10 minutes, plus 30 minutes to cool if using frosting** • Cook Time: **27 minutes**

6 tablespoons butter, melted but not hot

2 large eggs

1 teaspoon pure vanilla extract

½ cup solid-pack pumpkin puree

1 cup superfine blanched almond flour

⅓ cup granulated erythritol

¼ cup coconut flour

2 teaspoons baking powder

1 teaspoon ground cinnamon

¼ teaspoon ginger powder

¼ teaspoon xanthan gum

⅛ teaspoon ground cloves

⅛ teaspoon ground nutmeg

Pinch of kosher salt

1 cup Cream Cheese Frosting (page 326; optional)

1 Preheat the oven to 350°F. Place 8 cupcake liners in a standard-size 12-well cupcake pan.

2 Place the melted butter, eggs, vanilla extract, and pumpkin puree in a small blender and blend until smooth. Meanwhile, place the almond flour, sweetener, coconut flour, baking powder, cinnamon, ginger powder, xanthan gum, cloves, nutmeg, and salt in a medium-sized bowl and mix well.

3 Pour the wet ingredients from the blender into the bowl of dry mixed ingredients. Stir well until a thick batter has formed. Spoon the batter into the cupcake liners, filling each about two-thirds full. Bake for 27 minutes, or until a toothpick inserted in the center of a cupcake comes out clean.

4 Carefully remove the cupcakes from the pan and let cool on a baking rack for 30 minutes before frosting; if you're not using frosting, let cool for about 10 minutes to firm up before eating. When they're cool, spread or pipe about 2 tablespoons of the frosting onto each cupcake. Store in an airtight container in the refrigerator for up to 5 days or in the freezer for up to 3 months.

per cupcake, without frosting: Calories: 198 | Fat: 17g | Protein: 5g | Carbs: 6.75g | Fiber: 3.25g | Erythritol: 9g **Net Carbs: 3.5g**

per cupcake, with frosting: Calories: 298 | Fat: 28g | Protein: 6g | Carbs: 7.75g | Fiber: 3.25g | Erythritol: 18g **Net Carbs: 4.5g**

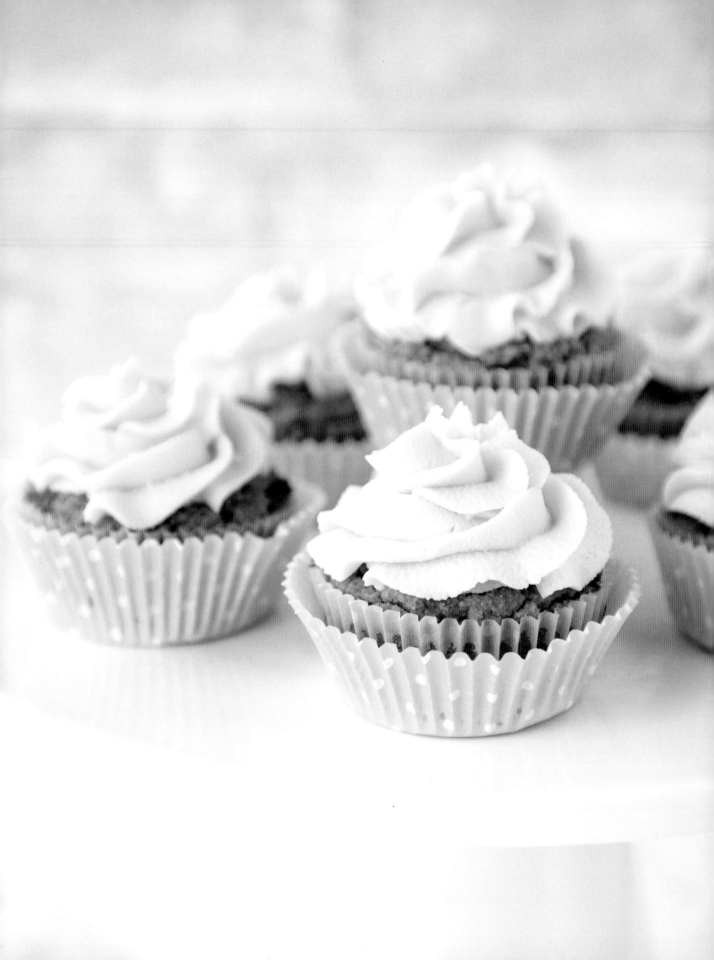

dairy-free egg-free nut-free vegetarian

No-Bake Sesame Cookies

I refer to these treats as cookies, but they have a nougat-like texture that is reminiscent of candy. Whatever you want to call them, they are easy and delicious! I prefer to eat them at room temperature, making them a great snack to take on the go. They will keep all day in your purse or in a lunch box for a quick and tasty pick-me-up that sustains you for hours.

Yield: **10 cookies** • Serving Size: **1 cookie** • Prep Time: **10 minutes**

¼ cup sesame seeds, toasted

⅓ cup powdered erythritol

⅓ cup tahini, room temperature

2 tablespoons butter, softened

2 tablespoons unsweetened, unflavored protein powder

½ teaspoon pure vanilla extract

Pinch of kosher salt

1   Pour the sesame seeds onto a small plate and set aside. Place the sweetener, tahini, butter, protein powder, vanilla extract, and salt in a food processor or small blender and blend until smooth.

2   Roll the mixture into 10 balls about 1½ inches in diameter. Roll each ball in the sesame seeds until coated, then flatten slightly. Store in an airtight container in the refrigerator for up to 1 week or in the freezer for up to 3 months.

> **Pro Tip:**
> *When tahini is stored, the oil will separate, so be sure to stir it well before you measure it out for this recipe.*

Calories: 92 | Fat: 9g | Protein: 4g | Carbs: 2g | Fiber: 1g | Erythritol: 8g | **Net Carbs: 1g**

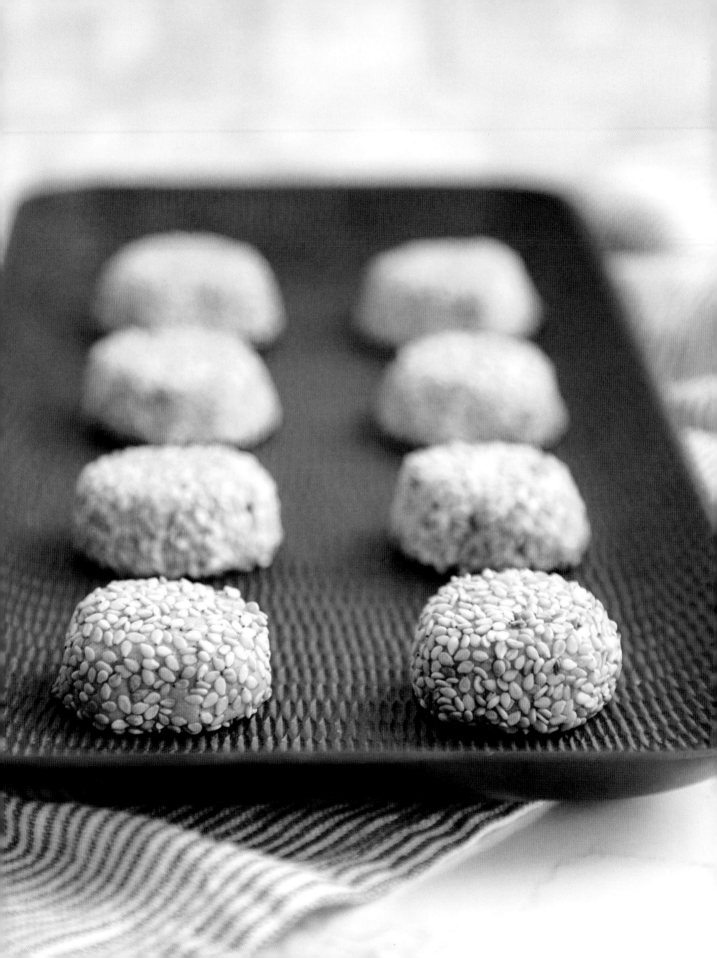

dairy-free egg-free nut-free vegetarian

Pecan Shortbread Cookies

When I was in my twenties, my favorite guilty pleasure was pecan sandies. I loved their buttery, nutty flavor and crunchy texture. This keto version is just as delicious, but without the carbs and sugar. It's also super easy to make, so double the batch and keep some in the freezer for snacking emergencies.

Yield: **16 cookies** ◆ Serving Size: **1 cookie** ◆ Prep Time: **5 minutes, plus 30 minutes to chill**

Cook Time: **12 minutes**

2 cups superfine blanched almond flour

½ cup chopped raw pecans

½ cup granulated erythritol

6 tablespoons butter, melted

1 teaspoon pure vanilla extract

1 Place all of the ingredients in a medium-sized bowl and mix well with a fork. Form the dough into a log and wrap tightly in plastic wrap. Chill for 30 minutes, or until firm.

2 Preheat the oven to 350°F. Line a 15 by 10-inch sheet pan with parchment paper.

3 Unwrap the dough and slice crosswise into ½-inch-thick rounds. Place the slices on the prepared sheet pan, spacing them about 1 inch apart. Bake for 12 minutes, or until golden brown on the edges.

4 Remove the cookies from the oven and place on a rack to cool. Store in an airtight container in the refrigerator for up to 3 days or in the freezer for up to 3 months.

Calories: 142 | Fat: 13g | Protein: 4g | Carbs: 4g | Fiber: 2g | Erythritol: 6g | **Net Carbs: 2g**

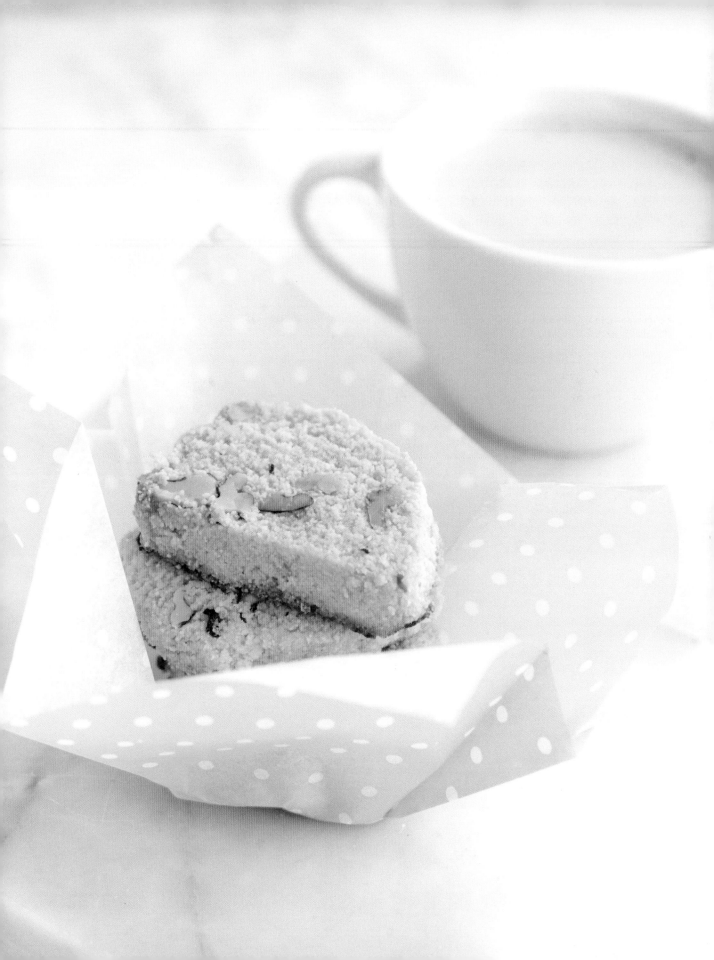

dairy-free egg-free nut-free vegetarian

Snickerdoodle Haystack Cookies

No-bake haystack cookies were one of my favorite treats when I was raw vegan about ten years ago. I made all kinds in my dehydrator, and they made the house smell so good! Unfortunately, it took at least twelve hours until they were ready to eat. I still love haystack cookies made with coconut, but now, on keto, I can add butter and cream cheese—and they are ready to eat in just minutes!

Yield: **10 cookies** • Serving Size: **1 cookie** • Prep Time: **5 minutes, plus 30 minutes to chill**

¼ cup (½ stick) unsalted butter, softened

2 ounces cream cheese (¼ cup), softened

⅓ cup powdered erythritol

1 teaspoon ground cinnamon

½ teaspoon pure vanilla extract

¼ teaspoon baking soda

2 cups unsweetened shredded coconut

1   Line a plate or small sheet pan with parchment paper.

2   Place the butter and cream cheese in a medium-sized bowl. Using an electric mixer, beat until smooth.

3   Add the sweetener, cinnamon, vanilla extract, and baking soda and beat for 10 seconds. Stir in the shredded coconut by hand until fully mixed.

4   Use a 1½-tablespoon cookie dough scoop to drop 10 mounded scoops onto the lined plate. Chill for 30 minutes before serving. Store in an airtight container in the refrigerator for up to 1 week or in the freezer for up to 3 months.

Calories: 181 | Fat: 18g | Protein: 2g | Carbs: 5g | Fiber: 3g | Erythritol: 6g | **Net Carbs: 2g**

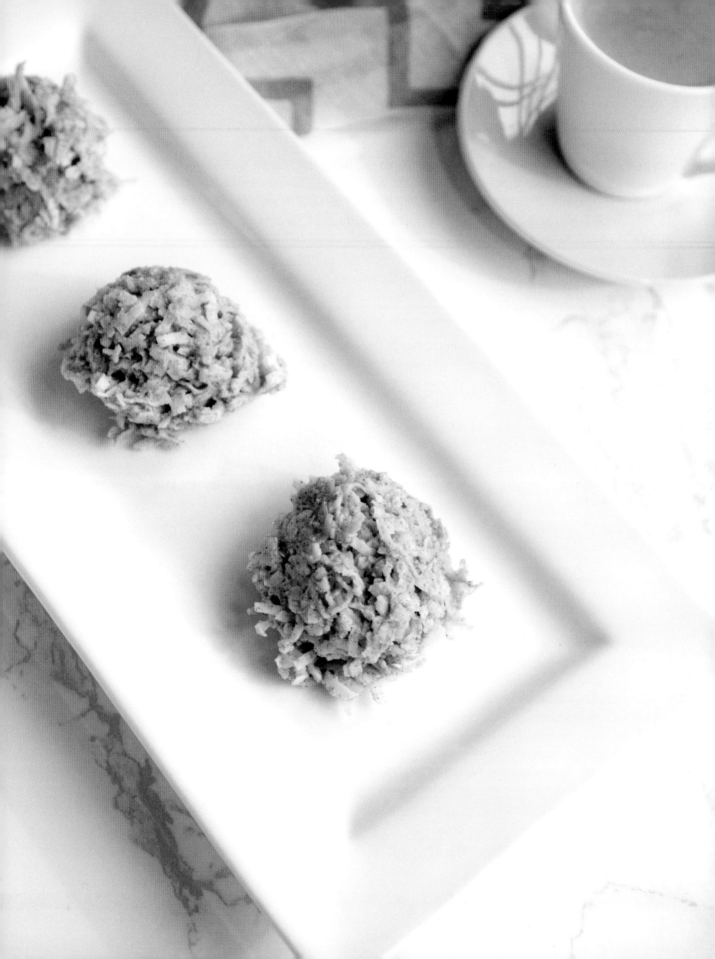

Raspberry Swirl Cheesecake

Impossibly smooth and creamy with a hint of bright raspberry flavor baked in, this cheesecake is a favorite in the Hungry household! It's made in a blender, so it's incredibly quick and easy to throw together; the hardest part is waiting for it to bake and chill before you can eat it. For even more raspberry flavor, serve it with a drizzle of my Raspberry Coulis.

Yield: one 8-inch cheesecake (10 servings) ◆ Serving Size: **1 slice**

Prep Time: **10 minutes, plus 1 hour to cool and 4 hours to chill** ◆ Cook Time: **1½ hours**

½ batch **Basic Shortbread Dough** (page 328)

3 (8-ounce) packages cream cheese, softened

3 large eggs

1 cup granulated erythritol

¼ cup heavy whipping cream

1½ teaspoons pure vanilla extract

¼ cup **Raspberry Coulis** (page 95), plus more for garnish if desired

Special equipment:

8-inch springform pan

> **Pro Tip:**
> *Because cheesecake can be tricky to cut due to its density, dip your knife in hot water for 10 seconds before slicing. Repeat before every other slice, being sure to wipe off the excess water with a towel before cutting into the cake.*

1 Preheat the oven to 350°F.

2 Press the shortbread dough into the bottom and halfway up the sides of an 8-inch springform pan. Par-bake for 8 minutes. Remove from the oven and let cool for 10 minutes. Reduce the oven temperature to 325°F.

3 While the crust is par-baking, make the filling: Place the cream cheese, eggs, sweetener, cream, and vanilla in a blender and blend until smooth, about 2 minutes.

4 Pour the filling over the par-baked crust and spread evenly. Spoon the raspberry coulis in circles on the top and swirl gently with a knife to mix it into the batter. Bake for 1 hour 20 minutes, or until the center barely moves when the pan is jiggled.

5 Turn off the oven and open the door partway, leaving the cheesecake in the oven to cool for 1 hour before removing. Place the cheesecake in the refrigerator to chill for at least 4 hours.

6 When ready to serve, run a knife around the inside edge of the pan, then release the clamp and remove the side of the pan. Cut the cheesecake into 10 even slices and spoon additional coulis over each slice, if desired.

7 Store in an airtight container in the refrigerator for up to 5 days or in the freezer for up to 3 months.

Calories: 334 | Fat: 28g | Protein: 9g | Carbs: 7.5g | Fiber: 1.5g | Erythritol: 23g | **Net Carbs: 6g**

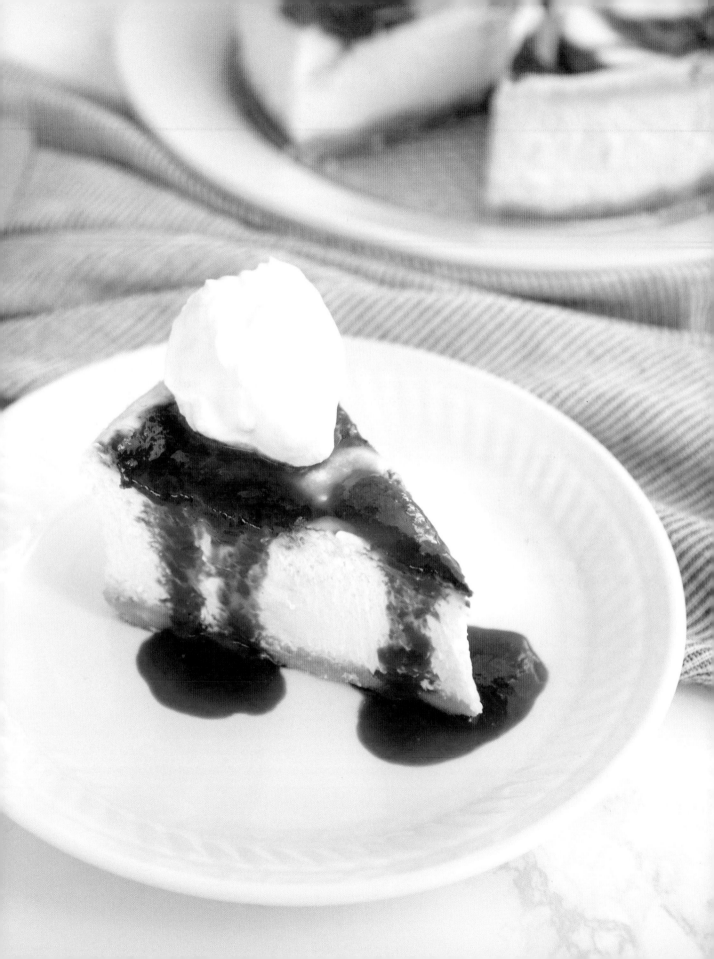

Triple Chocolate Cheesecake

dairy-free · egg-free · nut-free · vegetarian

If you're a chocolate lover, this chocolate-forward cheesecake is everything you've ever wanted in a dessert—chocolate in the crust and filling, along with a ganache topping. It's truly a dream dessert! A little goes a long way, so you may find that you have a lot left over. No problem; this cheesecake freezes perfectly! I've been enjoying a tiny slice here and there over the course of three months, and every bite is as good as the first!

Yield: **one 10-inch cheesecake (12 servings)** ◆ Serving Size: **1 slice**

Prep Time: **15 minutes, plus 1 hour to cool and 8 hours to chill** ◆ Cook Time: **1 hour 10 minutes**

For the crust:

2 cups superfine blanched almond flour

½ cup granulated erythritol

6 tablespoons butter, melted

3 tablespoons unsweetened cocoa powder

Pinch of kosher salt

For the filling:

4 (8-ounce) packages cream cheese, softened

1⅔ cups granulated erythritol

¼ cup unsweetened cocoa powder

5 large eggs

1 tablespoon pure vanilla extract

8 ounces unsweetened baking chocolate, melted

2 tablespoons heavy whipping cream

For the topping:

4 ounces unsweetened baking chocolate, chopped

¾ cup heavy whipping cream

3 tablespoons granulated erythritol

¼ teaspoon pure vanilla extract

1 Preheat the oven to 350°F.

2 Place all of the crust ingredients in a medium-sized bowl and mix well with a fork until pea-sized crumbs form. Transfer to a 10-inch springform pan and press the dough across the bottom and halfway up the sides of the pan. Par-bake for 8 minutes. Remove from the oven and let cool for 10 minutes. Reduce the oven temperature to 325°F.

3 Make the filling: Using an electric mixer and a large bowl, beat the cream cheese and sweetener until fluffy. Add the cocoa powder, eggs, and vanilla extract and beat until combined. Pour in the melted chocolate and cream and beat until the batter is smooth and thick, almost like frosting.

4 Spoon the batter into the springform pan, over the crust, and smooth the top with a metal spatula. Bake for 1 hour, or until the center barely moves when the pan is jiggled.

5 Turn off the oven and open the door partially, leaving the cheesecake in the oven for 1 hour before removing. Place the cooled cheesecake in the refrigerator to chill for 30 minutes.

6 Meanwhile, combine the topping ingredients in a medium-sized microwave-safe bowl. Microwave on high for 1 minute, then stir. Microwave for 30 seconds and stir. If the chocolate is still not fully melted, repeat one more time. Stir well until glossy and uniform in color. Set aside to cool for 15 minutes.

Special equipment:

10-inch springform pan

Calories: 398 | Fat: 39g | Protein: 13g | Carbs: 14g | Fiber: 8g | Erythritol: 38g | **Net Carbs: 6g**

7   Pour the topping over the center of the cheesecake and spread to about 1 inch from the edge, then place the cheesecake in the refrigerator to chill for at least 8 hours.

8   When ready to serve, run a knife around the inside edge of the pan, then release the clamp and remove the side of the pan. Cut the cheesecake into 12 even slices.

9   Store in an airtight container in the refrigerator for up to 1 week or in the freezer for up to 3 months.

Coconut Tarts

Coconut tarts are very popular here in the Caribbean, but of course this keto version is free of both gluten and sugar. It still has the same crunchy, chewy texture and sweetness, with a hint of nutmeg that perfectly complements the coconut filling and shortbread crust.

Yield: **six 4-inch tarts** • Serving Size: **1 tart** • Prep Time: **10 minutes** • Cook Time: **35 minutes**

½ batch Basic Shortbread Dough (page 328)

2 cups shredded unsweetened coconut

⅓ cup granulated erythritol

⅛ teaspoon ground nutmeg

¼ cup filtered water

3 tablespoons butter

1 large egg, beaten

2 tablespoons heavy whipping cream

Special equipment:

6 (4-inch) mini pie pans

1 Preheat the oven to 350°F.

2 Divide the shortbread dough between 6 mini pie pans (4 inches in diameter) and press evenly along the bottoms and up the sides. Par-bake the crusts for 8 minutes, or until lightly golden. Remove from the oven and set aside; leave the oven on.

3 Meanwhile, combine the coconut, sweetener, and nutmeg in a small saucepan over medium heat. Cook, stirring occasionally, for 5 minutes, or until lightly golden and fragrant. Add the water and butter and cook for 2 more minutes, or until the liquid is mostly absorbed.

4 Remove from the heat and stir in the beaten egg and cream. Divide the coconut mixture between the 6 par-baked crusts and spread evenly.

5 Bake for 20 minutes, or until both the crust and coconut filling are golden brown.

6 Remove from the oven and let cool for 20 minutes before serving. Serve the tarts in the pie pans so they hold together when warm; if you wish to unpan them, let them cool for at least 2 hours first to allow them to firm up. Store in an airtight container in the refrigerator for up to 5 days or in the freezer for up to 3 months.

Alternative Method:
If you don't want to mess with making individual tarts, you could make one 10-inch tart or pie. Complete the recipe as written but bake the tart or pie for 25 to 30 minutes to account for the larger size.

Calories: 437 | Fat: 42g | Protein: 7g | Carbs: 11g | Fiber: 7g | Erythritol: 16g | **Net Carbs: 4g**

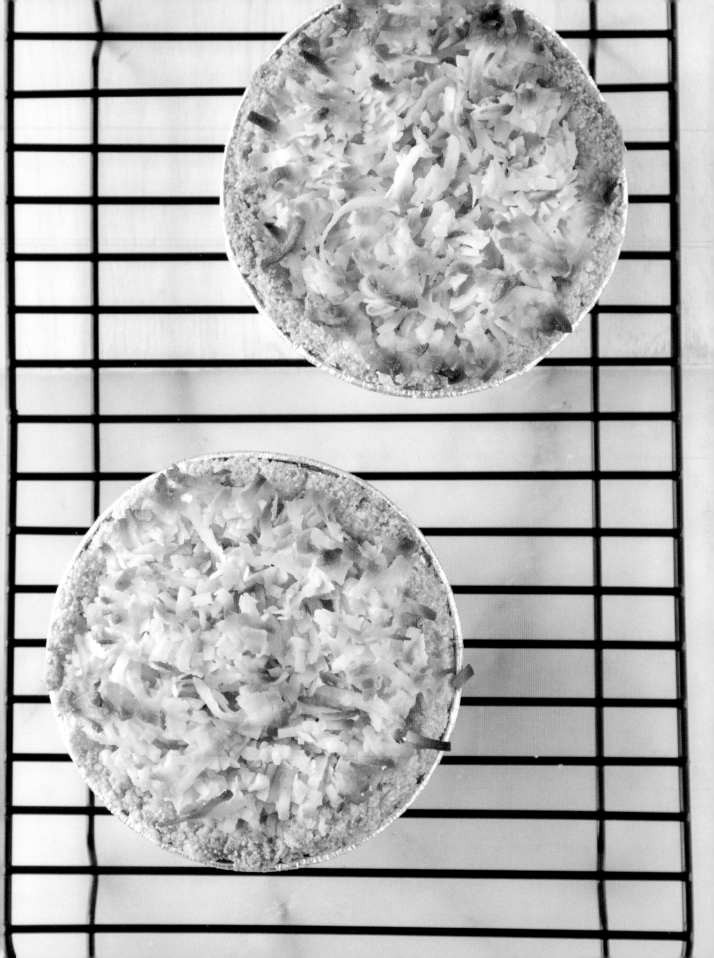

Coconut Paletas

In Belize, they sell paletas, or ice pops, in a wide variety of local flavors. Coconut is my favorite, but of course they are typically loaded with sugar. This keto version tastes as good as the real thing, without the extra carbs! You can customize these coconut paletas in lots of ways with chocolate, nuts, and toasted coconut.

Yield: **6 paletas** ◆ Serving Size: **1 paleta** ◆ Prep Time: **6 minutes, plus 3 to 4 hours to chill**

1 (14-ounce) can full-fat unsweetened coconut milk

3 tablespoons granulated erythritol

1 teaspoon pure vanilla extract

Melted chocolate, chopped almonds, and/or toasted shredded coconut, for topping (optional)

Special equipment:

6 (3-ounce) ice pop molds

1   Place the coconut milk, sweetener, and vanilla extract in a blender and blend for 30 seconds. Let the mixture rest for 5 minutes, then stir gently until any foam at the top has disappeared. Pour into 6 ice pop molds and freeze until firm, 3 to 4 hours. Store in the freezer until ready to eat.

2   Before serving, unmold the ice pops and sprinkle with chopped almonds or toasted coconut and drizzle with melted chocolate, if desired. Store in the freezer for up to 1 month.

Pro Tip:

If adding toppings to the frozen paletas, let the paletas sit at room temperature for about 2 minutes, then lightly press the toppings onto them and they should adhere just fine. Adding the melted chocolate last and then popping the paletas back in the freezer for 1 to 2 minutes will ensure that the toppings remain in place when you eat them. Also, chocolate as food "glue" is never a bad idea.

Variation:

Coconut-Rum Paletas. To make an adult version, add 2 ounces of white rum in place of the vanilla extract before freezing—just don't give them to the kids by mistake!

Calories: 100 | Fat: 10g | Protein: 0g | Carbs: 1g | Fiber: 0g | Erythritol: 6g | **Net Carbs: 1g**

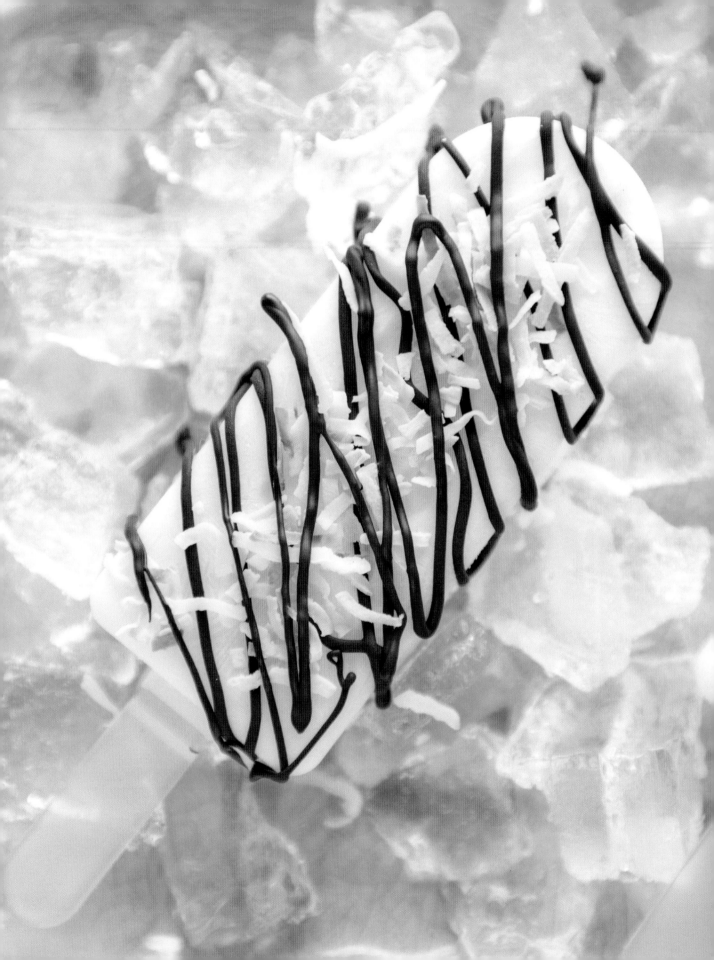

dairy-free egg-free nut-free vegetarian

Chocolate Ice Cream

Chocolate ice cream is one of my favorites. While it's delicious on its own, you can also use it as a base for all sorts of mix-ins. Add some chopped nuts, chunks of Triple Chocolate Cheesecake (page 346), dark chocolate shavings—you're limited only by your imagination.

Yield: **1 quart** ◆ Serving Size: **½ cup** ◆ Prep Time: **5 minutes, plus 30 minutes to chill base and 2 hours to freeze churned ice cream** ◆ Cook Time: **2 minutes**

1½ cups heavy whipping cream

1 cup unsweetened vanilla-flavored almond milk

3 large eggs

1 cup granulated erythritol

1 cup unsweetened cocoa powder

½ teaspoon xanthan gum

Pinch of salt

Special equipment:

Ice cream maker

1   Place the heavy cream, almond milk, eggs, sweetener, cocoa powder, xanthan gum, and salt in a blender and blend until smooth. Pour into a medium-sized microwave-safe bowl and microwave on high for 1 minute, then stir. Microwave for 30 seconds more and stir again. Microwave for another 30 seconds and stir. By now, the mixture should be thick enough to coat the back of a spoon. If it is still very runny, microwave for another 30 seconds and stir one more time.

2   Pour the ice cream mixture through a fine-mesh strainer to remove any lumps, then chill in the freezer for 30 minutes or in the refrigerator for 4 hours.

3   Pour the ice cream mixture into an ice cream maker and churn according to the manufacturer's instructions. Transfer to a freezer-safe container and freeze until firm, about 2 hours.

4   Store in an airtight container in the freezer for up to 1 month. For the best consistency, thaw for 10 minutes before serving.

Pro Tip:
If you wish to add mix-ins, add them during the final minute of churning, after the ice cream is mostly frozen. About ¾ cup of mix-ins is appropriate for this quantity of ice cream. No judgment here if you want to add more, though.

Calories: 155 | Fat: 14g | Protein: 5g | Carbs: 6.5g | Fiber: 3.5g | Erythritol: 24g | **Net Carbs: 3g**

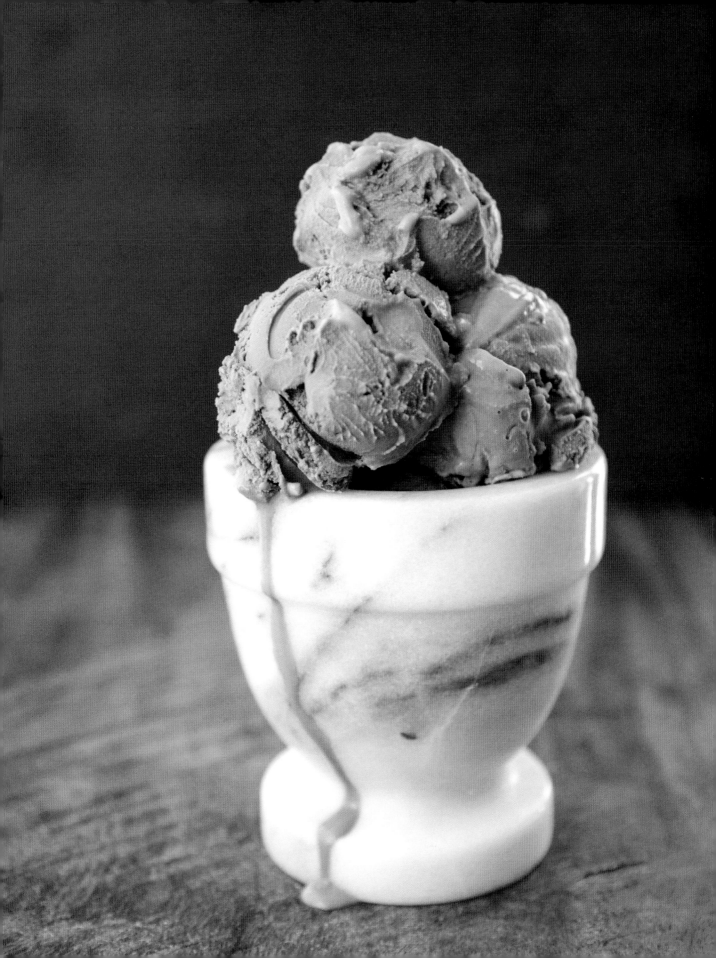

Vanilla Ice Cream

dairy-free *egg-free* *nut-free* *vegetarian*

Vanilla ice cream is a classic, but I enjoy it best paired with other desserts, like cobbler, brownies, or pie. I've kept it basic here so you can do the same, but like the Chocolate Ice Cream on page 352, this recipe can be customized in an unlimited number of ways with the mix-ins or toppings of your choice. Chopped nuts or chocolate, some of my Butter Rum Caramel Sauce (page 330) or Raspberry Coulis (page 95), or a handful of your favorite berries would work really well to dress it up.

Yield: **3 cups** ◆ Serving Size: **½ cup** ◆ Prep Time: **5 minutes, plus 30 minutes to chill base and 2 hours to freeze churned ice cream** ◆ Cook Time: **2 minutes**

2 cups heavy whipping cream

½ cup unsweetened vanilla-flavored almond milk

⅓ cup granulated erythritol

1 teaspoon pure vanilla extract

¼ teaspoon xanthan gum

⅛ teaspoon kosher salt

4 large egg yolks

Special equipment:

Ice cream maker

1 Place the cream, almond milk, sweetener, vanilla extract, xanthan gum, salt, and egg yolks in a blender and blend until smooth. Pour into a medium-sized microwave-safe bowl and microwave on high for 1 minute, then stir well. Microwave for 30 seconds, then stir. Microwave for 30 seconds more and stir again. At this point, the mixture should be thick enough to coat the back of a spoon. If it is still very runny, microwave for another 30 seconds and stir one more time.

2 Pour the ice cream mixture through a fine-mesh strainer to remove any lumps, then chill in the freezer for 30 minutes or in the refrigerator for 4 hours.

3 Pour the chilled ice cream mixture into an ice cream maker and churn according to the manufacturer's instructions. Transfer to a freezer-safe container and freeze until firm, about 2 hours.

4 Store in an airtight container in the freezer for up to 1 month. For the best consistency, thaw for 10 minutes before eating.

Pro Tip:
If you wish to add mix-ins, add them during the final minute of churning, after the ice cream is mostly frozen. About ½ cup of mix-ins is appropriate for this quantity of ice cream.

Calories: 301 | Fat: 29g | Protein: 2g | Carbs: 1g | Fiber: 0g | Erythritol: 11g | **Net Carbs: 1g**

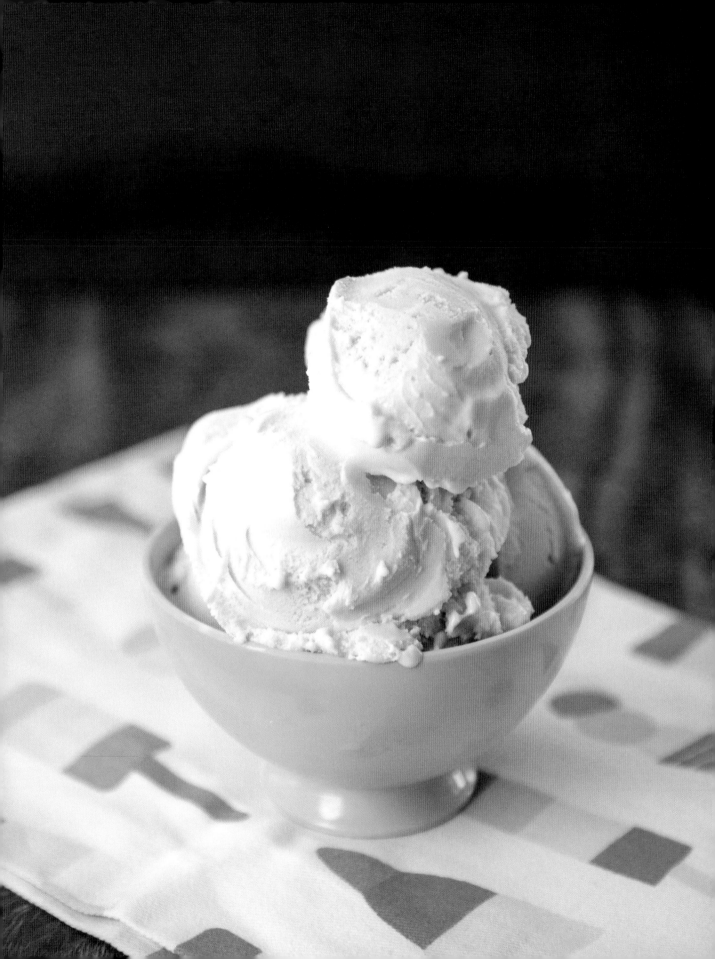

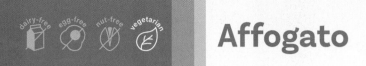

Affogato

The first time I had a real affogato was a few years ago at Eataly in New York City. Affogato is the perfect pairing of two of my favorite things—coffee and gelato. What's not to like? This version is made with my keto vanilla ice cream, and I think it's just as good.

Yield: **1 serving** ◆ Prep Time: **5 minutes**

½ **cup Vanilla Ice Cream (page 354)**

2 ounces hot brewed espresso

Scoop the ice cream into a heatproof cup or mug. Pour the hot espresso over the ice cream. Serve immediately.

Calories: 301 | Fat: 29g | Protein: 2g | Carbs: 1g | Fiber: 0g | Erythritol: 11g | **Net Carbs: 1g**

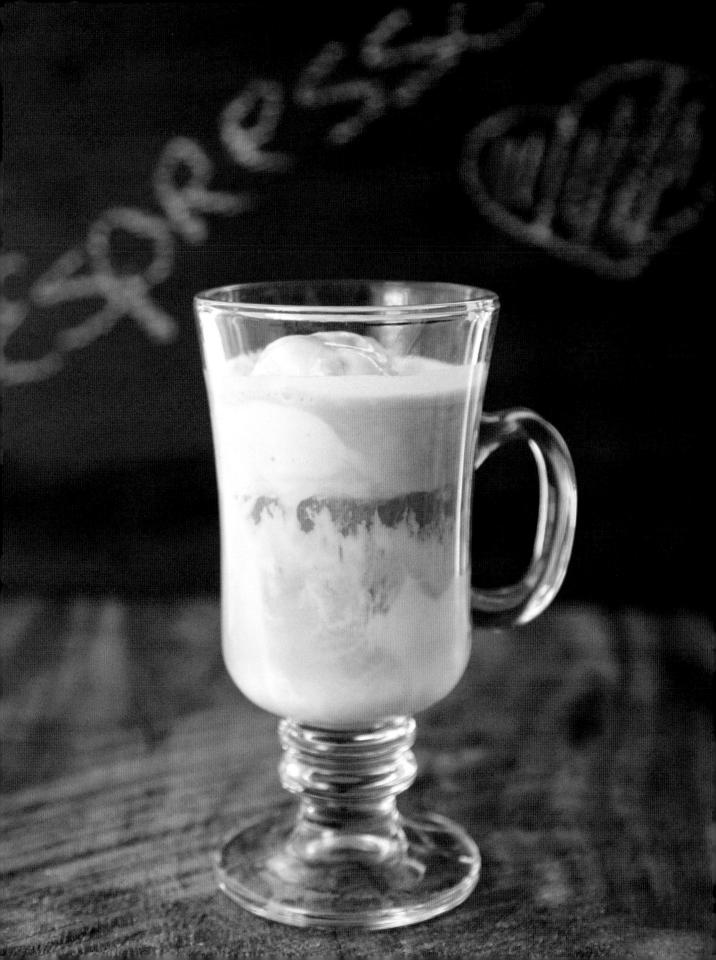

With Gratitude

To the fantastic team at Victory Belt: Thank you so much for your patience, encouragement, and hard work to make this book the best it could be! Holly and Pam, your thoughtful edits and suggestions will make me a better writer going forward, and I so appreciate you sharing your extensive knowledge of cooking and recipe writing with me during this process. I hope we'll get to work together again!

To Mr. Hungry: I could never have done this without your constant love, support, and encouragement. Thank you for being my best friend and companion for the last twenty-five years, and for being my tireless dishwasher over the past six months as I totaled the kitchen day after day to complete these recipes. Love you "many."

To Hungry Junior: I love you so much and can't wait to see what our next adventure as a family brings. I'm beyond thrilled that you have inherited my love of food, and I look forward to teaching you how to bring out the best of it in the coming years. Thank you for putting up with my many hours spent in the kitchen and on the computer to bring this book to life. I promise not to cook with cauliflower or broccoli for at least a week now that it's done. Love, Mom.

To my mom: Thank you for teaching me to cook at an early age and for letting me make huge messes in the pursuit of the perfect pie. You taught me to love food and that, even when you have very little to work with, you can still make it tasty. Also, and more importantly, you taught me by example how to be generous and kind and to be conscious of my spiritual need. I love you.

To my uncle, Chef Tom Perron: You were always more of a big brother than an uncle to me (mostly in that you tortured me mercilessly when we were younger, and of course I deserved it). I'm constantly in awe of your talent in the kitchen and the restaurant business in general. Thank you for teaching me how to cut an onion the right way, the value of a great knife, and to always push the limits of what is "normal" regarding flavor combinations. I still can't make a lobster bisque as good as yours, and I remain convinced that you left out a secret ingredient when you gave me your recipe, ha ha. I miss our cooking (and costly food shopping) sprees, and I hope that we'll be able to schedule one soon in spite of the challenges schedule and distance have posed. I've got a great kitchen and a guest room down here in Roatan, Honduras—just sayin'.

To my grandmother, Therese: You gave me my very first cookbook when I was four years old, and I still have it. It's stained and tattered from the many hours I spent in the kitchen poring over and cooking from it as a child. Thank you for getting me started on this road that led to writing a cookbook of my own, and for instilling a love of gardening and growing fresh ingredients as well. Some of my favorite food and family memories originated in your kitchens over the course of my life, and I am forever grateful for that.

To my in-laws, Moe and Elayne: Thanks for growing such an incredible son for me to marry, and for being an awesome extended family to me. Without your support, I never could have gotten to this point. Elayne, you were the first person I finally told when I started the blog and was embarrassed about it—your enthusiasm for it helped me get through those tough early months. I'll never forget being on the phone with you both when we watched that stat counter flying and celebrated my first million page views together all those years ago! Thank you for always being there when we needed you, and for supporting our decision to move out of the country for a while. I love you both very much.

To Stacey H.: Thank you for being such a good friend and an excellent assistant. You kept the blog and social media rolling while I was deep in the mental trenches of creating this book, and without you I don't think I could have done it! Only you and I truly know the endless tedium of calculating nutrition information for all of these recipes, so please believe that I very much appreciate you and your hard work to help me get them done on time. I still owe you a celebratory margarita by the pool!

To Judy, Karyn, Melissa, and Becky: You four stand out not only as wonderful friends over the years but also as my foodie-friend posse! We've shared recipes, cooked in each other's kitchens, enjoyed countless meals together, and always laughed our heads off. Even though we see each other rarely now that we're scattered around the globe, I love you and miss you all terribly! Thanks for always being there and for being an inspiration when it comes to a love of food, cooking, and entertaining. You guys are the best!

So many other friends and family have inspired and supported me through this process—unfortunately, too many to mention specifically by name here. You know who you are, and, more importantly, so do I. Please know that I appreciate and love all of you so very much!

Resources

Books I Recommend

The Carb Nite Solution by John Kiefer

The Complete Guide to Fasting by Jason Fung, MD, and Jimmy Moore

Craveable Keto by Kyndra D. Holley

Cultured Food for Health by Donna Schwenk

The Everyday Ketogenic Kitchen by Carolyn Ketchum

Keto Clarity by Jimmy Moore and Eric C. Westman, MD

The Keto Diet by Leanne Vogel

The Obesity Code by Jason Fung, MD

Simply Keto by Suzanne Ryan

The 30-Day Ketogenic Cleanse by Maria Emmerich

Keto Recipe Websites

Ibreatheimhungry.com

Alldayidreamaboutfood.com

Ditchthecarbs.com

Heyketomama.com

Kalynskitchen.com

Ketodietapp.com

Lowcarbmaven.com

Peaceloveandlowcarb.com

Sugarfreemom.com

Personalized Keto Coaching

Healthfulpursuit.com

Ketogenicgirl.com

Mariamindbodyhealth.com

Keto Forums and Other Helpful Resources

ibreatheimhungry.com/forums/forum/ibih-community-forum/

calorieking.com

facebook.com/groups/139715246632370/ (5 Day Keto Soup Diet Support Group)

facebook.com/groups/198008574075451/ (I Breathe I'm Hungry Facebook Community Group)

josepharcita.blogspot.co.uk/2011/03/guide-to-ketosis.html

keto-calculator.ankerl.com

livinlavidalowcarb.com

myfitnesspal.com

perfectketo.com/keto-macro-calculator/

reddit.com/r/intermittentfasting/

reddit.com/r/keto/

reddit.com/r/keto/wiki/faq

Food Brands I Recommend

I make many staple foods and condiments from scratch when there is time, but I purchase them for convenience's sake when there isn't. Some of these items have corresponding recipes in this book, but because you may not always have time to make them from scratch, either, I've included this list of my current favorite brands for reference. Also on this list are products that I use often as ingredients in my recipes. Be aware that not every brand will be available in your region, and some products may be discontinued after this book is printed. If you can't find the brands I recommend here, don't panic. Just read the product labels and find the brands in your store that contain the lowest amounts of carbohydrates.

Sugar-free pancake syrup—Maple Grove Farms, Log Cabin, Walden Farms, Cary's

Mayonnaise—Duke's, Hellmann's

Marinara sauce—Rao's, Organico Bello, Cucina Antica

Reduced-sugar ketchup—Heinz reduced sugar, Westbrae natural unsweetened, Real Good no sugar added

Salsa—Pace, Amy's Organic, Mateo's, 365 Everyday

Beef and chicken broth—Kirkland organic, Swanson, Pacific Foods, Kitchen Basics, College Inn

Unsweetened almond milk—Silk, Almond Breeze, Pacific Foods, Califia Farms

Kefir (always go for full-fat and unsweetened)—Lifeway, Maple Hill Creamery

Starter culture for vegetables—Cultures for Health, Body Ecology, Caldwell's

Kefir starter—Cultures for Health, Yogourmet, Body Ecology, Lifeway

Kombucha starter—Fermented Health, Fermentaholics, The Kombucha Shop

Recipe Index

basics

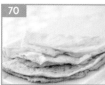

70 Cream Cheese Wraps

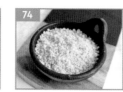

72 Cream Cheese Noodles

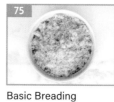

74 Keto Breadcrumbs

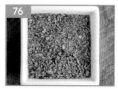

75 Basic Breading

76 Cajun Seasoning

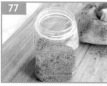

77 Chicken Seasoning

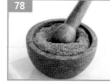

78 Blackening Seasoning

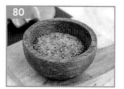

79 Jerk Seasoning

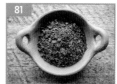

80 Beef Seasoning

81 Fish and Seafood Seasoning

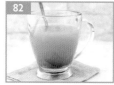

82 Easy Chicken Bone Broth

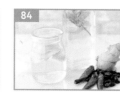

84 Simple Syrup— Basic and Flavored

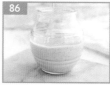

86 Creamy Basil- Parmesan Vinaigrette

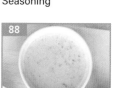

87 Strawberry Basil Vinaigrette

88 Ginger Scallion Dressing

89 Bacon & Tomato Dressing

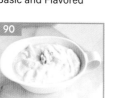

90 Creamy Blue Cheese Dressing

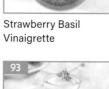

92 Creamy Lemon Caper Dressing

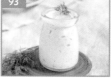

93 Tangy Feta & Dill Dressing

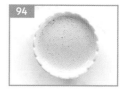

94 Tahini Lemon Dressing

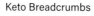
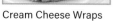
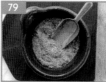
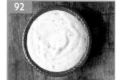

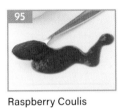

Raspberry Coulis

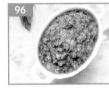

Easy Basil Pesto

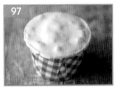

Basic Remoulade

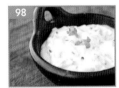

Cucumber Raita

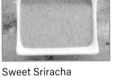

Sweet Sriracha
Dipping Sauce

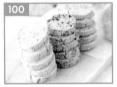

Compound Butter

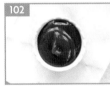

Keto Ketchup

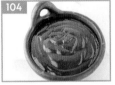

Easy Keto BBQ Sauce

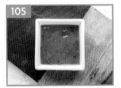

Sweet Chili Sauce

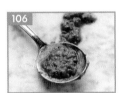

Easy No-Cook
Marinara

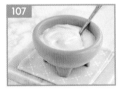

5-Minute Alfredo Sauce

fermented foods

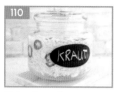
Spicy Sauerkraut

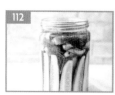
Easy Lacto-Fermented Half-Sour Pickles

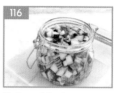
Quick Cucumber Pickles

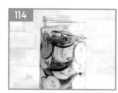
Cultured Red Onion Relish

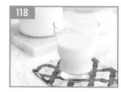
Homemade Dairy Kefir

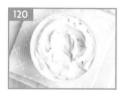
Herbed Kefir Cheese

Basic Kombucha

breakfast

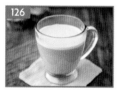
Bulletproof Pumpkin Spice Latte

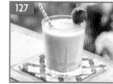
Kefir Strawberry Smoothie

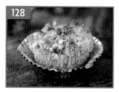
Cinnamon Walnut Streusel Muffins

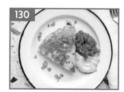
Spanish Tortilla with Chorizo

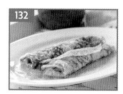
Snickerdoodle Crepes

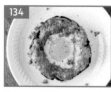
Sausage & Egg–Stuffed Portobello Mushrooms

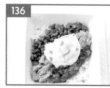
Savory Chorizo Breakfast Bowl

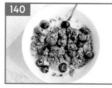
Cream Cheese Pancakes

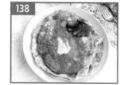
Cacao Coconut Granola

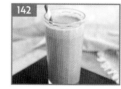
Chocolate Hemp Smoothie

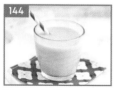
Pineapple Ginger Smoothie

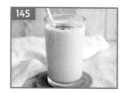
Coconut Chai Vanilla Smoothie

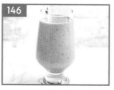
Raspberry Chia Smoothie

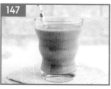
Moringa Super Green Smoothie

chicken

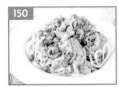

150
Chicken Tetrazzini

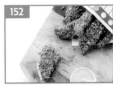

152
Pecan-Crusted
Chicken Fingers

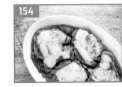

154
Chicken Parmesan

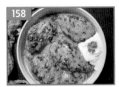

156
Green Chicken Enchilada
Cauliflower Casserole

158
Easy Salsa Chicken

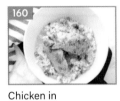

160
Chicken in
Coconut Broth

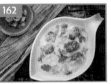

162
Green Chicken Curry

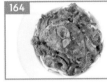

164
Chicken Cacciatore

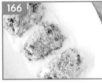

166
Cheesy Broccoli–
Stuffed Chicken

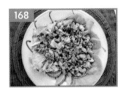

168
Chicken Larb

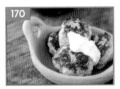

170
Tandoori Chicken
Meatballs

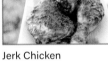

172
Jerk Chicken

beef

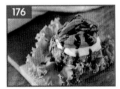

176
Caprese Burgers

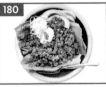

178
Marinated Skirt Steak

180
Easy No-Chop Chili

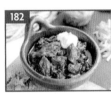

182
Chili con Carne

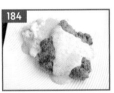

184
Chicken-Fried Steak
with Sour Cream Gravy

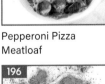

186
Pepperoni Pizza
Meatloaf

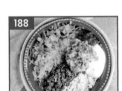

188
Beef Burrito Bowl

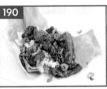

190
Korean BBQ
Beef Wraps

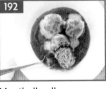

192
Meatballs alla
Parmigiana

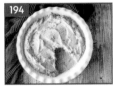

194
Cheesy Beef Stroganoff
Casserole

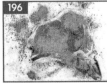

196
Coffee-Rubbed Rib-Eyes
with Balsamic Butter

pork

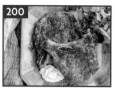
200
Cajun Pork Chops
with Aioli

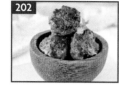
202
Sweet & Spicy
Asian Meatballs

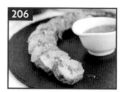
204
Pork Fried
Cauliflower Rice

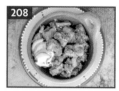
206
Mojo Pork Tenderloin

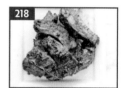
208
Pork Chili Verde

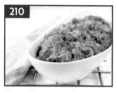
210
Easy Sausage &
Cauliflower Bake

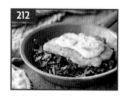
212
Schnitzel with Sour
Cream & Scallion Sauce

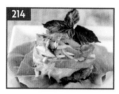
214
Bahn Mi Pork Burgers

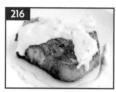
216
Pork Chops with
Dijon Tarragon Sauce

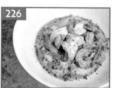
218
Easy Jerk Ribs

seafood

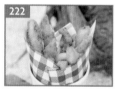
222
Cajun Fish Fingers

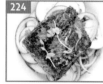
224
Blackened Snapper

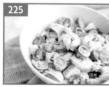
225
Shrimp Caprese Salad

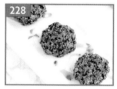
226
Shrimp & Grits

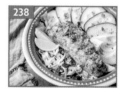
228
Spicy Tuna Cakes

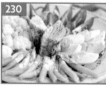
230
Niçoise Salad
with Seared Tuna

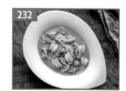
232
Shrimp Panang Curry

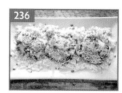
234
Smoked Salmon Stacks

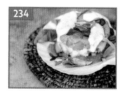
236
Baked Mahi Mahi in
Garlic Parsley Butter

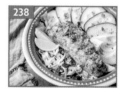
238
Fish Taco Bowl

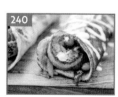
240
Shrimp Fajitas

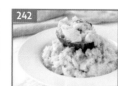
242
Creamy Lobster Risotto

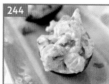
244
Spicy Shrimp-Stuffed
Avocados

veggie mains & sides

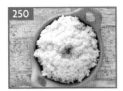
250
Basic Cauliflower Rice

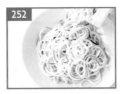
252
Basic Zucchini Noodles (Zoodles)

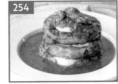
254
Eggplant Parmigiana

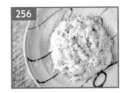
256
Cauliflower Risotto with Sherry & Hazelnuts

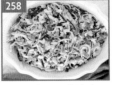
258
Vegetarian Pad Thai

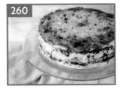
260
Vegetable Lasagna

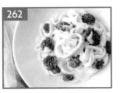
262
Faux-tuccini Alfredo with Broccoli

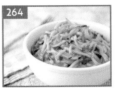
264
Zoodles with Creamy Roasted Red Pepper Sauce

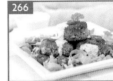
266
Faux-lafel

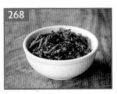
268
Braised Red Cabbage

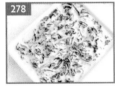
269
Cheesy Cauliflower Grits

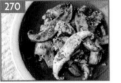
270
Marinated Portobello Mushrooms

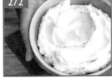
272
Cheesy Cauliflower Puree

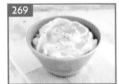
274
Sweet Sesame Glazed Bok Choy

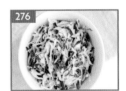
276
Orange & Tarragon Coleslaw

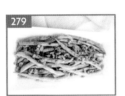
278
Creamed Spinach

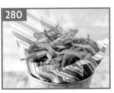
279
Sautéed Green Beans with Walnuts

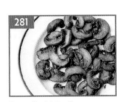
280
Spicy Jicama Shoestring Fries

281
Sautéed Mushrooms

snacks & appetizers

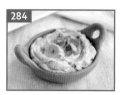
284
Jalapeño & Cilantro
Cauliflower Hummus

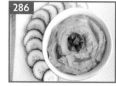
286
Roasted Red Pepper
Cauliflower Hummus

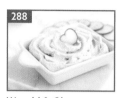
288
Wasabi & Ginger
Cauliflower Hummus

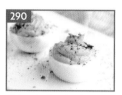
290
Chipotle Deviled Eggs

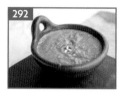
292
Restaurant-Style Salsa

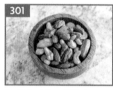
293
Easy Keto Guacamole

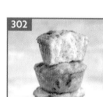
294
Easy Nacho Dip

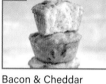
296
Broccoli Cheddar Puffs

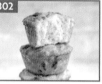
298
Parmesan Crisps

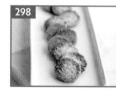
300
Keto Seed Crackers

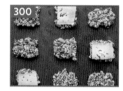
301
Buffalo Mixed Nuts

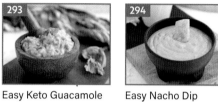
302
Bacon & Cheddar
Cornless Muffins

cocktails

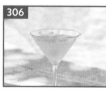
306
Pink Grapefruit Martini

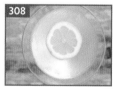
308
Lemon Drop Martini

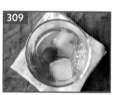
309
Old-Fashioned

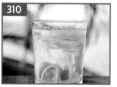
310
Caipirinha

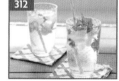
312
Classic Mojito

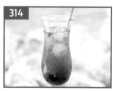
314
Blackberry Mojito

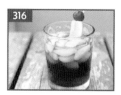
316
Bourbon Sweetie

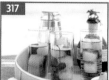
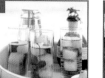
317
Whiskey Sour

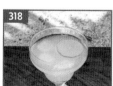
318
Margarita

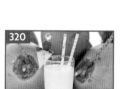
320
Piña Colada

desserts

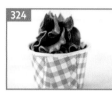

Chocolate Frosting

324

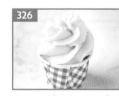

Cream Cheese Frosting

326

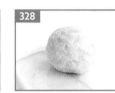

Basic Shortbread Dough

328

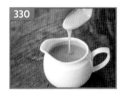

Butter Rum Caramel Sauce

330

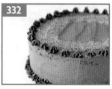

Epic Chocolate Crunch Layer Cake

332

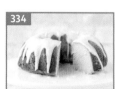

Lemon Sour Cream Bundt Cake

334

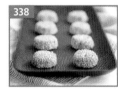

Pumpkin Spice Cupcakes

336

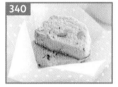

No-Bake Sesame Cookies

338

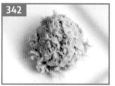

Pecan Shortbread Cookies

340

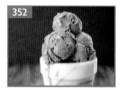

Snickerdoodle Haystack Cookies

342

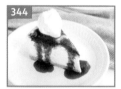

Raspberry Swirl Cheesecake

344

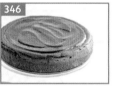

Triple Chocolate Cheesecake

346

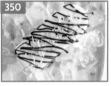

Coconut Tarts

348

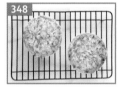

Coconut Paletas

350

Chocolate Ice Cream

352

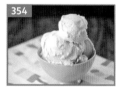

Vanilla Ice Cream

354

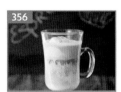

Affogato

356

Allergen Index

RECIPES	PAGE	dairy-free	egg-free	nut-free	vegetarian
Cream Cheese Wraps	70		✓		✓
Cream Cheese Noodles	72		✓		✓
Keto Breadcrumbs	74		✓		✓
Basic Breading	75		✓		✓
Cajun Seasoning	76	✓	✓	✓	✓
Chicken Seasoning	77	✓	✓	✓	✓
Blackening Seasoning	78	✓	✓	✓	✓
Jerk Seasoning	79	✓	✓	✓	✓
Beef Seasoning	80	✓	✓	✓	✓
Fish and Seafood Seasoning	81	✓	✓	✓	✓
Easy Chicken Bone Broth	82	✓	✓	✓	
Simple Syrup—Basic and Flavored	84	✓	✓	✓	✓
Creamy Basil-Parmesan Vinaigrette	86			✓	✓
Strawberry Basil Vinaigrette	87	✓	✓	✓	✓
Ginger Scallion Dressing	88	✓	✓	✓	
Bacon & Tomato Dressing	89	✓		✓	
Creamy Blue Cheese Dressing	90			✓	✓
Creamy Lemon Caper Dressing	92	✓		✓	✓
Tangy Feta & Dill Dressing	93			✓	✓
Tahini Lemon Dressing	94	✓	✓	✓	✓
Raspberry Coulis	95	✓	✓	✓	✓
Easy Basil Pesto	96		✓		✓
Basic Remoulade	97	✓		✓	✓
Cucumber Raita	98		✓	✓	✓
Sweet Sriracha Dipping Sauce	99	✓		✓	✓
Compound Butter	100		✓	✓	✓
Keto Ketchup	102	✓	✓	✓	✓
Easy Keto BBQ Sauce	104	✓	✓	✓	
Sweet Chili Sauce	105	✓	✓	✓	
Easy No-Cook Marinara	106	✓	✓	✓	✓
5-Minute Alfredo Sauce	107		✓	✓	✓
Spicy Sauerkraut	110	✓	✓	✓	✓
Easy Lacto-Fermented Half-Sour Pickles	112	✓	✓	✓	✓
Quick Cucumber Pickles	114	✓	✓	✓	✓
Cultured Red Onion Relish	116	✓	✓	✓	✓
Homemade Dairy Kefir	118		✓	✓	✓
Herbed Kefir Cheese	120		✓	✓	✓
Basic Kombucha	122	✓	✓	✓	✓
Bulletproof Pumpkin Spice Latte	126		✓	✓	✓
Kefir Strawberry Smoothie	127		✓		✓
Cinnamon Walnut Streusel Muffins	128				✓
Spanish Tortilla with Chorizo	130			✓	
Snickerdoodle Crepes	132			✓	✓
Sausage & Egg–Stuffed Portobello Mushrooms	134	✓		✓	
Savory Chorizo Breakfast Bowl	136			✓	
Cream Cheese Pancakes	138			✓	✓
Cacao Coconut Granola	140	✓			✓
Chocolate Hemp Smoothie	142		✓		✓
Pineapple Ginger Smoothie	144	✓	✓		
Coconut Chai Vanilla Smoothie	145		✓		✓
Raspberry Chia Smoothie	146		✓		✓
Moringa Super Green Smoothie	147	✓	✓		✓
Chicken Tetrazzini	150		✓		
Pecan-Crusted Chicken Fingers	152	✓			
Chicken Parmesan	154				
Green Chicken Enchilada Cauliflower Casserole	156		✓	✓	
Easy Salsa Chicken	158			✓	
Chicken in Coconut Broth	160	✓	✓	✓	

RECIPES	PAGE	dairy-free	egg-free	nut-free	vegetarian
Green Chicken Curry	162	✓	✓	✓	
Chicken Cacciatore	164	✓	✓	✓	
Cheesy Broccoli–Stuffed Chicken	166				
Chicken Larb	168	✓	✓	✓	
Tandoori Chicken Meatballs	170				
Jerk Chicken	172	✓	✓	✓	
Caprese Burgers	176			✓	
Marinated Skirt Steak	178	✓	✓	✓	
Easy No-Chop Chili	180		✓	✓	
Chili con Carne	182	✓	✓	✓	
Chicken-Fried Steak with Sour Cream Gravy	184				
Pepperoni Pizza Meatloaf	186				
Beef Burrito Bowl	188		✓	✓	
Korean BBQ Beef Wraps	190	✓	✓	✓	
Meatballs alla Parmigiana	192				
Cheesy Beef Stroganoff Casserole	194		✓	✓	
Coffee-Rubbed Rib-Eyes with Balsamic Butter	196		✓	✓	
Cajun Pork Chops with Aioli	200	✓		✓	
Sweet & Spicy Asian Meatballs	202	✓			
Pork Fried Cauliflower Rice	204	✓			
Mojo Pork Tenderloin	206	✓	✓	✓	
Pork Chili Verde	208	✓	✓	✓	
Easy Sausage & Cauliflower Bake	210		✓	✓	
Schnitzel with Sour Cream & Scallion Sauce	212				
Bahn Mi Pork Burgers	214	✓		✓	
Pork Chops with Dijon Tarragon Sauce	216		✓	✓	
Easy Jerk Ribs	218	✓	✓	✓	
Cajun Fish Fingers	222				
Blackened Snapper	224		✓	✓	
Shrimp Caprese Salad	225			✓	
Shrimp & Grits	226		✓		
Spicy Tuna Cakes	228	✓		✓	
Niçoise Salad with Seared Tuna	230	✓		✓	
Shrimp Panang Curry	232	✓	✓	✓	
Smoked Salmon Stacks	234	✓		✓	
Baked Mahi Mahi in Garlic Parsley Butter	236		✓		
Fish Taco Bowl	238	✓	✓	✓	
Shrimp Fajitas	240			✓	
Creamy Lobster Risotto	242		✓	✓	
Spicy Shrimp–Stuffed Avocados	244	✓		✓	
Basic Cauliflower Rice	250	✓	✓	✓	✓
Basic Zucchini Noodles (Zoodles)	252	✓	✓	✓	✓
Eggplant Parmigiana	254				✓
Cauliflower Risotto with Sherry & Hazelnuts	256		✓		✓
Vegetarian Pad Thai	258	✓	✓		✓
Vegetable Lasagna	260			✓	✓
Faux-tuccini Alfredo with Broccoli	262			✓	✓
Zoodles with Creamy Roasted Red Pepper Sauce	264		✓	✓	✓
Faux-lafel	266	✓			✓
Braised Red Cabbage	268		✓	✓	✓
Cheesy Cauliflower Grits	269		✓		✓
Marinated Portobello Mushrooms	270	✓	✓	✓	✓
Cheesy Cauliflower Puree	272		✓	✓	✓
Sweet Sesame Glazed Bok Choy	274	✓	✓	✓	✓
Orange & Tarragon Coleslaw	276	✓	✓	✓	✓
Creamed Spinach	278		✓	✓	✓
Sautéed Green Beans with Walnuts	279	✓	✓		✓
Spicy Jicama Shoestring Fries	280	✓	✓	✓	✓

RECIPES	PAGE	dairy-free	egg-free	nut-free	vegetarian
Sautéed Mushrooms	281		✓	✓	✓
Jalapeño & Cilantro Cauliflower Hummus	284	✓	✓	✓	✓
Roasted Red Pepper Cauliflower Hummus	286	✓	✓	✓	✓
Wasabi & Ginger Cauliflower Hummus	288	✓	✓	✓	✓
Chipotle Deviled Eggs	290	✓		✓	✓
Restaurant-Style Salsa	292	✓	✓	✓	✓
Easy Keto Guacamole	293	✓	✓	✓	✓
Easy Nacho Dip	294		✓	✓	✓
Broccoli Cheddar Puffs	296				✓
Parmesan Crisps	298		✓	✓	✓
Keto Seed Crackers	300	✓		✓	✓
Buffalo Mixed Nuts	301				✓
Bacon & Cheddar Cornless Muffins	302				
Pink Grapefruit Martini	306	✓	✓	✓	✓
Lemon Drop Martini	308	✓	✓	✓	✓
Old-Fashioned	309	✓	✓	✓	✓
Caipirinha	310	✓	✓	✓	✓
Classic Mojito	312	✓	✓	✓	✓
Blackberry Mojito	314	✓	✓	✓	✓
Bourbon Sweetie	316	✓	✓	✓	✓
Whiskey Sour	317	✓	✓	✓	✓
Margarita	318	✓	✓	✓	✓
Piña Colada	320		✓	✓	✓
Chocolate Frosting	324		✓	✓	✓
Cream Cheese Frosting	326		✓	✓	✓
Basic Shortbread Dough	328		✓		✓
Butter Rum Caramel Sauce	330		✓	✓	✓
Epic Chocolate Crunch Layer Cake	332				✓
Lemon Sour Cream Bundt Cake	334				✓
Pumpkin Spice Cupcakes	336				✓
No-Bake Sesame Cookies	338		✓	✓	✓
Pecan Shortbread Cookies	340		✓		✓
Snickerdoodle Haystack Cookies	342		✓	✓	✓
Raspberry Swirl Cheesecake	344				✓
Triple Chocolate Cheesecake	346				✓
Coconut Tarts	348				✓
Coconut Paletas	350	✓	✓	✓	✓
Chocolate Ice Cream	352				✓
Vanilla Ice Cream	354				✓
Affogato	356				✓

General Index

A

Affogato recipe, 356–357
alcohol, 30
Alldayidreamaboutfood (website), 360
allspice berries
  Cultured Red Onion Relish, 116–117
almond butter
  Vegetarian Pad Thai, 258–259
almond flour
  about, 32
  Bacon & Cheddar Cornless Muffins, 302–303
  Basic Breading, 75
  Basic Shortbread Dough, 328–329
  Broccoli Cheddar Puffs, 296–297
  Cacao Coconut Granola, 140–141
  Cheesy Cauliflower Grits, 269
  Cinnamon Walnut Streusel Muffins, 128–129
  Epic Chocolate Crunch Layer Cake, 332–333
  Keto Breadcrumbs, 74
  Lemon Sour Cream Bundt Cake, 334–335
  Meatballs alla Parmigiana, 192–193
  Pecan Shortbread Cookies, 340–341
  Pepperoni Pizza Meatloaf, 186–187
  Pumpkin Spice Cupcakes, 336–337
  Sweet & Spicy Asian Meatballs, 202–203
  Tandoori Chicken Meatballs, 170–171
  Triple Chocolate Cheesecake, 346–347

almond milk
  Bacon & Cheddar Cornless Muffins, 302–303
  Chocolate Hemp Smoothie, 142–143
  Chocolate Ice Cream, 352–353
  Cinnamon Walnut Streusel Muffins, 128–129
  Coconut Chai Vanilla Smoothie, 145
  Epic Chocolate Crunch Layer Cake, 332–333
  Kefir Strawberry Smoothie, 127
  Moringa Super Green Smoothie, 147
  Pineapple Ginger Smoothie, 144
  Raspberry Chia Smoothie, 146
  recommended brands, 361
  Vanilla Ice Cream, 354–355
almonds
  Faux-lafel, 266–267
  for snacking, 25
  Vegetarian Pad Thai, 258–259
arugula, 16
asparagus, 16
avocado oil, 35
avocados
  Bahn Mi Pork Burgers, 214–215
  Easy Keto Guacamole, 293
  Fish Taco Bowl, 238–239
  Pork Chili Verde, 208–209
  Shrimp Fajitas, 240–241
  Smoked Salmon Steaks, 234–235
  for snacking, 25
  Spicy Shrimp–Stuffed Avocados, 244–245

B

bacon
  Bacon & Cheddar Cornless Muffins, 302–303
  Bacon & Tomato Dressing, 89

Bacon & Cheddar Cornless Muffins recipe, 302–303
  Chili con Carne, 182–183
  Easy No-Chop Chili Soup, 180
  Pork Chili Verde, 208–209
Bacon & Tomato Dressing recipe, 89
Bahn Mi Pork Burgers recipe, 214–215
Bahn Mi Pork Salad recipe, 215
Baked Mahi Mahi in Garlic Parsley Butter recipe, 236–237
bakeware, 46
balsamic glaze, 176
bamboo shoots
  Green Chicken Curry, 162–163
Basic Breading recipe, 75
  Cajun Fish Fingers, 222–223
  Chicken Parmesan, 154–155
  Chicken-Fried Steak with Sour Cream Gravy, 184–185
  Eggplant Parmigiana, 254–255
  Schnitzel with Sour Cream & Scallion Sauce, 212–213
Basic Cauliflower Rice recipe, 250–251
  Beef Burrito Bowl, 188–189
  Cauliflower Risotto with Sherry & Hazelnuts, 256–257
  Creamy Lobster Risotto, 242–243
  Korean BBQ Beef Wraps, 190–191
  Savory Chorizo Breakfast Bowl, 136–137
Basic Kombucha recipe, 122–123
Basic Remoulade recipe, 97
  Cajun Fish Fingers, 222–223
Basic Shortbread Dough recipe, 328–329
  Coconut Tarts, 348–349
  Raspberry Swirl Cheesecake, 344–345

Basic Simple Syrup recipe
    Blackberry Mojito, 314–315
    Classic Mojito, 312–313
    Piña Colada, 320–321
Basic Zucchini Noodles recipe, 252–253
    Pepperoni Pizza Meatloaf, 186–187
    Zoodles with Creamy Roasted Red Pepper Sauce, 264–265
basil
    Bahn Mi Pork Burgers, 214–215
    Caprese Burgers, 176–177
    Chicken Cacciatore, 164–165
    Chicken Parmesan, 154–155
    Creamy Basil-Parmesan Vinaigrette, 86, 225
    Easy Basil Pesto, 96
    Easy Sausage & Cauliflower Bake, 210–211
    Eggplant Parmigiana, 254–255
    Roasted Red Pepper Cauliflower Hummus, 286–287
    Shrimp Caprese Salad, 225
    Strawberry Basil Vinaigrette, 87
beef
    Caprese Burgers, 176–177
    Cheesy Beef Stroganoff Casserole, 194–195
    Chicken-Fried Steak with Sour Cream Gravy, 184–185
    Chili con Carne, 182–183
    Coffee-Rubbed Rib-Eyes with Balsamic Butter, 196–197
    cube steaks, 184
    Easy Beef Bone Broth, 82–83
    Easy Nacho Dip, 294–295
    Easy No-Chop Chili, 180–181
    Korean BBQ Beef Wraps, 190–191
    Marinated Skirt Steak, 178–179
    Meatballs alla Parmigiana, 192–193
    Pepperoni Pizza Meatloaf, 186–187
Beef Burrito Bowl recipe, 188–189
    Easy Nacho Dip, 294–295
Beef Seasoning recipe, 80
bell peppers
    Chicken Cacciatore, 164–165
    Green Chicken Curry, 162–163

Shrimp Fajitas, 240–241
Shrimp Panang Curry, 232–233
Sweet & Spicy Asian Meatballs, 202–203
bitters
    Old-Fashioned, 309
Blackberry Mojito recipe, 314–315
Blackened Snapper recipe, 224
Blackening seasoning recipe, 78
Blackened Snapper, 224
blender, 43, 44
blue cheese
    Creamy Blue Cheese Dressing, 90–91
    tips for using, 90
bok choy
    about, 16
    Sweet Sesame Glazed Bok Choy, 274–275
books, recommended, 360
bourbon
    Old-Fashioned, 309
    Whiskey Sour, 317
Bourbon Sweetie recipe, 316
Braised Red Cabbage recipe, 266
broccoli
    about, 16
    Broccoli Cheddar Puffs, 296–297
    Cheesy Broccoli-Stuffed Chicken, 166–167
    Faux-tuccini Alfredo with Broccoli, 262–263
    Green Chicken Curry, 162–163
Broccoli Cheddar Puffs, 296–297
broth, recommended brands, 361
Brunch Buffet menu, 29
Brussels sprouts, 16
Buffalo Mixed Nuts recipe, 301
Bulletproof Pumpkin Spice Latte recipe, 126
butter
    about, 33–34
    compound, 31
    Gorgonzola Butter, 100–101
    Hotel Butter, 100–101
    Sun-Dried Tomato & Basil Butter, 100–101
butter lettuce, 16
Butter Rum Caramel Sauce recipe, 330–331

C
cabbage
    about, 16
    Braised Red Cabbage, 266
    Fish Taco Bowl, 238–239
    kimchee, 190
    Orange & Tarragon Coleslaw, 276–277
    Spicy Sauerkraut, 110–111
    Vegetarian Pad Thai, 258–259
Cacao Coconut Granola recipe, 140–141
cacao nibs
    Cacao Coconut Granola, 140–141
    Epic Chocolate Crunch Layer Cake, 332–333
Caipirinha recipe, 310–311
Cajun Fish Fingers recipe, 222–223
Cajun Pork Shops with Aioli recipe, 200–201
Cajun seasoning recipe, 76
    Basic Remoulade, 97
    Cajun Fish Fingers, 222–223
    Cajun Pork Shops with Aioli, 200–201
    Fish Taco Bowl, 238–239
    Spicy Jicama Shoestring Fries, 280
cakes and cupcakes
    Chocolate Frosting, 324–325
    Cream Cheese Frosting, 326–327
    Epic Chocolate Crunch Layer Cake, 332–333
    Lemon Sour Cream Bundt Cake, 334–335
    Pumpkin Spice Cupcakes, 336–337
    Raspberry Swirl Cheesecake, 344–345
    Triple Chocolate Cheesecake, 346–347
calorieking (website), 360
capers
    Basic Remoulade, 97
    Chicken Cacciatore, 164–165
    Creamy Lemon Caper Dressing, 92
Caprese Burgers recipe, 176–177

Carb Nite Solution, 12
The Carb Nite Solution (Kiefer), 360
carbohydrates
adding flavor instead of, 31
high-carb foods, 15
requirements for, 14
Casual Dinner with Friends menu, 30
cauliflower
about, 16
Basic Cauliflower Rice, 250–251
Cheesy Cauliflower Puree, 272–273
draining, 210
Easy Sausage & Cauliflower Bake, 210–211
Faux-lafel, 266–267
Green Chicken Enchilada Cauliflower Casserole, 156–157
Jalapeño & Cilantro Cauliflower Hummus, 284–285
Niçoise Salad with Seared Tuna, 230–231
Pork Fried Cauliflower Rice, 204–205
Roasted Red Pepper Cauliflower Hummus, 286–287
Wasabi & Ginger Cauliflower Hummus, 288–289
Cauliflower Risotto with Sherry & Hazelnuts recipe, 256–257
celery
about, 16
Easy Chicken Bone Broth, 82–83
for snacking, 25
Spanish Tortilla with Chorizo, 130–131
chai tea
Coconut Chai Vanilla Smoothie, 145
cheddar cheese
Bacon & Cheddar Cornless Muffins, 302–303
Beef Burrito Bowl, 188–189
Broccoli Cheddar Puffs, 296–297
Cheesy Cauliflower Grits, 269

Cheesy Cauliflower Puree, 272–273
Easy Nacho Dip, 294–295
Easy Salsa Chicken, 158–159
Green Chicken Enchilada Cauliflower Casserole, 156–157
Pork Chili Verde, 208–209
Savory Chorizo Breakfast Bowl, 136–137
cheesecake, slicing, 344
Cheesy Beef Stroganoff Casserole recipe, 194–195
Cheesy Broccoli–Stuffed Chicken recipe, 166–167
Cheesy Cauliflower Grits recipe, 269
Cheesy Cauliflower Puree recipe, 272–273
Cheesy Beef Stroganoff Casserole, 194–195
Cheesy Cauliflower Grits, 269
Pepperoni Pizza Meatloaf, 186–187
Shrimp & Grits, 226–227
chia seeds
Raspberry Chia Smoothie, 146
chicken
baking, 172
Cheesy Broccoli–Stuffed Chicken, 166–167
Chicken Cacciatore, 164–165
Chicken in Coconut Broth, 160–161
Chicken Larb, 168–169
Chicken Parmesan, 154–155
Chicken Tetrazzini, 150–151
Easy Chicken Bone Broth, 82–83
Easy Salsa Chicken, 158–159
Faux-tuccini Alfredo with Broccoli, 260
freezing, 150
Green Chicken Curry, 162–163
Green Chicken Enchilada Cauliflower Casserole, 156–157
Jerk Chicken, 172–173
Pecan-Crusted Chicken Fingers, 152–153
rotisserie, 150
shredding, 151

Tandoori Chicken Meatballs, 170–171
Chicken Cacciatore recipe, 164–165
Chicken in Coconut Broth recipe, 160–161
Chicken Larb recipe, 168–169
Chicken Parmesan recipe, 154–155
Chicken Seasoning recipe, 77
Chicken Tetrazzini recipe, 150–151
Chicken-Fried Steak with Sour Cream Gravy recipe, 184–185
Chili con Carne recipe, 182–183
chili peppers
Green Chicken Curry, 162–163
Shrimp Panang Curry, 232–233
Chili-Infused Simple Syrup recipe, 84–85
Chipotle Deviled Eggs recipe, 290–291
chocolate
about, 34
Chocolate Frosting, 324–325
Coconut Paletas, 350–351
Epic Chocolate Crunch Layer Cake, 332–333
Triple Chocolate Cheesecake, 346–347
Chocolate Frosting recipe, 324–325
Epic Chocolate Crunch Layer Cake, 332–333
Chocolate Hemp Smoothie recipe, 142–143
Chocolate Ice Cream recipe, 352–353
chorizo
Easy Nacho Dip, 294–295
Savory Chorizo Breakfast Bowl, 136–137
Spanish Tortilla with Chorizo, 130–131
Chunky Blue Cheese Dressing recipe, 90
cilantro
Bahn Mi Pork Burgers, 214–215
Beef Burrito Bowl, 188–189
Chicken in Coconut Broth, 160–161
Cucumber Raita, 98
Cultured Red Onion Relish, 116–117

cilantro (continued)
Easy Keto Guacamole, 293
Fish Taco Bowl, 238–239
Green Chicken Curry, 162–163
Green Chicken Enchilada
Cauliflower Casserole,
156–157
Jalapeño & Cilantro Cauliflower
Hummus, 284–285
Mojo Pork Tenderloin, 206–207
Pork Chili Verde, 208–209
Pork Fried Cauliflower Rice,
204–205
Quick Cucumber Pickles,
114–115
Restaurant-Style Salsa, 292
Savory Chorizo Breakfast
Bowl, 136–137
Shrimp Fajitas, 240–241
Shrimp Panang Curry, 232–233
Spanish Tortilla with Chorizo,
130–131
Spicy Shrimp–Stuffed
Avocados, 244–245
Vegetarian Pad Thai, 258–259
cinnamon
Cacao Coconut Granola,
140–141
Cinnamon Walnut Streusel
Muffins, 128–129
Coconut Chai Vanilla
Smoothie, 145
Cream Cheese Pancakes,
138–139
Snickerdoodle Crepes,
132–133
Cinnamon Walnut Streusel
Muffins recipe, 128–129
Classic Lasagna recipe, 259
Classic Mojito recipe, 312–313
cloves
Cultured Red Onion Relish,
116–117
club soda
Blackberry Mojito, 314–315
Classic Mojito, 312–313
coaching, 360
cocktail sauce, 102
cocoa powder
about, 34
Chocolate Hemp Smoothie,
142–143

Chocolate Ice Cream, 352–353
Coffee-Rubbed Rib-Eyes with
Balsamic Butter, 196–197
Epic Chocolate Crunch Layer
Cake, 332–333
Triple Chocolate Cheesecake,
346–347
coconut
about, 35
Cacao Coconut Granola,
140–141
Coconut Tarts, 348–349
Coconut-Rum Paletas, 350
Snickerdoodle Haystack
Cookies, 342–343
Coconut Chai Vanilla Smoothie
recipe, 145
coconut flour
about, 32
Bacon & Cheddar Cornless
Muffins, 302–303
Cinnamon Walnut Streusel
Muffins, 128–129
Easy Salsa Chicken, 158–159
Faux-lafel, 266–267
Lemon Sour Cream Bundt
Cake, 334–335
Pecan-Crusted Chicken
Fingers, 152–153
Pumpkin Spice Cupcakes,
336–337
Spicy Tuna Cakes, 228–229
coconut milk
Chicken in Coconut Broth,
160–161
Coconut Chai Vanilla
Smoothie, 145
Coconut Paletas, 350–351
Green Chicken Curry, 162–163
Moringa Super Green
Smoothie, 147
Piña Colada, 320–321
Pineapple Ginger Smoothie,
144
Raspberry Chia Smoothie, 146
Shrimp Panang Curry, 232–233
coconut oil, 36
Coconut Paletas recipe, 350–351
Coconut Tarts recipe, 348–349
Coconut-Rum Paletas recipe, 350
coffee
Affogato, 356–357

Bulletproof Pumpkin Spice
Latte, 126
Coffee-Rubbed Rib-Eyes with
Balsamic Butter, 196–197
Coffee-Infused Simple Syrup
recipe, 84–85
Coffee-Rubbed Rib-Eyes with
Balsamic Butter recipe, 196–197
collagen powder
about, 36
Pineapple Ginger Smoothie,
144
The Complete Guide to Fasting
(Fung and Moore), 12, 360
Compound Butter recipe, 100–101
compound butters, 31
cookies
No-Bake Sesame, 338–339
Pecan Shortbread, 340–341
Snickerdoodle Haystack,
342–343
cookware, 46
coriander seeds
Quick Cucumber Pickles,
114–115
Craveable Keto (Holley), 360
cream cheese
Cream Cheese Frosting,
326–327
Cream Cheese Noodles, 72–73
Cream Cheese Pancakes,
138–139
Cream Cheese Wraps, 70–71
Creamed Spinach, 278
Creamy Blue Cheese Dressing,
90–91
Easy Nacho Dip, 294–295
Green Chicken Enchilada
Cauliflower Casserole,
156–157
Herbed Kefir Cheese, 120–121
Raspberry Swirl Cheesecake,
344–345
Schnitzel with Sour Cream &
Scallion Sauce, 212–213
Snickerdoodle Crepes, 132–133
Snickerdoodle Haystack
Cookies, 342–343
Triple Chocolate Cheesecake,
346–347
Cream Cheese Frosting recipe,
326–327

Pumpkin Spice Cupcakes, 336–337

Cream Cheese Noodles recipe, 72–73

    Faux-tuccini Alfredo with Broccoli, 262–263

Cream Cheese Pancakes recipe, 138–139

Cream Cheese Wraps recipe, 70–71

    Shrimp Fajitas, 240–241

    Vegetable Lasagna, 260–261

Creamed Spinach recipe, 278

Creamy Basil-Parmesan Vinaigrette recipe, 86

    Shrimp Caprese Salad, 225

Creamy Blue Cheese Dressing recipe, 90–91

    Buffalo Mixed Nuts, 301

Creamy Lemon Caper Dressing recipe, 92

    Smoked Salmon Steaks, 234–235

Creamy Lobster Risotto recipe, 242–243

Creamy Shrimp Risotto recipe, 242

Creole Seasoning

    Easy Salsa Chicken, 158–159

    Shrimp & Grits, 226–227

cube steaks, 184

Cucumber Raita recipe, 98

cucumbers

    about, 16

    Cucumber Raita, 98

    Cultured Red Onion Relish, 116–117

    Easy Lacto-Fermented Half-Sour Pickles, 112–113

    Fish Taco Bowl, 238–239

    Quick Cucumber Pickles, 114–115

    Smoked Salmon Steaks, 234–235

Cultured Food for Health (Schwenk), 360

Cultured Red Onion Relish recipe, 116–117

D

daikon

    about, 16

Shrimp Panang Curry, 232–233

Vegetarian Pad Thai, 258–259

dairy products, 33

desserts

    Affogato, 356–357

    Basic Shortbread Dough, 328–329

    Butter Rum Caramel Sauce, 330–331

    Chocolate Frosting, 324–325

    Chocolate Ice Cream, 352–353

    Coconut Paletas, 350–351

    Coconut Tarts, 348–349

    Cream Cheese Frosting, 326–327

    Epic Chocolate Crunch Layer Cake, 332–333

    Lemon Sour Cream Bundt Cake, 334–335

    No-Bake Sesame Cookies, 338–339

    Pecan Shortbread Cookies, 340–341

    Pumpkin Spice Cupcakes, 336–337

    Raspberry Swirl Cheesecake, 344–345

    Snickerdoodle Haystack Cookies, 342–343

    Triple Chocolate Cheesecake, 346–347

    Vanilla Ice Cream, 354–355

dill

    Creamy Lemon Caper Dressing, 92

    Easy Lacto-Fermented Half-Sour Pickles, 112–113

    Tangy Feta & Dill Dressing, 93

dining out, 26–27

dips

    Easy Keto Guacamole, 293

    Easy Nacho Dip, 294–295

    Jalapeño & Cilantro Cauliflower Hummus, 284–285

    Restaurant-Style Salsa, 292

    Roasted Red Pepper Cauliflower Hummus, 286–287

    Wasabi & Ginger Cauliflower Hummus, 288–289

Ditchthecarbs (website), 360

dressings

    Bacon & Tomato Dressing, 89

    Chunky Blue Cheese Dressing, 90

    Creamy Basil-Parmesan Vinaigrette, 86

    Creamy Blue Cheese Dressing, 90–91

    Creamy Lemon Caper Dressing, 92

    Ginger Scallion Dressing, 88

    Strawberry Basil Vinaigrette, 87

    Tahini Lemon Dressing, 94

    Tangy Feta & Dill Dressing, 93

drinks

    Basic Kombucha, 122–123

    Blackberry Mojito, 314–315

    Bourbon Sweetie, 316

    Bulletproof Pumpkin Spice Latte, 126

    Caipirinha, 310–311

    Chocolate Hemp Smoothie, 142–143

    Classic Mojito, 312–313

    Coconut Chai Vanilla Smoothie, 145

    Homemade Dairy Kefir, 118–119

    Kefir Strawberry Smoothie, 127

    Lemon Drop Martini, 308

    Margarita, 318–319

    Moringa Super Green Smoothie, 147

    Old-Fashioned, 309

    Piña Colada, 320–321

    Pineapple Ginger Smoothie, 144

    Pink Grapefruit Martini, 306–307

    Raspberry Chia Smoothie, 146

    Whiskey Sour, 317

Dubliner cheese

    Cheesy Cauliflower Puree, 272–273

Dutch oven, 45

E

Easy Basil Pesto recipe, 96

Easy Beef Bone Broth recipe, 82–83

    Cheesy Beef Stroganoff Casserole, 194–195

Easy Beef Bone Broth (continued)
Chili con Carne, 182–183
Easy No-Chop Chili Soup, 180
Easy Chicken Bone Broth recipe, 82–83
Chicken Cacciatore, 164–165
Chicken in Coconut Broth, 160–161
Chicken Tetrazzini, 150–151
Easy Jerk Ribs recipe, 218–219
Easy Keto BBQ Sauce recipe, 104
Easy Jerk Ribs, 218–219
Jerk Chicken, 172–173
Easy Keto Guacamole recipe, 293
Beef Burrito Bowl, 188–189
Pork Chili Verde, 208–209
Savory Chorizo Breakfast Bowl, 136–137
Easy Lacto-Fermented Half-Sour Pickles recipe, 112–113
Easy Nacho Dip recipe, 294–295
Easy No-Chop Chili recipe, 180–181
Beef Burrito Bowl, 188–189
Easy No-Chop Chili Soup recipe, 180
Easy No-Cook Marinara recipe, 106
Chicken Parmesan, 154–155
Easy Sausage & Cauliflower Bake, 210–211
Eggplant Parmigiana, 254–255
Meatballs alla Parmigiana, 192–193
Pepperoni Pizza Meatloaf, 186–187
Vegetable Lasagna, 260–261
Easy Salsa Chicken recipe, 158–159
Easy Sausage & Cauliflower Bake recipe, 210–211
eating out, 26–27
Eggplant Parmigiana recipe, 254–255
eggs
Bacon & Cheddar Cornless Muffins, 302–303
Broccoli Cheddar Puffs, 296–297
Cacao Coconut Granola, 140–141
Cajun Fish Fingers, 222–223

Cheesy Broccoli–Stuffed Chicken, 166–167
Chicken Parmesan, 154–155
Chicken-Fried Steak with Sour Cream Gravy, 184–185
Chipotle Deviled Eggs, 290–291
Cinnamon Walnut Streusel Muffins, 128–129
Coconut Tarts, 348–349
Cream Cheese Noodles, 72–73
Cream Cheese Pancakes, 138–139
Cream Cheese Wraps, 70–71
Easy Salsa Chicken, 158–159
Eggplant Parmigiana, 254–255
Epic Chocolate Crunch Layer Cake, 332–333
Faux-lafel, 266–267
Keto Seed Crackers, 300
Lemon Sour Cream Bundt Cake, 334–335
Meatballs alla Parmigiana, 192–193
Niçoise Salad with Seared Tuna, 230–231
Pecan-Crusted Chicken Fingers, 152–153
Pepperoni Pizza Meatloaf, 186–187
poaching, 136
Pork Fried Cauliflower Rice, 204–205
Pumpkin Spice Cupcakes, 336–337
Raspberry Swirl Cheesecake, 344–345
Sausage & Egg–Stuffed Portobello Mushrooms, 134–135
Savory Chorizo Breakfast Bowl, 136–137
Schnitzel with Sour Cream & Scallion Sauce, 212–213
size of, 134
Snickerdoodle Crepes, 132–133
Spanish Tortilla with Chorizo, 130–131
Sweet & Spicy Asian Meatballs, 202–203
Tandoori Chicken Meatballs, 170–171

Triple Chocolate Cheesecake, 346–347
Vanilla Ice Cream, 354–355
Vegetable Lasagna, 260–261
electric mixer, 46
Emmerich, Maria, The 30-Day Ketogenic Cleanse, 360
entertaining, 27–30
Epic bars, 25
Epic Chocolate Crunch Layer Cake recipe, 332–333
equipment, 43–47
erythritol, 32–33
espresso
Affogato, 356–357

F
fasting, intermittent, 20
fat, requirements for, 18
Faux-lafel recipe, 266–267
Faux-tuccini Alfredo with Broccoli recipe, 262–263
feta cheese
Tangy Feta & Dill Dressing, 93
fish and seafood
Baked Mahi Mahi in Garlic Parsley Butter, 236–237
Blackened Snapper, 224
Cajun Fish Fingers, 222–223
Creamy Lobster Risotto, 242–243
Creamy Shrimp Risotto, 242
Fish Taco Bowl, 238–239
Niçoise Salad with Seared Tuna, 230–231
Shrimp Caprese Salad, 225
Shrimp Fajitas, 240–241
Shrimp & Grits, 226–227
Shrimp Panang Curry, 232–233
Smoked Salmon Steaks, 234–235
Spicy Shrimp–Stuffed Avocados, 244–245
Spicy Tuna Cakes, 228–229
Fish and Seafood Seasoning recipe, 81
fish sauce, 37
Fish Taco Bowl recipe, 238–239
5-Day Keto Soup Diet, 13, 360
5-Minute Alfredo Sauce recipe, 107
Faux-tuccini Alfredo with Broccoli, 262–263

flavor, adding, 31
flavored extracts/syrups, 37
flax seeds
Cacao Coconut Granola, 140–141
Keto Seed Crackers, 300
food processor, 44
foods
non-keto, 14–16
tracking, 19
forums, 360
french fries, swaps for, 22
fresh herbs, 35
Fung, Jason
The Complete Guide to Fasting, 12, 360
The Obesity Code, 360

G
Game Day menu, 29
ganache, 324
garlic
about, 94
Easy Lacto-Fermented Half-Sour Pickles, 112–113
Quick Cucumber Pickles, 114–115
garlic powder, 15
ginger
Chicken Larb, 168–169
Cultured Red Onion Relish, 116–117
Easy Chicken Bone Broth, 82–83
Ginger Scallion Dressing, 88
Korean BBQ Beef Wraps, 190–191
Pineapple Ginger Smoothie, 144
Pork Fried Cauliflower Rice, 204–205
Vegetarian Pad Thai, 258–259
Wasabi & Ginger Cauliflower Hummus, 288–289
Ginger Scallion Dressing recipe, 88
Ginger-Infused Simple Syrup recipe, 84–85
Girls' Night menu, 29
Gorgonzola Butter recipe, 100–101
Grapefruit-Infused Simple Syrup recipe, 84–85

Pink Grapefruit Martini, 306–307
grater, 46
Greek yogurt
Cucumber Raita, 98
Tandoori Chicken Meatballs, 170–171
green beans
Niçoise Salad with Seared Tuna, 230–231
Sautéed Green Beans with Walnuts, 279
Green Chicken Curry recipe, 162–163
Green Chicken Enchilada Cauliflower Casserole recipe, 156–157
green leaf lettuce, 16

H
hair loss, 19
hazelnuts
Cauliflower Risotto with Sherry & Hazelnuts, 256–257
Healthfulpursuit (website), 360
heavy whipping cream
Broccoli Cheddar Puffs, 296–297
Butter Rum Caramel Sauce, 330–331
Cheesy Cauliflower Puree, 272–273
Chicken Tetrazzini, 150–151
Chocolate Frosting, 324–325
Chocolate Hemp Smoothie, 142–143
Chocolate Ice Cream, 352–353
Coconut Tarts, 348–349
Creamy Blue Cheese Dressing, 90–91
Easy Sausage & Cauliflower Bake, 210–211
5-Minute Alfredo Sauce, 107
Piña Colada, 320–321
Pork Chops with Dijon Tarragon Sauce, 216–217
Raspberry Swirl Cheesecake, 344–345
Shrimp & Grits, 226–227
Tangy Feta & Dill Dressing, 93

Triple Chocolate Cheesecake, 346–347
Vanilla Ice Cream, 354–355
Zoodles with Creamy Roasted Red Pepper Sauce, 264–265
hemp protein, 142
Herbed Kefir Cheese recipe, 120–121
herb-infused oils, 31
Herb-Infused Simple Syrup recipe, 84–85
herbs, 35
Heyketomama (website), 360
high-carb foods, 15
Holley, Kyndra D., *Craveable Keto*, 360
Homemade Dairy Kefir recipe, 118–119
Herbed Kefir Cheese, 120–121
Kefir Strawberry Smoothie, 127
Hotel Butter recipe, 100–101

I
I Breathe I'm Hungry (blog), 5, 360
ice cream maker, 44
ice pop molds, 45
iceberg lettuce, 16
iced tea
Bourbon Sweetie, 316
immersion blender, 43
Instant Pot, 47
intermittent fasting, 20
Italian sausage
Classic Lasagna, 259
Easy Sausage & Cauliflower Bake, 210–211

J
Jalapeño & Cilantro Cauliflower Hummus recipe, 284–285
jalapeño peppers
Jalapeño & Cilantro Cauliflower Hummus, 284–285
Pork Chili Verde, 208–209
Restaurant-Style Salsa, 292
Shrimp Fajitas, 240–241
Spicy Sauerkraut, 110–111
Jerk Chicken recipe, 172–173
Jerk Seasoning recipe, 79
Easy Jerk Ribs, 218–219
Jerk Chicken, 172–173

jerky, for snacking, 25
jicama
    about, 16
    Spicy Jicama Shoestring Fries, 280
josepharcita (website), 360

K

kale, 15
Kalynskitchen (website), 360
kefir, recommended brands, 361
kefir grains, 118
Kefir Strawberry Smoothie recipe, 127
ketchup, recommended brands, 361
keto
    basics of, 14–20
    getting off track with, 21
    how it works, 8–11
    tips and tricks for, 22–30
Keto Breadcrumbs recipe, 74
    Baked Mahi Mahi in Garlic Parsley Butter, 236–237
    Cheesy Broccoli-Stuffed Chicken, 166–167
    Chicken Tetrazzini, 150–151
keto calculator, 360
Keto Clarity (Moore and Westman), 360
keto flu, 18
Keto Ketchup recipe, 102–103
    Caprese Burgers, 176–177
    Easy Keto BBQ Sauce, 104
Keto Seed Crackers recipe, 300
Ketodietapp (website), 360
Ketogenicgirl (website), 360
ketone test strips, 17
ketosis, getting into, 14
Ketostix, 17
The Keto Diet (Vogel), 360
kids, getting them involved, 24
Kiefer, John, 12
    The Carb Nite Solution, 360
kimchee, 190
kitchen scale, 47
knives, 45
kombucha, recommended brands, 361
Korean BBQ Beef Wraps recipe, 190–191

L

Lemon Drop Martini recipe, 308
Lemon Sour Cream Bundt Cake recipe, 334–335
Lemon-Infused Simple Syrup recipe, 84–85
    Bourbon Sweetie, 316
    Lemon Drop Martini, 308
    Whiskey Sour, 317
lemons
    about, 15
    Baked Mahi Mahi in Garlic Parsley Butter, 236–237
    Basic Remoulade, 97
    Bourbon Sweetie, 316
    Braised Red Cabbage, 266
    Creamy Basil-Parmesan Vinaigrette, 86
    Creamy Blue Cheese Dressing, 90–91
    Creamy Lemon Caper Dressing, 92
    fresh versus bottled, 334
    Lemon Drop Martini, 308
    Lemon Sour Cream Bundt Cake, 334–335
    Spicy Sauerkraut, 110–111
    Tahini Lemon Dressing, 94
    Tandoori Chicken Meatballs, 170–171
    Whiskey Sour, 317
lettuce
    about, 16
    Bahn Mi Pork Burgers, 214–215
    Caprese Burgers, 176–177
    Korean BBQ Beef Wraps, 190–191
    Niçoise Salad with Seared Tuna, 230–231
Lime-Infused Simple Syrup recipe, 84–85
    Caipirinha, 310–311
limes
    about, 15
    Bahn Mi Pork Burgers, 214–215
    Caipirinha, 310–311
    Cajun Fish Fingers, 222–223
    Chipotle Deviled Eggs, 290–291
    Easy Keto Guacamole, 293
    Fish Taco Bowl, 238–239
    Ginger Scallion Dressing, 88

Jalapeño & Cilantro Cauliflower Hummus, 284–285
Margarita, 318–319
Mojo Pork Tenderloin, 206–207
Pecan-Crusted Chicken Fingers, 152–153
Pork Fried Cauliflower Rice, 204–205
Restaurant-Style Salsa, 292
Roasted Red Pepper Cauliflower Hummus, 286–287
Spicy Shrimp-Stuffed Avocados, 244–245
Sweet Chili Sauce, 105
Sweet Sriracha Dipping Sauce, 99
Vegetarian Pad Thai, 258–259
Wasabi & Ginger Cauliflower Hummus, 288–289
livinlavidalowcarb (website), 360
lobster
    Creamy Lobster Risotto, 242–243
Lowcarbmaven (website), 360

M

macros, 18
magnesium, 42
mahi mahi
    Baked Mahi Mahi in Garlic Parsley Butter, 236–237
Manchego cheese
    Spanish Tortilla with Chorizo, 130–131
Margarita recipe, 318–319
Mariamindbodyhealth (website), 360
marinara sauce, recommended brands, 361
Marinated Portobello Mushrooms recipe, 270–271
Marinated Skirt Steak recipe, 178–179
mascarpone cheese
    about, 31
    Cauliflower Risotto with Sherry & Hazelnuts, 256–257
    Cheesy Broccoli-Stuffed Chicken, 166–167
    Creamy Lobster Risotto, 242–243

5-Minute Alfredo Sauce, 107
Zoodles with Creamy Roasted
Red Pepper Sauce,
264–265
mayonnaise, recommended
brands, 361
meal plans
Week 1, 50–53
Week 2, 54–57
Week 3, 58–61
Week 4, 62–64
Meatballs alla Parmigiana recipe,
192–193
menstruation, 19
microplane grater, 46
milk
Homemade Dairy Kefir,
118–119
mint
Bahn Mi Pork Burgers,
214–215
Blackberry Mojito, 314–315
Classic Mojito, 312–313
Cucumber Raita, 98
mixer, 46
mix-ins, for ice cream, 352, 354
Mojo Pork Tenderloin recipe,
206–207
molasses, 104
Moore, Jimmy
The Complete Guide to
Fasting, 12, 360
Keto Clarity, 360
moringa, 39, 147
Moringa Super Green Smoothie
recipe, 147
mozzarella cheese
Caprese Burgers, 176–177
Chicken Parmesan, 154–155
Easy Sausage & Cauliflower
Bake, 210–211
Eggplant Parmigiana, 254–255
Meatballs alla Parmigiana,
192–193
Pepperoni Pizza Meatloaf,
186–187
Shrimp Caprese Salad, 225
Vegetable Lasagna, 260–261
muddle, 310, 312, 314
muffins
Bacon & Cheddar Cornless,
302–303

Cinnamon Walnut Streusel,
128–129
mushrooms
about, 15
Cheesy Beef Stroganoff
Casserole, 194–195
Chicken Tetrazzini, 150–151
Marinated Portobello
Mushrooms, 270–271
Sausage & Egg-Stuffed
Portobello Mushrooms,
134–135
Sautéed Mushrooms, 281
Vegetable Lasagna, 260–261
myfitnesspal (website), 360

N
Niçoise Salad with Seared Tuna
recipe, 230–231
No-Bake Sesame Cookies recipe,
338–339
nut milks, 34
Nuts, Buffalo Mixed, 301

O
The Obesity Code (Fung), 360
oils, herb-infused, 31
Old-Fashioned recipe, 309
olive oil, 35
onions
about, 15
Cheesy Beef Stroganoff
Casserole, 194–195
Chicken Cacciatore, 164–165
Chicken Larb, 168–169
Chicken Tetrazzini, 150–151
Chili con Carne, 182–183
Cucumber Raita, 98
Cultured Red Onion Relish,
116–117
Easy Chicken Bone Broth,
82–83
Fish Taco Bowl, 238–239
Pork Chili Verde, 208–209
Quick Cucumber Pickles,
114–115
Restaurant-Style Salsa, 292
Shrimp Fajitas, 240–241
Smoked Salmon Steaks,
234–235
Spanish Tortilla with Chorizo,
130–131

Tandoori Chicken Meatballs,
170–171
Vegetable Lasagna, 260–261
Orange & Tarragon Coleslaw
recipe, 276–277
Orange-Infused Simple Syrup
recipe, 84–85
Margarita, 318–319
Old-Fashioned, 309
oranges
Mojo Pork Tenderloin, 206–207
Old-Fashioned, 309
oregano oil, 41
oyster mushrooms, 15

P
Pancakes, Cream Cheese, 138–139
pantry, staples for, 31–38
parchment paper, 47
Parmesan cheese
Basic Breading, 75
Cauliflower Risotto with Sherry
& Hazelnuts, 256–257
Cheesy Broccoli–Stuffed
Chicken, 166–167
Chicken Tetrazzini, 150–151
Creamed Spinach, 278
Creamy Basil-Parmesan
Vinaigrette, 86
Creamy Lobster Risotto,
242–243
Easy Basil Pesto, 96
Easy Sausage & Cauliflower
Bake, 210–211
5-Minute Alfredo Sauce, 107
Meatballs alla Parmigiana,
192–193
Parmesan Crisps, 298–299
Pepperoni Pizza Meatloaf,
186–187
Vegetable Lasagna, 260–261
Zoodles with Creamy Roasted
Red Pepper Sauce, 264–265
Parmesan Crisps recipe, 298–299
pasta
Chicken Cacciatore, 164–165
Cream Cheese Noodles, 72–73
Pepperoni Pizza Meatloaf,
186–187
swaps for, 22
Zoodles with Creamy Roasted
Red Pepper Sauce, 264–265

Patio Party menu, 30

Peaceloveandlowcarb (website), 360

peanut butter
    Shrimp Panang Curry, 232–233

peas
    Chicken Tetrazzini, 150–151
    Pork Fried Cauliflower Rice, 204–205

Pecan Shortbread Cookies recipe, 340–341

Pecan-Crusted Chicken Fingers recipe, 152–153

pecans
    Cacao Coconut Granola, 140–141
    Pecan Shortbread Cookies, 340–341
    Pecan-Crusted Chicken Fingers, 152–153

Pepperoni Pizza Meatloaf recipe, 186–187

perfectketo (website), 360

periods, 19

personal-sized blender, 43

pickle juice, 17

picky eaters, 22–23

Piña Colada recipe, 320–321

pine nuts
    Easy Basil Pesto, 96

pineapple
    Piña Colada, 320–321
    Pineapple Ginger Smoothie, 144

Pineapple Ginger Smoothie recipe, 144

Pink Grapefruit Martini recipe, 306–307

pistachios, for snacking, 25

PMS symptoms, 19

pork
    Bahn Mi Pork Burgers, 214–215
    Cajun Pork Shops with Aioli, 200–201
    Easy Jerk Ribs, 218–219
    Mojo Pork Tenderloin, 206–207
    Pork Chili Verde, 208–209
    Pork Chops with Dijon Tarragon Sauce, 216–217
    Pork Fried Cauliflower Rice, 204–205

Schnitzel with Sour Cream & Scallion Sauce, 212–213
    Sweet & Spicy Asian Meatballs, 202–203

Pork Chili Verde recipe, 208–209

Pork Chops with Dijon Tarragon Sauce recipe, 216–217

Pork Fried Cauliflower Rice recipe, 204–205

pork rinds
    about, 34
    for snacking, 25

potassium, 41

potatoes
    about, 15
    swaps for, 22

prebiotics, 40

probiotics, 40

protein, requirements for, 18

protein powder
    about, 36
    Cacao Coconut Granola, 140–141
    Chocolate Hemp Smoothie, 142–143
    Coconut Chai Vanilla Smoothie, 145
    No-Bake Sesame Cookies, 338–339
    Raspberry Chia Smoothie, 146

pumpkin
    Bulletproof Pumpkin Spice Latte, 126
    Pumpkin Spice Cupcakes, 336–337

pumpkin seeds
    Keto Seed Crackers, 300

Pumpkin Spice Cupcakes recipe, 336–337

Q

Quick Cucumber Pickles recipe, 114–115

R

radishes
    about, 16
    Bahn Mi Pork Burgers, 214–215
    Cultured Red Onion Relish, 116–117

Raspberry Chia Smoothie recipe, 146

Raspberry Coulis recipe, 95
    Raspberry Swirl Cheesecake, 344–345

Raspberry Swirl Cheesecake recipe, 344–345

recipes, guide to, 65

red curry paste
    Shrimp Panang Curry, 232–233

red peppers
    Roasted Red Pepper Cauliflower Hummus, 286–287
    Zoodles with Creamy Roasted Red Pepper Sauce, 264–265

Restaurant-Style Salsa recipe, 292
    Beef Burrito Bowl, 188–189
    Easy Keto Guacamole, 293
    Easy Nacho Dip, 294–295
    Easy No-Chop Chili, 180–181
    Easy Salsa Chicken, 158–159
    Savory Chorizo Breakfast Bowl, 136–137

rice, swaps for, 22

ricotta cheese
    Vegetable Lasagna, 260–261

Roasted Red Pepper Cauliflower Hummus recipe, 286–287

romaine lettuce
    about, 16
    Beef Burrito Bowl, 188–189

Romantic Dinner for Two menu, 29

rotisserie chicken, 150

rum
    Blackberry Mojito, 314–315
    Butter Rum Caramel Sauce, 330–331
    Classic Mojito, 312–313
    Coconut-Rum Paletas, 350
    Piña Colada, 320–321

Ryan, Suzanne, Simply Keto, 360

S

salads
    Bahn Mi Pork Salad, 215
    building, 248–249
    Niçoise Salad with Seared Tuna, 230–231
    Shrimp Caprese Salad, 225

salmon
  Smoked Salmon Steaks,
    234–235
salsa
  recommended brands, 361
  Spanish Tortilla with Chorizo,
    130–131
salsa verde
  Green Chicken Enchilada
    Cauliflower Casserole,
    156–157
Shrimp Fajitas, 240–241
salt
  about, 38
  for lacto-fermenting, 112
salted rim, 318
sauces
  Basic Remoulade, 97
  Butter Rum Caramel Sauce,
    330–331
  Cucumber Raita, 98
  Easy Basil Pesto, 96
  Easy Keto BBQ Sauce, 104
  Easy No-Cook Marinara, 106
  5-Minute Alfredo Sauce, 107
  Keto Ketchup, 102–103
  Raspberry Coulis, 95
  Sweet Chili Sauce, 105
  Sweet Sriracha Dipping
    Sauce, 99
Sausage & Egg–Stuffed
  Portobello Mushrooms recipe,
  134–135
Sautéed Green Beans with
  Walnuts recipe, 279
Sautéed Mushrooms recipe, 281
Savory Chorizo Breakfast Bowl
  recipe, 136–137
scale, 47
scallions
  Bahn Mi Pork Burgers, 214–215
  Creamy Lobster Risotto,
    242–243
  Creamy Shrimp Risotto, 242
  Ginger Scallion Dressing, 88
  Korean BBQ Beef Wraps,
    190–191
  Pork Fried Cauliflower Rice,
    204–205
  Schnitzel with Sour Cream &
    Scallion Sauce, 212–213
  Shrimp & Grits, 226–227

Sweet & Spicy Asian
  Meatballs, 202–203
Schnitzel with Sour Cream &
  Scallion Sauce recipe, 212–213
Schwenk, Carolyn, Cultured Food
  for Health, 360
SCOBY (Symbiotic Culture of
  Bacteria and Yeast)
  Basic Kombucha, 122–123
seasoning mixes
  Beef Seasoning, 80
  Blackening Seasoning, 78
  Cajun Seasoning, 76
  Chicken Seasoning, 77
  Fish and Seafood Seasoning, 81
  Jerk Seasoning, 79
seltzer water
  Blackberry Mojito, 314–315
  Classic Mojito, 312–313
sesame seeds
  Cacao Coconut Granola,
    140–141
  Keto Seed Crackers, 300
  No-Bake Sesame Cookies,
    338–339
  Spicy Tuna Cakes, 228–229
  Sweet Sesame Glazed Bok
    Choy, 274–275
  Vegetarian Pad Thai, 258–259
sherry
  Cauliflower Risotto with
    Sherry & Hazelnuts,
    256–257
  Chicken Tetrazzini, 150–151
  Creamy Lobster Risotto,
    242–243
  Schnitzel with Sour Cream &
    Scallion Sauce, 212–213
shiitake mushrooms, 15
shopping lists
  Week 1, 52–53
  Week 2, 56–57
  Week 3, 60–61
  Week 4, 64
shortcuts, 24–25
shredding chicken, 151
shrimp
  Creamy Shrimp Risotto, 242
  removing tails from, 226
  Shrimp Caprese Salad, 225
  Shrimp Fajitas, 240–241
  Shrimp & Grits, 226–227

Shrimp Panang Curry, 232–233
Spicy Shrimp-Stuffed
  Avocados, 244–245
Shrimp Caprese Salad recipe, 225
Shrimp Fajitas recipe, 240–241
Shrimp & Grits recipe, 226–227
Shrimp Panang Curry recipe,
  232–233
side dishes, swaps for, 22
Simple Syrup—Basic and
  Flavored recipe, 84–85
simple syrups, 31, 85
Simply Keto (Ryan), 360
slow cooker, 43
Smoked Salmon Steaks recipe,
  234–235
snacks, tips for, 25
Snapper, Blackened, 224
Snickerdoodle Crepes recipe,
  132–133
Snickerdoodle Haystack Cookies
  recipe, 342–343
sodium, 17
sour cream
  Beef Burrito Bowl, 188–189,
    294–295
  Cheesy Beef Stroganoff
    Casserole, 194–195
  Chicken-Fried Steak with
    Sour Cream Gravy, 184–185
  Cucumber Raita, 98
  Green Chicken Enchilada
    Cauliflower Casserole,
    156–157
  Lemon Sour Cream Bundt
    Cake, 334–335
  Pork Chili Verde, 208–209
  Schnitzel with Sour Cream &
    Scallion Sauce, 212–213
  Shrimp Fajitas, 240–241
  Spanish Tortilla with Chorizo,
    130–131
  Tangy Feta & Dill Dressing, 93
soy sauce, 37
Spanish Tortilla with Chorizo
  recipe, 130–131
Spicy Jicama Shoestring Fries
  recipe, 280
Spicy Sauerkraut recipe, 110–111
Spicy Shrimp–Stuffed Avocados
  recipe, 244–245
Spicy Tuna Cakes recipe, 228–229

spinach
about, 16
Creamed Spinach, 278
Vegetable Lasagna, 260–261
spiral slicer, 45
sports drinks, 17
spring greens, 16
Sriracha sauce
Spicy Tuna Cakes, 228–229
Sweet Sriracha Dipping Sauce, 99
starter culture
Cultured Red Onion Relish, 116–117
Homemade Dairy Kefir, 118–119
recommended brands, 361
Spicy Sauerkraut, 110–111
strawberries
Kefir Strawberry Smoothie, 127
Strawberry Basil Vinaigrette, 87
Strawberry Basil Vinaigrette recipe, 87
Sugarfreemom (website), 360
Sun-Dried Tomato & Basil Butter recipe, 100–101
sunflower seeds
Keto Seed Crackers, 300
supplements, 39–42
Sweet Chili Sauce recipe, 105
Spicy Tuna Cakes, 228–229
Sweet Sesame Glazed Bok Choy recipe, 274–275
Sweet & Spicy Asian Meatballs recipe, 202–203
Sweet Sriracha Dipping Sauce recipe, 99
sweeteners, 32–33
syrup, recommended brands, 361
syrups, simple, 31, 85

T
tahini
Jalapeño & Cilantro Cauliflower Hummus, 284–285
No-Bake Sesame Cookies, 338–339
Roasted Red Pepper Cauliflower Hummus, 286–287
storing, 338
Tahini Lemon Dressing, 94

Wasabi & Ginger Cauliflower Hummus, 288–289
Tahini Lemon Dressing recipe, 94
Tandoori Chicken Meatballs recipe, 170–171
Tangy Feta & Dill Dressing recipe, 93
tarragon
Orange & Tarragon Coleslaw, 276–277
Pork Chops with Dijon Tarragon Sauce, 216–217
tea. See also iced tea
Basic Kombucha, 122–123
tequila
Margarita, 318–319
The 30-Day Ketogenic Cleanse (Emmerich), 360
Thousand Island dressing, 102
tips and tricks, 22–30
tomatoes
Bacon & Tomato Dressing, 89
Caprese Burgers, 176–177
Chicken Cacciatore, 164–165
Easy No-Cook Marinara, 106
Faux-lafel, 266–267
Niçoise Salad with Seared Tuna, 230–231
Restaurant-Style Salsa, 292
Shrimp Caprese Salad, 225
tools, 43–47
tortillas, swaps for, 22
tracking food, 19
traveling, 27
tricks and tips, 22–30
Triple Chocolate Cheesecake recipe, 346–347
truffle salt, 31
tuna
Niçoise Salad with Seared Tuna, 230–231
Spicy Tuna Cakes, 228–229
turmeric
Pineapple Ginger Smoothie, 144

V
vacationing, 27
Vanilla Ice Cream recipe, 354–355
Affogato, 356–357
Vegetable Lasagna recipe, 260–261

vegetables, carbohydrates in, 16
Vegetarian Pad Thai recipe, 258–259
vodka
Lemon Drop Martini, 308
Pink Grapefruit Martini, 306–307
Vogel, Leanne, The Keto Diet, 360

W
walnuts
Cacao Coconut Granola, 140–141
Cinnamon Walnut Streusel Muffins, 128–129
Sautéed Green Beans with Walnuts, 279
wasabi, 228, 288–289
Wasabi & Ginger Cauliflower Hummus recipe, 288–289
water, requirements for, 17
water chestnuts
Sweet & Spicy Asian Meatballs, 202–203
websites, recommended, 360
Week 1 meal plan, 50–53
Week 2 meal plan, 54–57
Week 3 meal plan, 58–61
Week 4 meal plan, 62–64
Westman, Eric C., Keto Clarity, 360
Whiskey Sour recipe, 317
white wine
Chicken Cacciatore, 164–165
Shrimp & Grits, 226–227

X
xanthan gum, 36

Z
Zoodles with Creamy Roasted Red Pepper Sauce recipe, 264–265
Zoodles with Zesty Roasted Red Pepper Sauce recipe, 264
zucchini
Basic Zucchini Noodles, 252–253
Chicken Tetrazzini, 150–151
Vegetable Lasagna, 260–261